THE

NEGATIVE

CALORIE
DIET

FROM ROCCO TO:

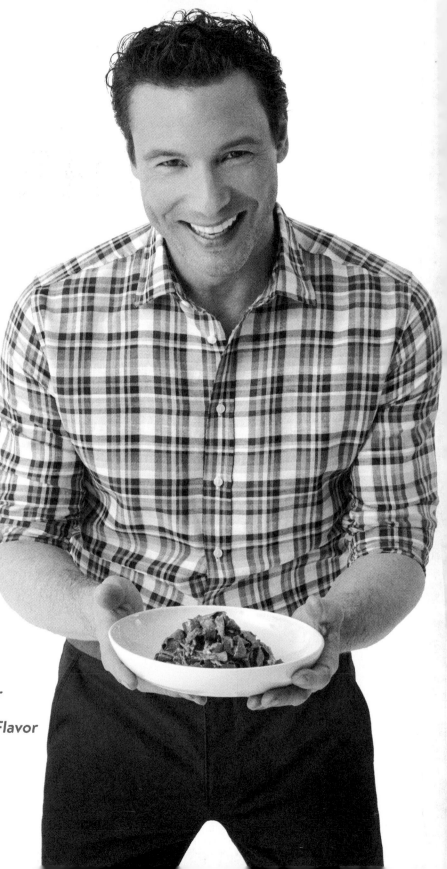

ALSO BY ROCCO DISPIRITO

Cook Your Butt Off!

The Pound a Day Diet

Now Eat This! Italian

Now Eat This! Quick Calorie Cuts

Now Eat This! Diet

Now Eat This!

Rocco Gets Real

Rocco's Real Life Recipes

Rocco's Five Minute Flavor

Rocco's Italian-American Flavor

Flavor

THE
NEGATIVE
CALORIE
DIET

LOSE UP TO 10 POUNDS IN 10 DAYS WITH
10 ALL YOU CAN EAT FOODS

ROCCO DISPIRITO

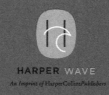

HARPER WAVE

An Imprint of HarperCollinsPublishers

HarperCollins books may be purchased for educational, business, or sales promotional use. For information, please e-mail the Special Markets Department at SPsales@harpercollins.com.

FIRST EDITION

Designed by Hsu + Associates

Photographs on pages ii, x, 32, 64, 228, 230, and 277 by Christopher Testani. All other photographs courtesy of Rocco DiSpirito.

Library of Congress Cataloging-in-Publication Data has been applied for.

ISBN: 978-0-06-237813-2

16 17 18 19 20   OV/RRD   10 9 8 7 6

CONTENTS

Introduction viii

PART I

THE NEGATIVE CALORIE DIET

CHAPTER ONE It's Not About the Calories 3

CHAPTER TWO Meet the 10 Negative Calorie Foods 11

CHAPTER THREE Eat Real, Feel Great, Lose Weight 25

CHAPTER FOUR The 10-Day Negative Calorie Cleanse 33

CHAPTER FIVE The 20-Day All You Can Eat Plan 45

PART II

THE NEGATIVE CALORIE RECIPES

CHAPTER SIX Smoothies 67

CHAPTER SEVEN Breakfast 99

CHAPTER EIGHT Soups and Salads 119

CHAPTER NINE Mains 151

CHAPTER TEN Snacks 197

CHAPTER ELEVEN Desserts 215

PART III

THE NEGATIVE CALORIE LIFESTYLE

CHAPTER TWELVE Going Meatless 231

CHAPTER THIRTEEN The Family Plan 241

CHAPTER FOURTEEN Eating Out and On the Go 247

CHAPTER FIFTEEN Maintain—The Negative Calorie Way 257

Index 267

NEGATIVE CALORIE DIET RECIPE INDEX

SMOOTHIES

Cucumber-Strawberry Green Smoothie	68
Spinach, Pineapple, Lime, and Mint Smoothie	70
Apple-Lime-Cilantro Protein Smoothie	72
Green Goddess Smoothie	74
Tropical Sunrise Smoothie	76
"Dillicious" Green Smoothie	78
Lemon-Ginger Smoothie	80
Orange Greensicle Smoothie	82
Sangrita Tomato, Orange, and Red Pepper Smoothie	84
The Virgin Mary Smoothie	86
Strawberry Shortcake Smoothie	88
Almond Vanilla Protein Smoothie	90
Spiced Apple Pie Smoothie	92
Blueberry-Basil Smoothie	94
Citrus-Berry Smash Smoothie	96

BREAKFAST

Apple and Cinnamon Breakfast "Risotto" with Oat Bran and Almonds	100
Blueberry and Quinoa Porridge with Mint	102
Breakfast Citrus Salad with Cucumbers and Basil	104
Breakfast Pizza with Mushrooms and Broccoli	106
Kale, Red Onion, and Tomato Frittata	108
Avocado Toast with Spinach and Tomatoes	110
Mexican Cauliflower Chili Scramble	112
Breakfast Bowl with Quinoa and Berries	114
Spinach and Mushroom Omelet	116

SOUPS AND SALADS

Charred Thai-Style Broccoli Salad with Almonds and Lime	120
Crabmeat Salad with Apple, Celery, and Leafy Greens	122
Chicken Soup with Escarole and Leeks	124
Shrimp and Cucumber Salad with Red Onion and Poblanos	126
Flank Steak Salad with Horseradish and Apple	128
Mixed Leafy Green Soup "Caldo Verde" with Chickpeas	130
Rocco's Chef Salad	132
Seared Tuna Tataki Salad with Citrus, Tofu, and Watercress	134
Asian Curry Mussel Soup	136
Shaved Brussels Sprouts with Warm Toasted Garlic, Almond, and Lemon Dressing	138
Strawberry and Spinach Salad with Almonds and Basil	140
Swiss Chard Turkey Salad with Golden Raisins and Capers	142

The Grate Salad Bowl with Chia Seed
Dressing   144

Mushroom Bouillon with Leeks, Tofu,
and Wasabi   146

Leafy Green Salad with Creamy Almond
Dressing and Radishes   148

Shrimp and Cabbage Hot Pot
with Chile Peppers   184

Shrimp with Mustard Greens,
Mushrooms, and Miso   186

Sliced Pepper Steak with Swiss Chard
and Mushrooms   188

Spinach Pesto Pasta with Tomatoes   191

MAINS

Almond-Encrusted Flounder
with Chopped Spinach and Clam Broth   152

Baked Chicken with Sweet-and-Sour
Red Cabbage   156

Vegetable Pot-au-Feu   158

Beef-Stuffed Cabbage with Pepper
and Tomato Goulash   160

Chicken with Mustard Greens, Quinoa,
and Oranges   162

Eggplant Roll-Ups   164

Filet of Beef with Braised Kale
and Black Olives   167

Flounder "a la Plancha"
with Catalonian Eggplant Relish   170

Grilled Shrimp with Marinated Cucumbers,
Kale, and Cauliflower   172

Meatballs with Mushroom
and Spinach Gravy   174

"Pappardelle" of Chicken with Winter Pesto   177

Roasted Cauliflower with Green Peppers,
Almond Curry, and Lime   180

Shiitake and Bok Choy Stir-Fry   182

SNACKS

Cucumber and Almond Rice Sushi   198

No-Sugar-Added Organic Cranberry Sauce   200

Cauliflower and Apples
with Thai Almond Butter Sauce   202

Eggplant and Almond Dip with Celery   204

Peanutty Apple Slices   206

Red Ants on a Log   208

Apple, Cranberry, and Almond Bars   210

Rocco's Raw Apple Sauce   212

DESSERTS

Chocolate and Almond Butter Truffles   216

Chocolate-Dipped Strawberries
with Crushed Almonds   218

Cocoa-Dusted Almonds   220

Instant Almond Cake with Mixed Berries   222

Crepes Suzette with Oranges
and Vanilla Cream   224

Citrus and Mixed Berry Bowl
with Whipped Topping   226

INTRODUCTION

Many years ago, I made a *kerplunk* in the cooking world by re-creating "comfort foods" like fried chicken, cheeseburgers, mac and cheese, and ice cream, devising recipes that were still delicious but lower-calorie, lower-fat versions of the originals. I didn't think anything of using processed cheese, artificial sweeteners, packaged pudding mixes, and zero-calorie additives to do so. The results tasted fantastic.

Then I was hit with some major backlash from my readers and clients: "It's not okay to cook with fake sweeteners, fake fat, or fake *any-thing*!" they protested. I heard everyone loud and clear. I educated myself about what goes into processed foods and began to dismantle my nutritional orthodoxies faster than a car thief stripping a Porsche on a New York City side street at three a.m. I realized that I needed more than my longtime strategy of downsizing calories and fat in order to stabilize my own weight and achieve excellent health. So I started to incorporate more organic, whole foods into my diet, namely in the form of fresh veggies and fruit and lean, clean sources of protein.

The arrival point of my adventure turned out to be a whole new way of cooking that is even more delicious and satisfying than the "fake food"

methods I had relied on in the past. Not only did I finally lose the extra 10 pounds I'd been carrying around, but I've found that eating whole foods actually makes me *feel* better than ever.

With every book I write, my food philosophy continues to evolve. My nutritional recommendations have become a bit purer. I've become a stronger proponent of eating organic foods rather than mass-produced stuff grown in toxic soils, adulterated with chemicals, and concocted mostly for profit by our nation's big food manufacturers. In many ways, I've come full circle: The way I cook now is a total throwback to how I watched my mother and grandmother cook when I was a kid, using home-grown foods picked from our family's garden.

Soon after I started eating this way, people I met through television appearances and other ventures began asking me to make and deliver healthy meals for them. I obliged, and before I knew it, I had the happy accident of a brand-new business. Over the last few years, I've started to run a kitchen where a small staff and I cook organic, gluten-free, sugar-free, nutrient-dense meals for a handful of clients who receive customized programs based on their medical and nutritional needs. It's like running a restaurant again, but without some of the inherent hassles—and with *much* more nutritious menu items! The business has grown so fast that we recently moved into a larger facility with a bigger kitchen, and we can barely keep up with the demand.

The meals we make were initially based on the recipes from one of my recent books, *The Pound a Day Diet,* but then gradually evolved to incorporate more and more negative calorie foods. In the time since we launched, I've observed amazing successes with our eating plans: Not only have my clients lost weight, but they love the food. Some have made such positive strides in their health that they were able to stop taking diabetes medications. Others report that their energy levels have skyrocketed and they're less reliant on caffeine to get through the day. A few of my clients even asked if I was lacing their meals with energy drink additives!

Through it all, I witnessed another little miracle: The Negative Calorie Diet had staying power. No one was falling off the wagon. This was unusual, since there is a very high attrition rate associated with many weight-loss programs. Several years ago, the *International Journal of Obesity* reported that of the more than 60,000 dieters enrolled in a large commercial weight-loss pro-

gram, only 13,000 people were still hanging in there at 26 weeks, and after a year, only 3,900 dieters were left. That's a pretty high dropout rate, if you ask me.

I don't have 60,000 dieters under my wing (at least not yet!), but those who are enrolled in my home food delivery program have a remarkable level of adherence. Most are still following the principles of my eating plan well into their second year—and maintaining their weight loss without feeling that they're on a "diet."

Clearly, the Negative Calorie Diet is more than just a 30-day program; it is a whole new lifestyle. At the end of 30 days, you can expect to be thinner—by 10 to 20 pounds—look younger, have more energy, and feel healthier. Based on what I've seen with my clients, you should also see measurable improvements in your digestion, blood pressure, blood sugar control, energy level, and laboratory blood tests (including cholesterol).

I've spent several years tweaking and evolving this eating plan and my negative calorie recipes, using myself and my clients as guinea pigs. Luckily, it won't take you that long because I've tested everything for you. All you have to do is keep turning the pages!

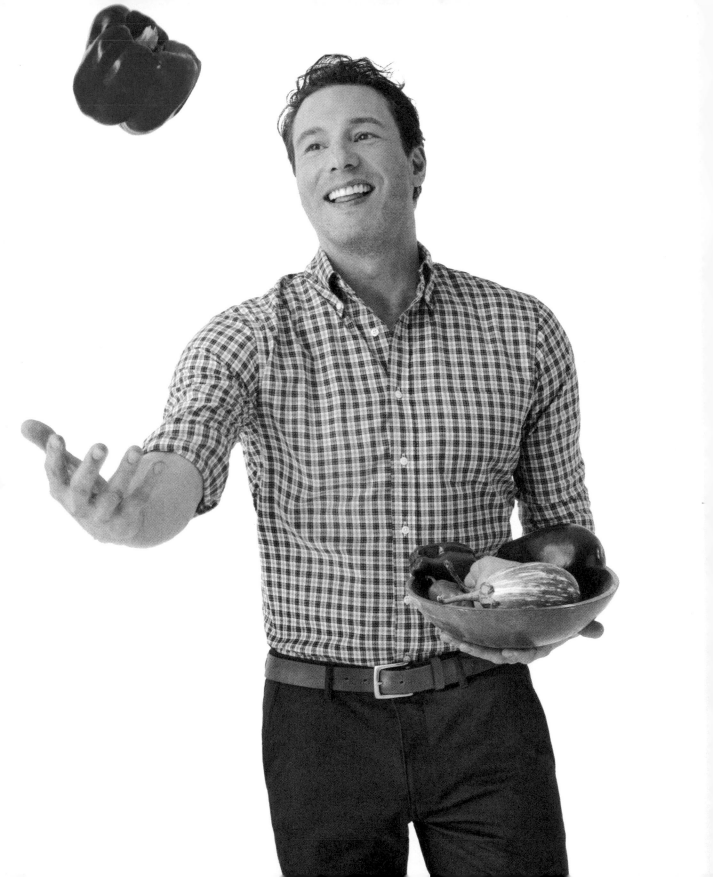

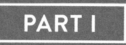

PART I

THE NEGATIVE CALORIE DIET

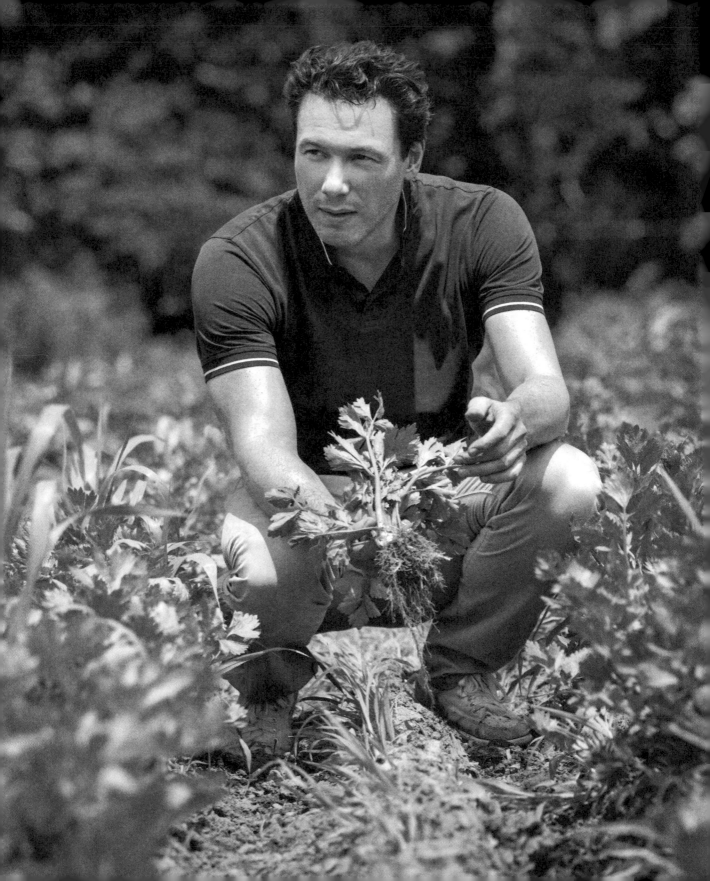

CHAPTER ONE

IT'S NOT ABOUT THE CALORIES

FROM now on, you're going to ask yourself one question before you eat anything: *"Is this a negative calorie food?"*

If the answer is *"yes,"* then you know you can eat it because you know that the food in question is something that will nourish your body, supplying the energy and nutrients you need to stay healthy. You don't have to count how many calories it contains or portion out minuscule amounts of it. You can eat it. It's that simple.

If the answer is *"no,"* then you want to put that food back on the grocery store shelf, remove it from your pantry or fridge, or skip over it on a restaurant menu, because it is *not* going to provide nourishment for your body. And it's certainly not going to help you lose weight.

So what is a "negative calorie" food? That's what I'm going to show you in this book. You're about to learn how simple and delicious it is to eat foods that naturally support your weight-loss efforts. Negative calorie foods can help your body

burn fat and lose weight. They can boost the rate at which your body burns calories, both temporarily and in the long run. And they can help you feel full after you eat them—so you actually eat less food overall.

GOOD CALORIES, BAD CALORIES

If you want to get in shape, you need to lose fat and build muscle. In order to burn that fat, you've got to maintain a "negative calorie balance," which means that you consume fewer calories than you expend. Traditionally, a negative calorie balance is achieved by cutting calories so that your body taps into stored fat for energy. But this approach, unfortunately, requires tedious calorie-counting and hunger-producing food restriction. In other words: a short-term diet that is doomed to fail.

I wanted to figure out a better strategy for losing weight and reducing body fat. I wondered: What if there was a way to create a negative calorie balance without cutting calories but instead, eating as much as you want?

Well, it turns out there is—and the secret is eating real, wholesome foods. Negative calorie foods.

Now, I'm not a big calorie advocate—I will never suggest that you count or track every calorie you eat. But calories are a useful measure when we're looking at how food impacts weight loss and gain. So what is a calorie? Technically, a calorie is the measurement of the approximate amount of heat (energy) needed to raise 1 gram of water 1 degree Celsius. By that definition, calories are the same, regardless of whether they come from fat, protein, or carbohydrate. That may be true in theory—but could it be true that your body processes all calories equally?

Let's use the example of a large orange. It has about 100 calories. So does a small chocolate candy bar. But do these foods have the same effect on your weight? No! The candy bar has no nutritive value and gets stored by the body as fat, whereas the orange contains vitamins and minerals, and fiber, which actually help control your weight.

From my own experience, I know that I pack on weight when I regularly wolf down a greasy slice of pizza for dinner, but when I eat healthier meals that contain roughly the same amount of calories—such as a large piece of grilled tuna and some vegetables—my weight stays stable. You don't have to be a nutrition expert to realize that there's a huge difference, nutritionally, between the pizza and the fish dinner. Bottom line: It's not how *many* calories you eat (quantity), but the *types* of calories you eat (quality).

I credit eating negative calorie foods as the first step on my road to staying in shape. Actually, let me retract that. The first step was the one where I got tired of gaining and losing the same 10 pounds about a million times in the last few years. If you added up all of my discarded weight, I've probably lost an entire person or two!

ALL CALORIES ARE NOT CREATED EQUAL

Eating *high-quality* calories fuels your metabolism and helps your body to burn fat, while eating *low-quality* calories is linked to weight gain and poor health. But don't take it from me—there's plenty of scientific proof to back this up! Here are a few examples:

• University of Connecticut researchers compared two groups of dieters: those who ate quality foods such as vegetables, salads, nuts, seeds, lean beef, poultry, and chicken; and those who ate lower-quality foods like bread, pasta, fruit juices, and dairy foods. The dieters in the high-quality-food group consumed 300 more calories each day than the dieters in the low-quality group, but burned more body fat! Published in *Nutrition and Metabolism* in 2004, this study showed that quality calories (and more of them) give you a metabolic advantage when it comes to weight loss.

• Investigators at the University of Pennsylvania placed study participants in one of two groups: dieters who ate high-quality foods such as fresh fruits and vegetables that were naturally high in fiber; and dieters who were allowed to eat a range of foods, including 5 to 6 daily servings of bread and rolls, pasta, bagels, cereals, unsalted pretzels, and popcorn (lower-quality calories!). Over the course of the 6-month study, dieters in the high-quality-calorie group ate a total of 9,500 more calories than the other group and lost 200 percent more weight!

• Researchers compared the results of dieters adhering to a low-fat diet (which typically includes lower-quality calories from processed carbohydrates) versus a low-carbohydrate diet (which typically includes lots of high-quality protein and fresh vegetables) for 12 weeks. On the low-carb diet, women ate 1,500 calories daily; men, 1,800 calories daily. A second group of low-carb dieters was allowed to eat 300 extra calories a day; the women ate 1,800 calories; the men, 2,100 calories. As for the low-fat diet, the women ate 1,500 calories a day; the men, 1,800 calories daily. The average amount of weight lost was as follows: the low-carb diet, 23 pounds; the low-carb diet plus 300 daily calories, 20 pounds; and the low-fat diet, 17 pounds. Okay, run through those numbers again: More weight was lost on low-carb plus 300 calories diet (a higher-calorie diet!) than the low-fat diet that controlled calories and fat.

How are study results like these possible? Two reasons: First, a calorie is *not* a calorie. Some calories are more "fattening" than others. Second, some calories—which I call negative calories—put your body into a negative calorie balance, and help you lose weight.

In a scientific paper published in 2014 titled "How Calorie-Focused Thinking About Obesity and Related Diseases May Mislead and Harm Public Health," the authors used the example of four specific types of food, each with the same amount of calories, to demonstrate how differently each one impacts body weight and body fat when consumed: salmon (a protein), olive oil (a fat), white rice (a refined carbohydrate), and vodka (mostly alcohol).

Salmon, the protein, helps you feel full, because protein satiates you, mostly by suppressing various gut hormones involved in regulating appetite.

Then there's the fat, olive oil. Fat calories are usually more fattening. Why? Your body doesn't need to use much energy to convert food fat into body fat. Your body burns up 20 times more energy digesting protein compared with the energy it needs to digest fats.

As for the white rice, it gets rapidly absorbed and quickly converted into sugar in the bloodstream. Unless that blood sugar gets burned up quickly or enters cells, it is likely to be stored as fat. For sure, the quick spike in sugar will be followed by a fast crash, leaving you with cravings for more food.

Oh—and the alcohol. It increases your hunger. What's more, it is also recognized by the body as a sugar, and thus is quickly converted to fat that becomes padding around your tummy and hips.

As you can see, calorie per calorie, each of these foods impacts your body differently. So while calories can be helpful to use as a rough measure when you're looking to lose weight, it is essential to bear in mind that not all calorie sources are the same. The great thing about negative calorie foods is that they are a high-quality calorie source, so you can eat as much of them as you want. I know it sounds too good to be true, but I can assure you it's not. It worked for me and it's working for so many of my clients every day.

So, what is a negative calorie food? Here are the criteria by which we can assess any food and determine whether or not it's a negative calorie food. It must meet all three of the following guidelines:

1: THE WHOLE FOODS FACTOR

Negative calorie foods are *whole foods*—those that have not been altered from their original state, or have been modified only slightly, for example, through cooking. Calories from whole foods are high-quality calories.

By contrast, foods that have been substantially altered are considered processed foods, and they contain low-quality calories. Take the potato, for example: Potatoes are a whole food. Potato chips are a processed food.

To burn fat, you must limit the amount of processed food you eat, and foods like cookies, chips, and other packaged foods are processed. They definitely don't grow in the form in which you buy them. Ever seen a potato chip plant? I didn't think so.

The beauty of eating whole foods is that the calories they contain do not get stored as fat like calories from processed foods and junk foods. You can eat more calories from whole foods and still lose weight.

A case in point: Scientists at the City of Hope Medical Center (Duarte, California) analyzed two groups of heavy people, who were all on a medically supervised, calorie-restricted liquid diet. For a snack, half the dieters included 3 ounces of almonds (a whole food that contains quality calories) in their daily diet, while the other half included the same amount of calories in the form of processed foods like popcorn and wheat crackers. Both groups consumed 1,000 calories daily. Over the course of 24 weeks, the almond-eaters lost more weight than the processed snack-eaters even though they ate the same number of calories. Again, high-quality calories won out.

When you eat whole foods–particularly the 10 foods I'll be emphasizing here—they help put your body in fat-burning, weight-losing mode.

2: THE FAT BURN FACTOR

One of the keys to burning fat and losing weight is to boost your metabolism—your body's food-to-fuel process. The more efficient your metabolism, the more fat your body burns.

There are a number of ways to rev up your metabolism. One is to exercise, especially with strength training, because it builds muscle. Muscle is metabolically active—it is your body's primary fat-burning tissue. Another way is to periodically detox (which you'll do on this plan), because detoxing helps cleanse your liver—your body's primary fat-burning organ—allowing it to function more efficiently.

The third way is to choose "thermogenic" foods. Okay, this term may sound complicated, but it simply refers to the heat that is generated by the body as you digest a meal. This process boosts your metabolism and burns calories. In fact, the Mayo Clinic says that thermogenesis can account for 100 to 800 of the calories you expend each day.

Certain foods are more thermogenic than others, namely cruciferous vegetables like broccoli and cauliflower, and all sorts of proteins. You automatically create a negative calorie balance when you eat these foods.

3: THE FULL FACTOR

Negative calorie foods are "satiating," which means that they fill you up. Think of this as like a natural form of gastric bypass, with no surgery needed; negative calorie foods make you feel full more quickly so you automatically eat less of them. The reason these foods are so satiating is that they're high in water and loaded with fiber (think fruits and vegetables), or are rich in protein (think lean meats).

If you've ever tried (and failed at) dieting, it's likely that hunger was your number one pitfall. Calorie-based diets don't take satiety into account. Maybe you stuck to your meal plan for a week or two, but you were always hungry. Who wants to feel like that all the time? Our bodies and our brains were not designed to ignore hunger. In fact, we're evolutionarily wired to seek out high-calorie foods when we feel that we're starving. That's why, when you're on a diet, and you're constantly hungry, all you want to do is make a beeline to the nearest hot fudge sundae.

Another reason many diets leave you feeling hungry is that they include processed carbohydrates such as breakfast cereals, white bread, or white rice. All of these carbs are composed of starch molecules, which your body converts into sugar moments after you eat. That quick digestion causes a spike in glucose (blood sugar), followed by a fast crash.

Think back on a time when you had a muffin for breakfast and got a rush of energy, only to feel a steep drop and a major sugar craving by noon. That's what the other side of sugar feels like. By contrast, negative calorie foods provide a steady source of fuel, keeping you energized with no spikes or crashes. So: no more urges to overnosh or binge, as long as you've got high-quality, negative calorie foods on your side.

There you have it: Negative calorie foods contain whole-food calories that fill you up and help your body to burn fat instead of store it. The net result is real, sustainable weight loss without deprivation.

METABOLIC SECRETS REVEALED

The Negative Calorie Diet is based on putting your body in a negative calorie balance naturally, without counting calories or obsessing over them. You can eat with impunity—all you want—as long as you ensure that every meal includes at least one or more of the 10 negative calorie foods. In fact, the more of these foods you eat, the more weight you are likely to lose. (I'll unveil these foods in the next chapter; if your curiosity gets the best of you, I give you permission to turn to page 11 and take a peek now).

But piling on negative calorie foods isn't the only tool in my chef's bag. I also went hunting for the 10 best fat-burning proteins on the planet to make tasty and filling meals. Protein is harder for the body to break down than other macronutrients such as carbohydrates or fats, and, hence, requires more energy to do so. In a meal that includes protein, up to 25 percent of its calories may be burned off by thermogenesis. Again, do the math: If you eat a 400-calorie meal that includes a serving of protein such as meat, chicken, or fish, you can expect to expend 100 calories (25 percent of the total calories in the meal) just digesting it. Voilà! Protein also helps you to feel full and satisfied, plus it contains essential substances called amino acids that help your body repair and rebuild muscle.

Adding spices to your meals also creates a thermogenetic effect. I've identified the top 10 spices that help to increase thermogenesis and boost metabolism (see page 17)—and I'll show you how to use them to create healthy, flavorful food. So just think: protein + negative calorie foods + spices = a delicious way to burn fat and lose weight!

EATING PLAN ESSENTIALS

My eating plan is built around a 30-day period. Once you cycle through the first 30 days, my hope is that you'll continue to implement these healthy lifestyle changes for the long haul. Here's a breakdown of those first 30 days:

• **A 10-day cleanse** centered on 10 negative calorie foods. In these first 10 days you can reasonably expect to lose up to a pound a day for a potential total of 10 pounds in 10 days. Read that again: 10 pounds in 10 days. Nice, isn't it?

There's nothing draconian about this cleanse: You'll enjoy three delicious detox drinks and one solid meal, either a filling salad or a satiating soup, daily. One reason the cleanse works so well is that it detoxes you off the Really Bad Stuff: refined and added sugar, bleached white flour, gluten, hydrogenated fats, alcohol, genetically modified food, and chemicals in our foods that can disrupt metabolism and make the liver less efficient, and thus pack on body fat.

My cleanse scrubs this stuff away and gently supports the body's own detoxification processes. It's also an excellent way to kick off the rest of the Negative Calorie Diet and ultimately transition to better long-term eating habits.

• **The 20-day eating plan** in which you'll eat protein, supplemented by negative calorie foods, spices, and an array of superfoods bursting with flavor and health-promoting, fat-burning benefits. On the 20-day plan, you'll be able to enjoy dining out, too. Unlike most diets, the Negative Calorie Diet makes it easy to dine outside the home. And what a relief that you don't have to count calories, carbs, or fat grams; guess at serving sizes; measure out portions; or add up points at every meal. How satisfying—to eat as much as you want, as long as you choose high-quality foods!

After a few days on the program, you may notice that you've stopped craving junk food and sweets, and you no longer feel the urge to overeat. As your body begins to feel deeply satisfied and nourished from the nutrients you're providing it, you will actually start to crave the foods that are making it feel so good.

Your palate will begin to adjust to the subtle sweetness of fresh, organic fruits and vegetables, and you'll notice a difference in quality and flavor when you cook with proteins devoid of nasty stuff like antibiotics and hormones. As you drop pounds, your energy will soar. You may experience fewer aches and pains and better skin, and your immunity will be supercharged. You won't want to return to the land of the Really Bad Stuff—no more beelines to an ice cream sundae for you.

- **70 Negative Calorie Recipes.** Here's where you'll find easy-to-make recipes that emphasize fresh, whole foods that are minimally processed, locally grown, and organic—real food with real ingredients. In general, each recipe uses no more than 10 ingredients, not including seasonings, of course, with short prep times. After cooking in restaurants for nearly twenty-five years, I've spent the last several years cooking for myself, my friends, and my clients. I quickly found that cooking like an everyday home cook can be time-consuming and incompatible with my crazy-busy life. So I figured out how to create amazing, nutritious meals using fewer ingredients. These simple meals come together easily and save you money!

When it came to creating these recipes, there was a huge element of exploration involved. But because I'm a naturally curious person who never tires of new experiences, I welcomed the adventure. Through it all, I narrowed my universe of flavorings down to a few that I know are natural and organic. If an ingredient was even minimally processed, it was off the table. I use organic cocoa powder, monk fruit extract, and coconut nectar for sweet; citrus fruits, tart fruits, and flavored vinegars for sour; seaweed and unprocessed Celtic sea salt for salty; and organic mustards for bitter, thereby covering the landscape of the four tastes that bring food to life.

Now if you're ready, I'd like to show you how to navigate away from the foods making you fat, tired, and unhappy . . . and lead you into the world of wholesome foods that will help you get healthy and lose weight for good.

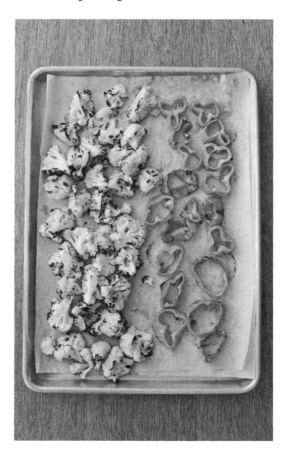

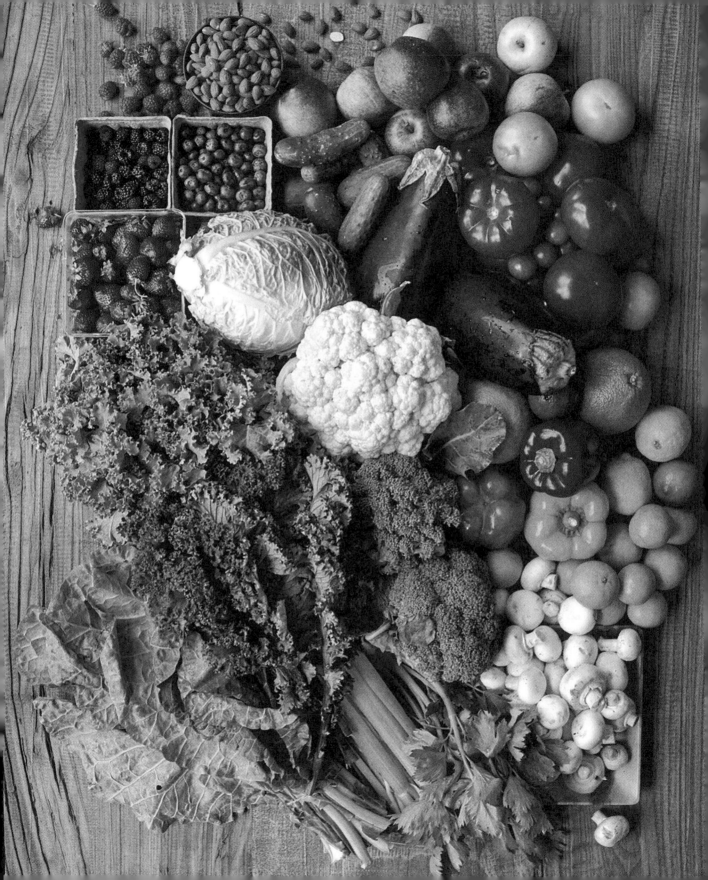

CHAPTER TWO

MEET THE 10 NEGATIVE CALORIE FOODS

CERTAINLY there are tons of healthy, nutrient-dense foods on the planet. But for the purposes of this eating plan, I've selected the top 10 negative calorie foods that I believe will help you meet your weight-loss goals. How did I select these 10 foods, you ask? Easy:

- SCIENCE Each of these foods is backed by credible research showing that it is satiating, is thermogenic, and contains quality whole-food calories.

- NUTRITION These foods are high in important nutrients, including fiber, vitamins, and minerals that not only help to support a robust metabolism, but also support overall health!

- VERSATILITY I'm a chef. I know good food, and I know the obstacles that keep people from cooking at home. To that end, all 10 foods that I've selected are easy to source at your local

grocery store or farmers' market; they are simple to cook with; and most of all, they are delicious.

So without further ado, here are the 10 negative calorie foods that you will be incorporating into your diet. Let's go at this alphabetically.

1. ALMONDS

In my opinion, there are few better things in life than a handful of almonds. These amazing nuts do everything for your body except sweat or wash your exercise clothes. They're high in protein and fiber, which means that a small handful really does satisfy.

Research suggests that eating almonds helps aid your weight-loss efforts, too. In a study published in the *European Journal of Clinical Nutrition*, folks who snacked on 1.5 ounces of almonds (about 30 nuts) every day felt more satiated throughout the day and ate less calories at other times. In other words, a daily almond snack made it easier to avoid overeating throughout the day. And in another study, published in the *Journal of the American College of Nutrition*, volunteers who regularly snacked on a mere 6 almonds daily were 4 pounds lighter, with an 0.8-inch-smaller waist circumference, as compared with non-almond eaters.

USE IT TO LOSE IT Almonds are a great snack option for weight loss. Try eating a handful of almonds about 20 minutes before a meal to control your appetite and help you eat less overall. Or enjoy them as a snack anytime. Many of my recipes use almonds in creative ways, too—check out the Almond Vanilla Protein Smoothie (page 90), Apple and Cinnamon Breakfast "Risotto" with Oat Bran and Almonds (page 100), or Cucumber and Almond Rice Sushi (page 198).

2. APPLES

I'm rewording an old adage: "An apple a day keeps the *fat* away."

How so? In a word: polyphenols. These are natural and beneficial plant compounds found in apples that have been shown to help reduce body fat—and, specifically—belly fat.

Scientists at the Nippon Sport Science University in Tokyo conducted a study of 71 obese men and women and asked them to consume 600 milligrams (about 3 apples' worth) a day of either apple polyphenols or a placebo for 3 months. The participants' total cholesterol, LDL (bad) cholesterol, body weight, and belly fat were all measured before and after the experiment. At the end of the study, the researchers found that the people who supplemented with apple polyphenols had the best reductions and improvements in all of these measurements, as compared with those on the placebo.

But polyphenols are not the only "magic bullets" in apples. They also contain pectin, a slow-digesting fiber in their skin that tames appetite and makes you feel full by keeping food in your stomach longer—a fact also confirmed by various studies. One study reported that people ate 15 percent fewer calories after eating an apple prior to a meal. Pectin is also thought to limit how much fat your cells can absorb, and has been shown to help lower "bad" or LDL cholesterol and boost the beneficial HDL cholesterol our body needs. And while it's true that apples are high in sugar, the presence of fiber and pectin means that eating an apple (as opposed to drinking apple juice) won't cause a spike in your blood sugar.

USE IT TO LOSE IT On days when you don't want to snack on almonds, try an apple. Like almonds, an apple will help fill you up. Try having a few apple slices about 15 minutes before a meal to help tame your appetite and capitalize on the benefits of this versatile fruit. Or get your apple fix from my Crabmeat Salad with Apple, Celery, and Leafy Greens (page 122), Spiced Apple Pie Smoothie (page 92), or Peanutty Apple Slices (page 206).

3. BERRIES

Sure, they look gorgeous and taste delicious—but did you know that berries are also some of the top fat-burning fruits you can eat?

For starters, berries are naturally satiating because they're loaded with fiber. With a food I adore, like fresh blueberries, I've been known to eat beyond a feeling of fullness for the sake of sheer tastiness. But it's actually pretty tough to overindulge in berries. When's the last time you ate an entire pint of strawberries or raspberries? Probably never . . . because at a certain point, you felt too full to keep eating.

Next, there's the thermogenic effect of berries. These tiny fruits contain a compound called resveratrol (also found in grapes and red wine) that increases heat in the body (thermogenesis), boosting metabolism and burning calories in the process.

Berries go a step further in the weight-control arena. They help regulate leptin, a hormone produced by our fat cells. Named for the Greek word *leptos*, meaning "thin," leptin is released into the bloodstream after you eat. It heads to the brain, where it helps blunt the sensation of hunger, which is why it is sometimes referred to as the "satiety hormone." Having high levels of leptin in your body is a good thing, because your hunger stays in check, and you're less likely to overeat.

Berries also contain carnitine, which is considered a fat burner because it helps carry fat into the energy factories of cells—the mitochondria. If carnitine is in short supply, most fats can't get into the mitochondria to be burned for fuel.

There are lots of other benefits to eating berries. They help to detoxify the body (which is why they're front and center on my cleanse) and to lower cholesterol and blood sugar levels. Plus, they are sometimes referred to as "brain berries" because they help to boost cognitive function and protect against age-related memory loss.

USE IT TO LOSE IT Enjoy a daily dose of berries in smoothies, stirred into a bowl of oatmeal, in salads, or all by themselves.

4. CELERY

I know celery gets a bad rap as a "diet food," but as a chef, I love this versatile veggie. It has such a wonderful flavor profile, and real knockout potential when used in various dishes. In fact, the veggie

THE ONE TRUE NEGATIVE CALORIE FOOD

The big reveal: It's water.

Water contains zero calories and is also a huge factor in stimulating thermogenesis. In research conducted at Humboldt State University in Arcata, California, drinking a little over two 8-ounces glasses of water was shown to increase metabolic rate by 30 percent in just 10 minutes.

Water also satisfies both thirst and hunger signals. Researchers at Virginia Tech found that people who drank water before meals lost more weight than those who did not. Often, thirst pangs are mistaken for hunger—so the next time you find yourself craving a snack in your mid-afternoon slump, drink a large glass of water first and see how you feel. The oxygen content in water (H_2O) also offers your brain and body a mini energy boost, and aids in detoxification.

For a significant fat burn, let's all raise our water glasses!

basket at the bottom of my fridge looks like it's growing celery sticks!

I also love celery because it is so filling. That's because it's high in fiber (its stringiness tells you that) and water. This means you can fill up on it without consuming a lot of calories.

USE IT TO LOSE IT There are hundreds of ways to use celery: Eat it with abandon as a snack. Toss it into stews, soups, and salads. Juice it with apples for a power beverage that will give you vital nourishment to lose weight and prevent illnesses. It has barely any calories per stalk, so you can definitely eat or juice as much celery as you want.

5. CITRUS FRUITS

Or shall I say "nature's diet pills"? The vitamin C found in citrus fruits—oranges, lemons, grapefruits, and others—helps the body burn fat for fuel, especially if you work out. In 2005, research published in the *Journal of the American College of Nutrition* found that people with adequate vitamin C levels burn 30 percent more fat during a moderate exercise bout than people with low vitamin C levels. Other research published since then has reported similar findings that marginal vitamin C status hinders weight loss.

Scientists believe that the mechanism behind the vitamin's effect on fat burning is linked to the role it plays in the manufacture of carnitine. As I explained earlier, carnitine shuttles fatty acids to the machinery in cells that burns them for fuel.

Remember the infamous grapefruit diet from back in the '80s? While I would never suggest something as extreme as eating only grapefruit every day for days on end, there have been some interesting studies conducted on the effectiveness of consuming grapefruit to aid in weight loss. In a 2006 article published in the *Journal of Medicinal Food*, scientists divided 91 obese patients into four groups. Each group was given either: (1) a placebo capsule and 7 ounces of apple juice, (2) a grapefruit capsule and 7 ounces of apple juice, (3) a placebo capsule and 8 ounces grapefruit juice, or (4) a fresh grapefruit. The study lasted 12 weeks.

Of the four groups, those eating the fresh grapefruit whittled off the most weight. One possible reason is that grapefruit also contains a natural compound called naringenin. It helps regulate blood sugar levels and helps prevent metabolic syndrome—a precursor to diabetes—by assisting the liver in burning up excess fat.

All citrus fruits, including lemons, limes, and oranges, contain a natural compound called limonene, which is found in the rind of the fruit. Limonene helps the liver neutralize toxins and carcinogens. Of course, we don't normally eat the bitter rind, so the best way to get this benefit is to simply use a fine, handheld grater to zest your citrus. I don't know many dishes that aren't improved by the addition of a little lemon or lime zest!

USE IT TO LOSE IT An orange makes a great snack—or dessert—when you're craving something sweet. Add lemon and lime slices to your water for some extra fat-burning benefits, and use a Microplane or another fine grater to add citrus zest to salads, smoothies, and yogurt to get the maximum benefit from these power-packed fruits. You'll find even more delicious ways to use citrus fruits in my recipes—such as Breakfast Citrus Salad with

Cucumbers and Basil (page 104), Citrus-Berry Smash Smoothie (page 96), and Seared Tuna Tataki Salad with Citrus, Tofu, and Watercress (page 134).

6. CRUCIFEROUS VEGETABLES

These are basically your cabbage-family veggies such as broccoli, cabbage, cauliflower, and Brussels sprouts. I'm often asked why they bear the name "cruciferous," so I looked it up! It turns out they were named for their "cross-shaped" flower petals.

I tagged these veggies as negative calorie foods for a couple of reasons. First, they contain indole-3-carbinol (I3C), a natural compound that stops the growth and expansion of fat cells, as stated in a 2013 study published in the *International Journal of Obesity*. It works primarily by reducing a bad form of estrogen that can lead to fat accumulation and can interfere with muscle development.

And second, cruciferous vegetables contain a natural ingredient called 3,3'-diindolylmethane, or DIM for short, that helps to destroy synthetic estrogens in the body. These estrogens come from various sources, including gasoline fumes, plastics, medicines, pesticides, and perfumes—any product that comes from petrochemical manufacturing. Foreign estrogens also come from our food supply. The hormones fed to cows and chickens (in order to fatten them up) contain estrogen. When we consume the meat or milk of animals that are fed hormones, those hormones get passed to us—and they have the same effect on humans, causing us to store fat.

USE IT TO LOSE IT Eat cruciferous vegetables daily, as much as you want—raw as snacks, in stir-fries and salads, or as side dishes seasoned with spices or peppers. Or get your dose in my Charred Thai-Style Broccoli Salad with Almonds and Lime (page 120), Shaved Brussels Sprouts with Warm Toasted Garlic, Almond, and Lemon Dressing (page 138), or Mexican Cauliflower Chili Scramble (page 112).

7. CUCUMBERS

Cucumbers are packed with insoluble fiber, a form of fiber than does not dissolve in water. As it passes through your intestinal tract, it maintains its form and speeds up the passage of food and waste. (The phrase "laxative effect" springs to mind.) Insoluble fiber also slows the body's digestion of starch (thus delaying the absorption of glucose, or sugar, that gets stored as fat), and helps to scrub away unwanted bacteria from your GI system.

Now for some cucumber trivia: This vegetable is rich in what little-known antioxidant now considered a strong anticancer compound?

Stumped? The answer is fisetin. According to a 2012 report in *Antioxidants and Redox Signaling*, the fisetin in cucumbers helps the body prevent the development of cancer and memory loss. Two other negative calorie foods high in fisetin are apples and strawberries.

USE IT TO LOSE IT I love cucumbers for their flavor and texture, and I use them in practically everything: salads, soups, snacks, juices, and, yes, sandwiches. Try starting your meals with a cucumber-based salad. You can't gulp it down; it will take a while to chew. With cucumbers, you'll be burning calories, getting full, and cleansing your digestive system all in one.

8. GREEN LEAFY VEGETABLES

Are you in the habit of stuffing yourself at meals? Do buffet restaurants send you thank-you cards?

Control the urge to splurge by starting your meals with a big green salad (but hold the cheese, creamy dressing, and croutons!). In a study of 42 women at Penn State University, those who had a large green leafy salad for their first course ate 12 percent less of a high-carb pasta entrée even though they were offered unlimited portions. The volume of a predinner salad fills you up before you even get started on your entrée.

What do I mean by "green leafy vegetables"? Think lettuce, spinach, kale, arugula, turnip and mustard greens, and Swiss chard. All leafy greens are chock-full of valuable phytonutrients and are brimming with fiber.

One group of those phytonutrients—thylakoids—are used in plant cells during photosynthesis, the process by which plants make their own food by converting sunlight into energy. Primarily found in the leaves of plants, thylakoids have been found to stabilize appetite-regulating hormones, normalize cholesterol and triglycerides, and decrease body weight in animals and humans. In a Swedish study, a group of 15 people who took supplemental thylakoids reported that it was easier to resist the temptation to eat between meals. Thylakoids slow down the digestion of fat, tricking stomachs into believing they have eaten enough.

Foods containing thylakoids also prevent your body from releasing very high amounts of insulin when you eat a high-fat meal, according to a study published in the *Scandinavian Journal of Gastroenterology*. This is an important finding, since chronically high levels of insulin can lead to fat gain and health risks such as diabetes.

How do you know if a veggie is high in thylakoids? If it's green, it's got 'em.

USE IT TO LOSE IT Make room for at least one moderately sized mixed salad every day. And don't forget the celery and cucumbers! Toss handfuls of spinach or kale into your smoothies, too; you'll never taste the spinach in my Orange Greensicle Smoothie (page 82), but it's there! Anytime you increase your intake of leafy greens, you will see your efforts reflected on the scale.

9. MUSHROOMS

I've always insisted on mushrooms on my pizza, but little did I know that those sliced fungi could be burning off the fat I was gaining by eating that pizza!

Here's the scoop (slice?):

Mushrooms are unique in that they're the only nonanimal source of vitamin D. They actually absorb this vitamin in the same way we do: from the sun. People with inadequate blood levels of vitamin D are at risk for developing obesity, and may be more at risk for mood disorders.

Ever wonder what gives mushrooms their meaty texture and taste? They contain an amino acid also found in animal protein called glutamate. This amino acid is thought to impart the distinctive flavor that chefs refer to as *umami*—often

TOP 10 FAT-BURNING CONDIMENTS AND SPICES

Negative calorie foods aren't the only way to capitalize on the negative calorie effect. Spices also offer a variety of fat-burning and health-promoting benefits. Here are my favorite negative calorie condiments and spices:

1. **Cayenne pepper:** Regarded across various cultures as a medicinal food for at least 9,000 years, cayenne pepper can rev up metabolism and boost fat-burning by up to 25 percent. Just remember: a little goes a long way!

2. **Black pepper:** This kitchen staple has a thermogenic effect and has been shown to help alleviate sluggish digestion. I strongly encourage you to keep a pepper mill filled with peppercorns and grind your pepper fresh for each use.

3. **Turmeric:** This bright orange spice has been valued for its medicinal properties for centuries. It has been shown to reduce triglyceride levels, boost fat-burning, keep blood sugar steady, and fight inflammation in the body.

4. **Mustard:** Whole-grain mustard (not honey mustard or any other sweetened mustards) adds flavor to many dishes and helps you feel full. Among condiments it has one of the highest thermogenic effects.

5. **Horseradish:** Oh, the things you can do with horseradish. I love it in a Bloody Mary, paired with roast beef, and stirred into cocktail sauce. I love it even more now that I know it can help to increase my fat burn and boost my metabolism.

6. **Cinnamon:** This sweet spice may delay the rate at which your stomach empties, meaning it can make you feel fuller for longer. It also lessens the production of insulin after you eat. Insulin is the hormone that turns excess sugar into fat. Tamping down insulin production can mean less weight gain. Cinnamon is a natural way to sweeten your food, too, so you don't have to rely on added sugar.

7. **Ginger:** In research, ginger has been shown to enhance thermogenesis and reduce feelings of hunger. Fresh is best. I prefer young ginger, which is just-harvested and moist with a pink tinge and mellow flavor. Look for it in Chinese markets in the spring and early summer. At other times, any fresh ginger from the supermarket will do.

8. **Garlic:** This common cooking ingredient is thermogenic, and thus helps speed up your metabolism. It can also cut blood pressure and does so by generating a substance called nitrous oxide, which can relax vessels, leading to decreased blood pressure in both people with normal blood pressure and those with hypertension. Garlic also helps normalize cholesterol; it acts like a natural detergent in the arteries by breaking up fat molecules.

9. **Cardamom:** This is a terrific detox spice. Cardamom, which can be bought ground or in pod form, has long been used in Ayurvedic medicine as a natural detoxifier, as a digestive aid, and even as an immunity booster. It tastes like a cross between citrus and pepper and is delicious in baked goods and Indian dishes.

10. **Cumin:** Popular in Indian, Mexican, South American, and Middle Eastern cuisines, cumin is one of the spices you will find in any curry blend. It has long been used as a digestive aid and adds a delicious, mildly spicy flavor to many dishes.

considered the fifth flavor of food, just past sweet, salty, bitter, and savory. Mushrooms also contain molecules called "beta-glucans." These are branches of glucose that can't be dismantled by the digestive system because of their biochemical shape. Upon reaching the intestine, beta-glucans morph into a gel that slows the passage of food through the gastrointestinal tract. The gel also binds to dietary cholesterol, preventing it from being absorbed and thus lowering blood cholesterol levels. These actions are believed to promote satiety and weight loss.

Who knew mushrooms had so much going for them?

USE IT TO LOSE IT Enjoy mushrooms sprinkled on salads, incorporated into stir-fries and soups, tucked into an omelet, or as toppings for meat, chicken, and fish dishes. I encourage you to branch out from regular old button mushrooms, too, and sample different varieties. They each have their own unique flavor profiles, but they all share the common denominator of helping you shed pounds.

10. NIGHTSHADES

The word *nightshades* sounds a bit spooky and ominous, but there's nothing scary about this plant family, which includes tomatoes, red and green bell peppers, and "hot" peppers such as chiles and jalapeños, and eggplant. So why are they called nightshades? Because unlike most plants, which grow in the sunlight of daytime, these veggies have the ability to grow at night.

Nightshades bring a lot to the weight-control table. Tomatoes, bell peppers, and eggplant have a high water volume, so they help you feel full. They are also packed with fiber. Hot peppers like habaneros, jalapeños, and chipotles not only add a flavorful kick to almost any dish, they are also proven fat burners.

How can hot peppers help you lose weight? The secret is in a natural chemical they contain called capsaicin. Capsaicin has two things going for it. First, it's thermogenic, meaning that it activates the natural process that converts food to heat. Capsaicin offers an even greater thermogenic benefit if you exercise. Researchers at Kyoto University in Japan conducted a study to assess the thermogenic

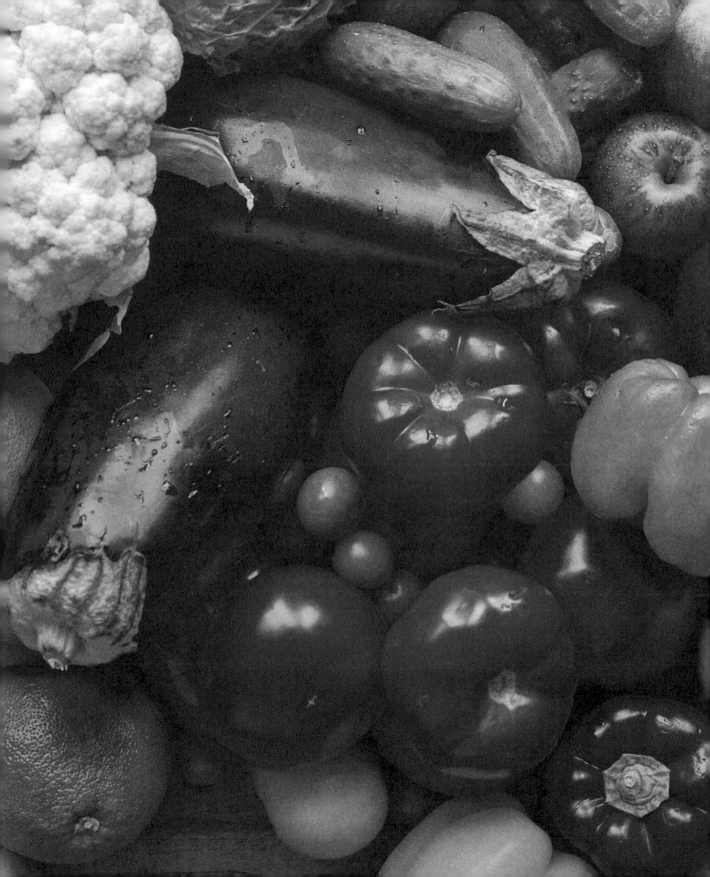

effect of capsaicin and exercise. They recruited 10 men to take either 150 milligrams of capsaicin, or a placebo, one hour before they worked out, and tested them afterward. It turned out that capsaicin significantly increased the body's ability to burn fat as energy (compared with the placebo). These findings suggest that capsaicin encourages the use of fats as fuel during rest and exercise, and may boost weight loss when you diet and exercise regularly.

Second, capsaicin is satiating and helps curb your appetite so that you eat fewer calories. Studies show that when people eat a chile-spiked meal, they tend to eat much less later in the day. USE IT TO LOSE IT Be sure to add nightshades to your shopping cart: tomatoes and peppers for salads, eggplant for Italian dishes, and hot peppers for Mexican food. Here are three more easy and delicious ways to eat your nightshades: Eggplant Roll-Ups (page 164); Kale, Red Onion, and Tomato Frittata (page 108); and Beef-Stuffed Cabbage with Pepper and Tomato Goulash (page 160).

PROTEIN

Lean protein is a key component of the Negative Calorie Diet, as it, too, is a fat burner. For one thing, protein is a highly thermogenic macronutrient. Protein may even help you spot-reduce your tummy. In a number of studies, people who increased their intake of lean proteins to 25 to 30 percent of their total diet shed more belly fat than people who ate less protein.

Additionally, protein gives you that lasting feeling of being full and satisfied after a meal. It also prevents hunger pains, because you digest it relatively slowly, keeping hunger hormones at bay.

It's important to choose wisely when it comes to protein. Here are my top 10 favorite sources, all of which you will enjoy on your 20-day plan:

1. BEEF (LEAN CUTS SUCH AS FLANK STEAK AND LEAN GROUND BEEF)

I want to set the record straight here: there is no compelling health or weight-loss reason to cut red meat out of your diet completely. Beef is high in protein, plus it delivers B vitamins, iron, zinc, and other essential minerals. From a fat-burning perspective, lean beef also ranks well, as it stimulates the production of leptin.

Whenever possible, opt for grass-fed beef. Grass-fed lean beef contains a unique nutrient called conjugated linoleic acid (CLA) that promotes fat metabolism. CLA burns fat and prevents fat absorption from the gut. Grass-fed beef also contains fewer calories than industrially raised meat—and it tastes a lot better.

Remember: not all red meat is "bad"; the key is to select leaner cuts, such as flank steak and 96-percent-lean ground beef. Avoid beef that is marbled with fat—I'll show you plenty of ways to add flavor without depending on excess fat.

2. CHICKEN

In a 2011 study published in *Biological Trace Element Research*, eating four 7-ounce portions of chicken during the week, while following a 10-week controlled diet, helped 24 volunteers lose weight, most of which was body fat.

Chicken has a built-in thermogenic effect

that burns calories and depletes fat stores, so it makes sense that these volunteers would lose fat on a diet rich in this animal protein. Just be sure to look for humanely raised, organic chicken that was raised without antibiotics, hormones, or other drugs. The quality of the chicken you'll find at your local grocery store really does vary, and it is worth the extra dollars to get the cleanest possible protein source.

I know that chicken bores many dieters, but don't worry. I'm not going to ask you to grill a plain chicken breast and pair it with a side of steamed vegetables every night. I've created some chicken recipes for this book that are huge on flavor—just you wait.

3. CLAMS

Clams are always a "yes" for me—that is, unless they're swimming in a bowl of creamy chowder, or served as part of a fried seafood platter. Clams are one of the best sources available of vitamin B_{12}, which is involved in regulating metabolism. Try steaming them for a simple, easy, and delicious source of protein.

4. CRABMEAT

Besides being sweetly delicious and filling, crabmeat contains iodine, which helps to support healthy thyroid function. Located in the middle of your lower neck, the thyroid churns out hormones (T3 and T4) that regulate your metabolism. If your thyroid is underactive (hypothyroidism), your metabolism will be slow, and you can gain weight; this is why you want an optimally functioning thyroid. One way to help your thyroid along is to eat foods naturally high in iodine, a mineral that is essential for the production of thyroid hormones that regulate the metabolism. Crabmeat is one of the few foods that offer a naturally concentrated source of iodine. Be sure to buy only the real thing—not that imitation stuff, which is full of chemicals and tastes nothing like real crabmeat!

5. EGGS

In a 2007 study, researchers found that when obese men and women ate 2 eggs for breakfast as part of a calorie-reduced diet instead of a bagel breakfast with equal calories and weight (mass), they lost 6 pounds compared with 3.5 pounds over an 8-week period. While this study was done with whole eggs rather than just the whites (which I prefer and use in my egg-based recipes), researchers theorize it is mainly the protein in the eggs that promotes satiety.

Buy the highest-quality eggs you can afford—as close to the farm as possible. The best eggs have a bright orange yolk, not a pale yellow one. Again, as with all proteins, the way the animal is raised has a real impact on both flavor and nutrition.

6. FLOUNDER

Fish, in general, is considered a high-quality source of protein with low saturated fat, nutritious trace minerals, and vitamins D and B. It also contains omega-3 fatty acids, which can be very helpful in preventing weight gain.

A 2009 study in the *British Journal of Nutrition* supports this fact: Australian researchers assigned 124 men and women of different weights to three groups: normal weight, overweight, and

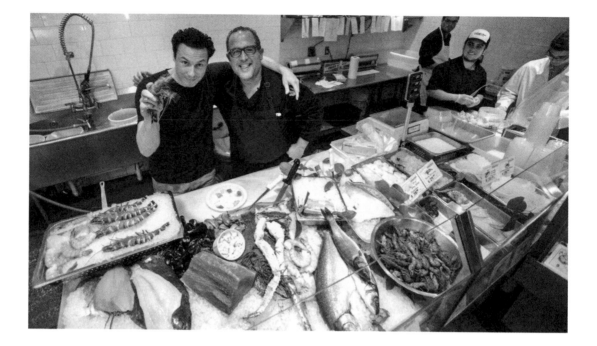

obese. Blood samples were drawn after the individuals had fasted for 10 hours. Then, the researchers measured the levels of omega-3 fatty acids in the subjects' blood. They found that the lower the subjects' omega-3 levels were, the higher their weights, the fatter their tummies, and the wider their hips. Why was this? Researchers think that omega-3 fatty acids work by helping increase lean muscle, which boosts metabolism.

It's important to eat a wide variety of fish. Salmon, herring, tuna, cod, and flounder are great choices. I particularly like flounder because it is so versatile, easy to cook, and rich in nutrients.

7. MUSSELS

Mussels are one of the cheapest and tastiest forms of animal protein available, and because of their natural filtration system, they are virtually immune to toxins in the environment. They get microscopic nutrients directly from the water in which they live.

Plus, they are delicious and healthful and easy to prepare. And when they're ladled into my mussel soup with their glistening blue-black shells, they are definitely beautiful.

Mussels and other shellfish also contain tyrosine, which is important in the synthesis of thyroid hormones. Tyrosine is also converted by the brain into dopamine and norepinephrine—two brain chemicals that promote a feeling of well-being.

8. SHRIMP

Shrimp is among the most versatile of all proteins. It works deliciously in Italian foods such as scampi, Greek dishes like kebabs, Mexican entrées like fa-

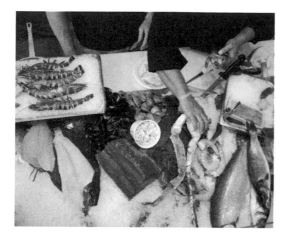

jitas, and Asian stir-fries—not to mention that it's fabulous over salads or served as shrimp cocktail for an appetizer.

Beyond all this, shrimp is an excellent weight-loss food. Like other shellfish, it's high in iodine. It's also high in calcium, known for its fat-burning benefit. Buy wild-caught shrimp when you can find it—it tastes better and offers more nutrients than farmed shrimp.

9. TUNA

Tuna is loaded with omega-3 fatty acids. As I've mentioned, these special fats boost the metabolism by helping the body form muscle. They also help improve transmission of mood-regulating brain chemicals. In addition, omega-3 fats increase oxygenation of the blood, which means better delivery of nutrients to your muscles for growth and repair after exercising.

The easiest way to buy tuna is canned (water-packed), and it tastes delicious in salads and sandwiches. If you want to get off that hook, buy fresh, wild-caught sushi-grade tuna, such as ahi tuna.

You can also purchase it frozen. Bake it, grill it, or panfry it, and you won't be disappointed.

If you go the fresh route, eat it within a day of buying it. Frozen tuna is best consumed within 3 months of purchase.

10. TURKEY

White-meat turkey contains less fat and cholesterol than many other animal proteins, and skinless turkey breast offers a cornucopia of vitamins and minerals, including niacin, vitamins B_6 and B_{12}, iron, selenium, and zinc.

As for weight control, turkey contains an amino acid called tryptophan, a substance used by your body to make serotonin, a mood-enhancing, stress-relieving chemical. When your stress levels go down, production of the appetite-suppressing hormone leptin goes up.

Clearly, negative calorie foods, combined with protein, have a powerful effect on metabolism, weight loss, and appetite. You're going to love this amazing new way of eating.

Before I show you how to eat more to lose more, let's talk about how to choose the very best negative calorie foods to fuel your weight loss.

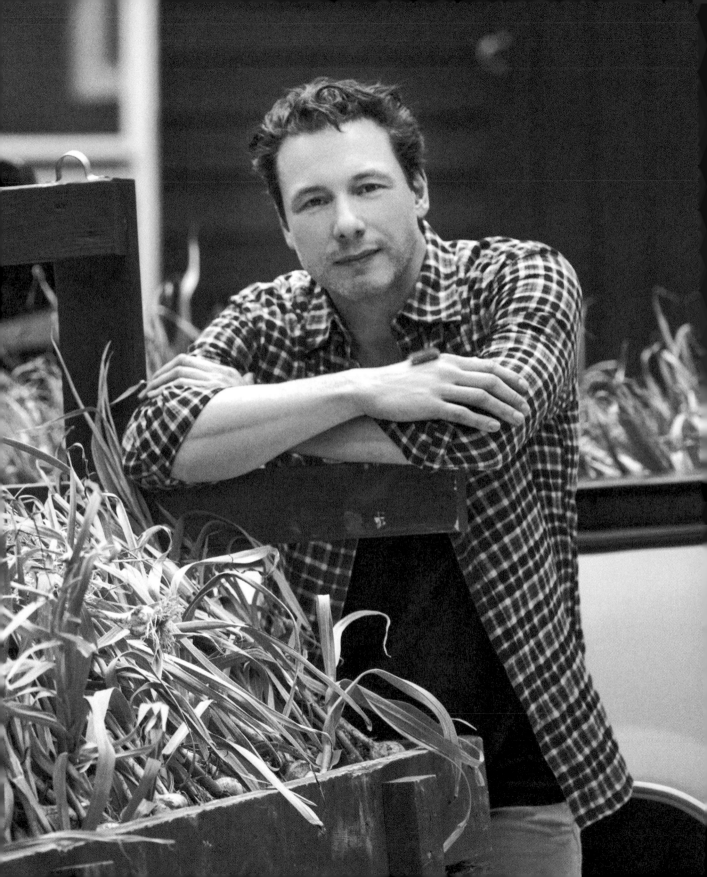

CHAPTER THREE

EAT REAL, FEEL GREAT, LOSE WEIGHT

AS a child, I spent a lot of time at my grandmother's house on Long Island. It was actually a working farm, with livestock, and fruit and vegetable crops planted as far as my eyes could see. There were fig trees, blackberry brambles, peach trees, plum trees, apple trees, and grapes growing on arbors. She grew a variety of lettuces—escarole, arugula, and romaine—as well as red and white onions, broccoli, carrots, parsley, tomatoes, cabbages, peas, peppers, and more. Everywhere you looked, something was growing, and Grandmother's gardens were always beautiful and fruitful. We ate according to season, a concept that has long been a reality for farmers but only recently has become a hot gastronomic trend. We also preserved some vegetables, like tomatoes and peppers, so we could eat them all winter long. Even as a kid I could taste the difference between store-bought canned tomatoes and the tomatoes my grandmother canned herself. When I eat organic food today, it takes me right back to those happy days.

But as I got older and immersed myself in the culinary world, I veered away from the fresh, healthy eating of my childhood. When I was the chef of a three-star restaurant in New York City, my only focus was on making food that tasted good. I didn't care about organics, genetically modified food, calories, or carbs. Fat was my best friend. I used to research ways to get as much fat—think goose fat, bacon fat, and lard—into my food as possible.

Then I learned I had high cholesterol and high blood pressure. Soon the weight listed on my driver's license seemed to be accurate for only the left side of my body. I had to make some tough choices. Imagine a chef giving up all the culinary tricks learned over a lifetime and having to learn how to cook a whole new way: with health at the forefront of his priorities. It wasn't easy but I did it. If a chubby chef who relied on fat more than kids rely on ketchup can do it, so can you.

THE ORGANIC SOLUTION

The term "organic," as you may know, refers to the farming practice of growing crops in sync with the seasonal cycles and without applying herbicides, fungicides, pesticides, or synthetic fertilizers. In my view, the organic method is the traditional way of farming; it's the so-called "conventional" type of farming that is actually a modern invention. Eating fresh, local, organic food is very important to me, and it's important to this eating plan. I'll admit I'm pretty strict about it, but that's because it is just plain better for you—and your waistline. Organic foods offer more nutrients and they're free of chemicals like pesticides, which have been linked to all sorts of health issues, and connected to obesity.

In addition to selecting organically grown produce, I also recommend choosing organic protein sources. As you saw in my top protein choices in Chapter 2, I am picky about the quality of my protein. I always try to cook with farm-raised poultry and meats. Chickens and turkeys with this designation are typically raised without the regular use of antibiotics. And organic birds can't be fed "poultry litter," which is a feed mixture that includes droppings (blech!).

Similar rules apply to organic cattle. Beef labeled "organic" has been raised without routine usage of antibiotics or hormones. Also look for the terms "American Grass-Fed Approved" or "USDA Process Verified Grass-Fed." This certification guarantees that the cow was raised on a diet of 99 percent grass and had seasonal access to a pasture.

When it comes to choosing organic protein sources, seafood presents a bit of a challenge. Organic labels on fish and shellfish don't mean much, because to date the FDA has not approved organic standards for fish or shellfish. Seafood might be labeled as either "wild" or "farm-raised," however. Farm-raised fish are grown in an environment that is rarely ideal. They are often hatched in overcrowded pens, which are frequently infested with sea lice. Farmers use pesticides to treat these infestations. Farmed fish may also be treated with growth hormones and antibiotics, and their diet isn't so great either—they are sometimes fed pellets made from cornmeal, soy, genetically modified canola oil, and other nasty ingredients. Some farmed salmon are even fed artificial coloring agents to mimic wild salmon's deep pink color! Farmed salmon also just doesn't taste as good as wild-caught salmon—it tends to have a spongy texture and a bland flavor. Watch out for farmed shrimp, too. It's frequently treated with antibiotics and can contain high levels of contaminants.

THE ATTACK OF THE OBESOGENS

Unless you're eating mostly organic whole foods, you've probably been exposed to obesogens, also called endocrine disrupters. These are chemical substances—dietary, pharmaceutical, and industrial compounds—that may interfere with the production or activity of the hormones produced by your endocrine system. Obesogens "trick" our bodies into thinking they are natural hormones—a process that can increase fat-forming estrogens in the body and thwart the function of metabolic-boosting thyroid hormones. They also lower the body's regulation of leptin (which, as you'll remember from page 13, helps to keep us from overeating). In short, obesogens encourage our bodies to store fat and predispose us to weight gain.

The list of obesogens is ever-evolving, but currently includes food additives such as high-fructose corn syrup and MSG, as well as pesticides and BPA, a chemical compound found in some plastics used in food packaging.

So in addition to choosing negative calorie foods, you've got to avoid obesogens. It's not quite as simple as reading labels (though that helps tremendously—bye-bye, high-fructose corn syrup!), but if you're aware of where obesogens lurk, you can avoid them. The primary sources of these chemicals are:

Nonorganic meat. As we discussed in Chapter 2, conventionally raised cattle are fattened up with hormones: hormones that are similar to steroids taken by bodybuilders and athletes. Other cattle are given female hormones like estrogen. In male cattle, this synthetic estrogen chemically castrates the animal, enabling it to grow faster. In female cattle, estrogen shuts down the menstrual cycle, thereby devoting more of the cow's energy to growth (as in bulk).

Besides the hormones that we ingest when we eat our steaks and burgers, a substantial portion of these hormones literally passes through the cattle into their poop and ends up in the soil. When we consume hormone-injected meat or foods grown in hormone-contaminated soil, those chemical substances enter our bloodstream, where they can wreak havoc.

Take these actions to reduce your exposure to obesogens in your meat:

- Buy the leanest cuts of meat you can, since hormones get stored in the fat of beef.

- Purchase only organic or grass-fed meat, poultry, and eggs.

- Choose meat and poultry labeled "no antibiotics added" or "certified organic."

- Start incorporating more meatless mains into your diet. Pick one or two days a week to eat only plant-based meals.

Nonorganic dairy. Dairy foods also carry obesogens, mostly from female cows that are fed hormones to increase their milk production. To avoid obesogens in dairy, one solution is to go dairy-free, or at least milk-free. Some suggestions:

- Opt for nondairy milks made from nuts such as almond milk or coconut milk; from grains, like rice milk; or from vegetables such as hemp. (I try to stay away from soy milk, though; highly processed soy is an endocrine disrupter.)

- Get your calcium from nondairy sources. Leafy greens such as kale and collard greens, as well as cruciferous veggies like Brussels sprouts and cauliflower, are great sources of calcium, as are sardines, chickpeas, beans, and figs.

- Still love dairy? Purchase only organic, grass-fed milk products.

Pesticides. Pesticides and fungicides are sprayed on conventionally grown produce and can be found in farm-raised fish because of contaminated groundwater. Here are some of the best ways to avoid ingesting them:

- Buy organic foods. Remember: They haven't been treated with pesticides, fungicides, or other chemicals.

- Purchase fish raised in environmentally healthy environments, or certified as wild-caught. A good Web site to consult as you make seafood choices is: www.seafoodwatch.org.

High-fructose corn syrup (HFCS). This chemically altered version of corn syrup (already a highly processed food) is a big-time obesogen. Most of the places you'll find HFCS are pretty unsurprising—it's typically present in packaged bread, crackers, candy, and cookies as well as soda and sugary drinks. But food manufacturers also sneak HFCS into seemingly "healthy" foods like granola bars, yogurt, frozen entrées, tomato sauce, condiments, and even nut mixes. It's important to always read the label carefully when you buy packaged foods and make sure HFCS is not listed in the ingredients.

The body metabolizes HFCS differently from other sugars, converting it straight into fat. This conversion process may also elevate levels of triglycerides (fat in the blood), and high triglycerides are linked to heart disease. Eliminating HFCS from your diet may help you drop excess pounds and improve your overall health. Here's my advice on how to start:

- Read food labels and avoid foods containing HFCS. This will be easy if you're eating more whole foods and eliminating gluten and refined sugar from your diet.

- Break the fast food habit. Fast foods often contain HFCS, even if they don't taste sweet.

- Eliminate all sugary beverages from your diet. Focus on drinking more water, and choose seltzer, green tea, or herbal tea when you want something with a little flavor.

GO NON-GMO

GM (genetically modified) foods are created when genetic engineers insert genes from one living thing (say, a bacterium or a virus) into the DNA of a completely unrelated living thing (say, corn), in order to create a food product—a genetically modified organism, or GMO—that is more tolerant of frost or weed killers, resistant to pests, or more shelf stable. You may have seen the controversy about GMOs in the news lately. Though the debate between biotech companies, the food industry, environmental watchdogs, and the government is ongoing, my personal vote is to steer clear of all genetically engineered foods.

In fact, scientists from our own Food and Drug Administration (FDA) caution that GM foods could give rise to new toxins and new allergens and need to undergo more rigorous testing to ascertain their long-term effects. But unfortunately, they've also stated that GM foods are "substantially equivalent" to conventional foods and do not currently require safety testing or special labeling.

I object to GM foods for several reasons. First,

I love pure food, and I don't want to eat "frankenfoods." Second, GM foods pose a real environmental hazard and threaten to wipe out some heirloom crops. The wind can easily pick up GM seeds and scatter them into fields that grow organic and non-GMO crops.

Third, I definitely want to avoid health-destroying, fat-producing pesticides. More than 80 percent of all GM crops are engineered for "herbicide tolerance." This means they've been bred with a gene that ensures the crop will survive when sprayed with a weed killer. A major problem, however, has resulted from this practice: There's now an epidemic of herbicide-resistant "super weeds" growing all over the place, which has led to crops being treated with more weed killers than ever. In fact, more than 500 million pounds of herbicides have been used since GM crops were first introduced in the '90s. That, of course, means more toxic herbicide residues end up on our foods.

Fourth, I want to protect my health. The American Academy of Environmental Medicine (AAEM) has enumerated the potential health risks posed by eating GM foods: infertility, weakened immunity, accelerated aging, poor insulin control, abnormal cholesterol, and gastrointestinal issues, among others. In 2009, the AAEM urged doctors to recommend non-GMO diets, emphasizing that doctors are probably seeing illnesses in their patients right now that are linked to ingesting GM foods.

Finally, I have an ethical issue with companies that produce GM seeds. Huge agrochemical conglomerates like Monsanto are buying seeds, genetically modifying them, patenting them, and selling them to farmers. Other farmers are then sued if patented GM seeds are found accidentally growing in their fields because of wind drift.

I won't spend a nickel on products made by companies that use such business practices. With the buying decisions we make every single day, we have the opportunity to vote with our wallets by not purchasing GM foods. How can you be sure you are avoiding GMOs?

- Check the PLU code on the sticker of fresh produce. Any code beginning with an 8 indicates that it is a genetically modified food. Fortunately, most American-grown produce is still GMO-

BUY LOCAL

What if a food doesn't have a label or a sticker?

In the absence of any labeling, the best solution is to find out where the item was grown or raised. A lot of the food you'll find on the shelves of your grocery store has been trucked in from thousands of miles away, or imported from foreign countries. How do you think fruits and vegetables could possibly survive a several-thousand-mile trip? They're shot up with and bathed in a variety of chemicals to help them stay (or at least appear to stay) fresh.

Buy local if you can—and support your local farmers' markets. If you're a New Yorker, and the food was grown in Pennsylvania or Vermont or upstate New York, it's local to you. It wasn't grown in Belgium or China or Mexico. It didn't travel from California to get to you, and it's still food—whole food that's loaded with flavor and nutrition.

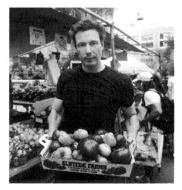

free. Exceptions are corn, soybeans, sugar beets, zucchini, yellow summer squash, and papaya.

- Buy organic (I'll say it again!). Certified organic products cannot intentionally contain any GMOs, so look for labels with "100 percent organic" or "made with organic ingredients."

- Avoid buying a lot of packaged foods and, when you do buy them, always read the label and look for organic varieties and brands that are stamped with the blue-and-green Project Verified NonGMO label.

STOP EATING YOUR WAY TO INFLAMMATION

When you choose organic, non-GMO whole foods, you're not only avoiding obesogens and maximizing your nutrition—you're also helping to prevent one of the most insidious underlying causes of poor health: inflammation.

Inflammation is a natural process; it's the way your body responds to stress or trauma, and it's not always a bad thing. When you have an injury, such as a cut or a sprain, or an illness brought on by germs, your body sends in a squad of healers: enzymes, antibodies, white blood cells, and nutrients to fight the infection and remove the germs. This inflammatory response is why you'll notice swelling after an injury or a fever when you're sick. Once healing is under way, the inflammation subsides—the swelling goes down, the fever reduces.

But your body also becomes inflamed when it's under attack from poor nutrition, accumulated toxins, stress, and environmental toxins—over time, that inflammation can become chronic. You may not notice it, since it's happening on the inside, but chronic inflammation can ultimately lead to many illnesses such as diabetes, hypertension, cardiovascular disorders, dementia, arthritis, eczema, and even cancer. In a report published in the *Journal of Epidemiology*, researchers found that of more than 80,000 people studied, those who developed cancer had significantly higher markers for inflammation than their disease-free counterparts.

Mounting evidence shows that good nutrition and stress reduction strategies can help prevent chronic inflammation. Here are some everyday steps you can take:

- Eat organic fruits and veggies. They are loaded with disease-fighting antioxidants and health-promoting phytochemicals, all of which fight inflammation. Cruciferous vegetables—broccoli, cabbage, Brussels sprouts, kale, and cauliflower—are especially rich in these inflammation-fighting compounds. Choosing organic produce also reduces your exposure to pesticides—an instigator of inflammation in the body.

- Kick out refined carbs and all processed foods. I'm talking about foods made with white flour, added sugar, and high-fructose corn syrup. These unhealthy carbs promote inflammation.

- Choose healthful fats. These include extra-virgin olive oil and moderate amounts of avocados, nuts, and seeds. Healthy fats counter inflammation.

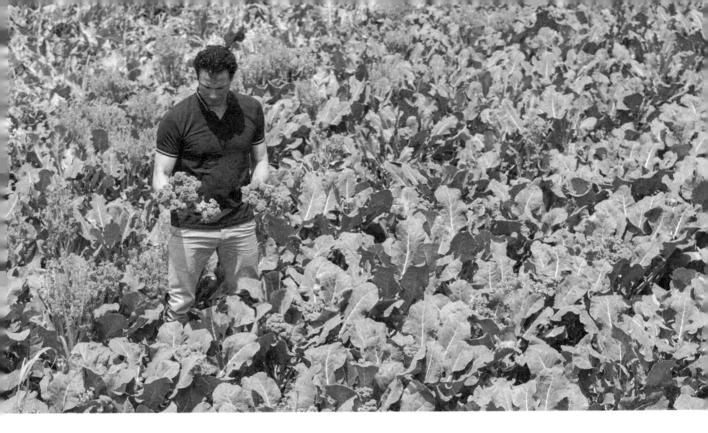

• Eat wild-caught fish a couple of times a week. The omega-3 fats present in high quantities in fish like tuna, mackerel, sardines, and salmon can help reduce inflammation.

• Spice it up. As you know from page 17, spices are more than just flavoring agents—they also have fat-burning power. On top of that, spices are full of phytochemicals that fight inflammation. Two of the best anti-inflammatory spices are ginger and turmeric.

• Eliminate possible allergens from your diet. Ignoring an intolerance or sensitivity to gluten, lactose, or other substances may worsen chronic inflammation. When the body recognizes these allergens as hostile invaders, the immune system revs up and increases the circulation of inflammatory compounds.

• Watch your weight. Putting on excess pounds can promote inflammation. Dropping just 5 to 10 percent of your body weight can have a huge impact with respect to lowering inflammation. The Negative Calorie Diet will help you reach, and maintain, your ideal weight.

I really love feeling good, and when I eat whole foods, I feel good. My mind and body feel alive and vibrant. My spirit thrives because I feel that I'm not only doing something healthy for myself, but also doing something healthy for the planet.

You can choose to do the same. It all starts with eating clean. Let's get started . . .

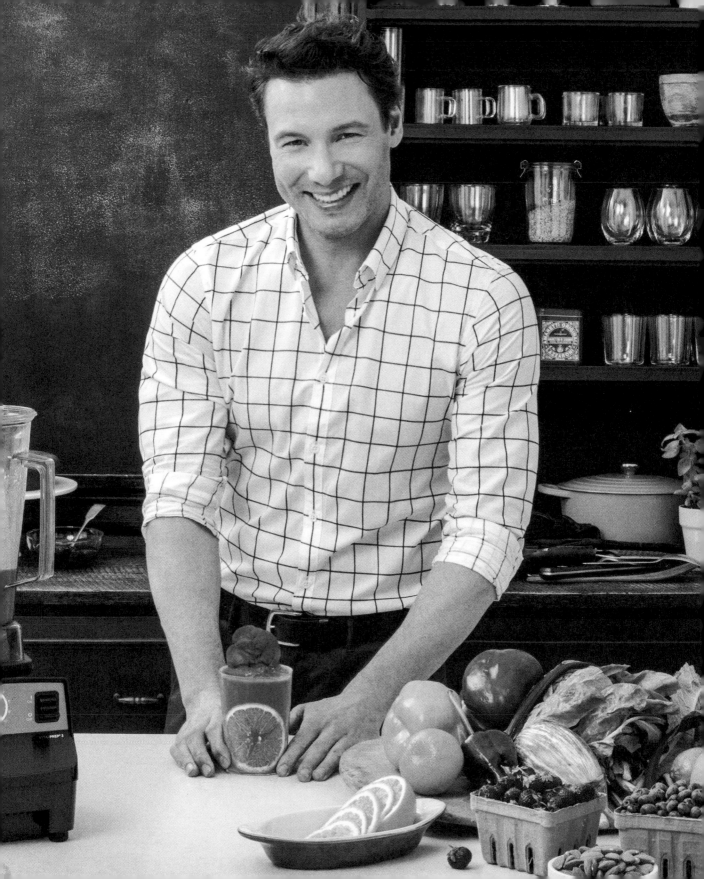

CHAPTER FOUR

THE 10-DAY NEGATIVE CALORIE CLEANSE

YOU'VE probably heard a lot about cleansing (also called "detoxing"), which has become a big trend lately. Maybe you've read interviews with celebrities who swear by juice cleanses, or seen expensive kits for sale online, or spoken with a friend or coworker who's extolled the virtues of the latest "detox." You might be wondering: What exactly is a cleanse, and why do our bodies need to be "cleansed," anyway?

Every cell in your body produces waste that has to be eliminated. Every one of us has had, and will continue to have, some level of exposure to toxins via pesticides, radiation, chemicals and preservatives, and other chemical by-products in our water, our food, and our air. Toxic exposure can harm the body and places a big burden on our bodies' natural detoxification organs, namely the skin, kidneys, bowels, and liver.

We can give those organs a hand by eating whole foods, drinking pure water, and exercising regularly. All of these measures are essential to helping our organs efficiently and effectively eliminate toxins from the body. I like to think of detoxification as an internal housecleaning that gets the body back to optimal functioning.

Weight loss is another pleasant side effect of the Negative Calorie Diet cleanse. In fact, many people lose up to a pound a day on this part of the program. Do the math: That's 10 pounds in 10 days! Because you're eating mostly negative calorie foods and eliminating sugar and processed carbs from your diet—two categories of food that promote weight gain—your body will naturally be in a state of negative calorie balance. Plus, you'll be eating and drinking plenty of fiber, which stimulates weight loss by moving excess fat and calories out of your body. And consuming more liquids—a key part of this cleanse—also helps to accelerate weight loss and fat burn.

And with this plan—unlike some popular fasts and juice cleanses—you won't feel hungry while you're cleansing, because you'll be eating negative calorie foods that are wholesome and satiating. So you can go on with your life as usual—working, exercising, running around with your kids—without feeling fatigued. There's no putting your life on hold, postponing activities, or canceling events. You can "do life" with absolutely no downtime.

SMOOTHIES, SOUPS, AND SALADS

On this cleanse, you'll enjoy a trio of meal options: smoothies, soups, and salads, for a total of four meals a day. Of those four meals, three are smoothies, and the fourth is either a soup or a salad. There's a reason for this structure.

SMOOTHIES

First, each smoothie is made with two or more negative calorie foods, so you get a concentrated infusion of nutrients that will help accelerate your metabolism. Second, my smoothies are high in water and fiber, so you'll get more bang for your buck from a fullness standpoint. Finally, you'll be fortifying your smoothies with protein powder. And as you know by now, protein boosts your fat burn, helps to build metabolically active muscle, and enhances satiety.

SOUPS

There's nothing I love more than a bowl of hearty, homemade soup. It's true comfort food. But soup has another merit, which is backed up by a mountain of research: It can help you drop pounds and keep them off. That's because even though it's mostly water, soup is immensely satisfying.

More than two decades of studies show that soup increases satiety, eases hunger, and keeps us from overeating. The reason: Soup is a bona fide "low energy-dense food," which means that it gives you more food and nutrition for fewer calories, so you ultimately feel fuller. And, like the smoothies, my soups are loaded with negative calorie foods.

SALADS

Fruits and veggies are particularly effective for detox purposes when consumed raw—that way, all of their natural fiber and nutrients are intact. The vitamins, minerals, and antioxidants can only do you good, and the natural sugars in the fruit will help reduce cravings for sweets. Salads are an especially enjoyable way to get your daily dose of vitamins. You might be skeptical that your appetite will be satisfied by a salad, but trust me, it will. To create a salad that will fill you up and burn fat, it's important to add some protein to your salad bowl—I've given you recipes that include plant and animal protein.

Cleansing is about more than what you're putting *in* your body. Just as important, you need to address what stays *out* of it! Here's my three-step approach for preparing to detox:

STEP 1: KICK OUT THE TOXINS

Every day, we're exposed to harmful, health-robbing toxins in our environment and our food and even in the air we breathe, and they can accumulate in the liver, the body's main detox organ. How do you know if your liver is overburdened with toxins? Major signs include chronic fatigue, headaches, allergies, bloating, skin problems, moodiness, and "brain fog."

The simplest way to reduce your exposure to environmental toxins (particularly those in food) is to focus on eating whole foods and drinking pure water daily, both of which you'll do on this plan!

STEP 2: DECONTAMINATE YOUR DIET

Here's what you'll need to skip—and why.

- **Added Sugar and Sweeteners.** Sugar is highly addictive; some experts have said that it is the hardest addiction to kick, perhaps six to eight times harder than cocaine. One downside of sugar is that it imparts a "natural high" by triggering the brain to pump out the "feel good chemical," serotonin. You want that feeling, so you eat more sugar. Researchers at Yale University found that when a group of women were shown photographs of a milk shake made with chocolate ice cream, they displayed brain activity on a par with addicts who craved drugs or alcohol.

Of course, consuming a lot of the sweet stuff can also contribute to obesity, diabetes, and cardiovascular problems. Sodas are obviously banned on this cleanse; 12 ounces of cola have roughly 12 teaspoons of sugar. Also banned are bottled smoothies, store-bought fruit and vegetable juices, sweetened coffees, and any bottled beverage that lists high-fructose corn syrup on the label. Artificial sweeteners are also banned—so no diet soda!

- **Processed Foods.** These include processed grains and many foods that come in a box. Processed foods contain not only added sugar, but also other additives and preservatives. They're like pollution in your body. When they linger in fat cells, they can cause problems, such as interfering with blood sugar levels, triggering inflammation, and slowing down metabolism. Give them a rest and you'll notice an immediate difference: you'll feel lighter, more energetic, and mentally sharper.

- **Dairy.** Commercially produced dairy contains common allergens that can tax your immune system if you're sensitive to them. Many people with dairy sensitivities regularly experience symptoms related to lactose intolerance, such as diarrhea and bloating, but don't make the connection until they steer clear of milk products for a bit and their symptoms disappear. On the cleanse, we're going to give dairy a rest for 10 days. Be sure to note how you feel before and after; sometimes food sensitivities are masked because we consume a food so regularly, it's only when we take a break that we notice how much better we feel when we're not eating it.

- **Gluten.** Gluten is a plant protein found in grains including wheat, barley, and rye. Many people are intolerant of gluten and suffer digestive unrest after eating it. About 1 in 133 people in the United States is actually allergic to gluten. This allergy is called celiac disease, a severe immune reaction that occurs in the small intestine after ingestion of gluten and can lead to nutrient deficiencies.

There's nothing inherently wrong with eating grains; whole grains are high in fiber, and many offer important vitamins and minerals, such as folic acid. But for the most part in the United States, we're eating GMO wheat and grains, which contain very high levels of gluten. A lot of my gluten-free clients report that when they travel abroad—to Italy, for example—they enjoy pasta and have no problems at all. I tell them that's because the wheat in Italy and other European countries hasn't changed in more than 500 years, and European countries ban GMO foods.

If you stop eating grains—at least for a while—you can expect to lose weight. Why? Because we eat a ridiculous amount of these foods in this country, and they are loaded with calories. Once you cut gluten-containing grains out of your diet, you'll start feeling better and looking a whole lot trimmer.

- **Hydrogenated Oils.** I strongly encourage you to shun foods or food products that contain "partially hydrogenated vegetable oils," a source of trans fats. (You should do this whether you're cleansing or not!) Trans fats effectively decelerate your metabolism and make your body more resistant to insulin. Always check the ingredients list at the bottom of a food label; anything "hydrogenated" must be avoided.

- **Alcohol.** Let's just get this out of the way: nothing—*nothing*—washes down a great meal better than a hearty glass of red wine. But while you're on the cleanse, alcoholic beverages are out of the question. Yes, I know that giving up your nightly cocktail may be among the toughest sacrifices. But alcohol stresses the liver, slows the metabolism by depressing the central nervous system, and adds extra calories to your day. Heavy drinking also stops your body's fat-burning power and creates excess belly fat, so you want to keep the booze out of your system while you're giving your body time to heal itself through a detox.

- **Coffee.** Here's something I'm going to leave up to you, but with some caveats. I don't have a problem with coffee in theory, but I have a problem with brewed coffee. Studies have demonstrated that brewed coffee contains so much acid that it causes inflammation, and therefore can be harmful.

Another reason to ditch coffee: several studies suggest that regular caffeine intake may lead to insulin resistance, causing a possible increase in your risk for diabetes, as well as making it easier for you to put on extra weight.

If you're a serious caffeine junkie, I suggest that you switch to my favorite pick-me-up: espresso (just one a day during the cleanse!). Because it is such a small, concentrated amount of coffee, it is less likely to cause inflammation than consuming large cups of brewed coffee. You might also consider switching to green tea or matcha; both have proven fat-burning power. Or choose herbal teas or coffee substitutes. Some good ones are Pero, Roma, Cafix, and Teeccino. Another option is to try maca tea, the legendary Peruvian superfood and energy and endurance booster.

STEP 3: PREP THE DAY BEFORE THE CLEANSE

Before you detox your body, you will need to detox your fridge and pantry. Toss out anything that might derail your cleanse, including everything listed in Step 2. Tell your family and friends that you'll be cleansing and not available to go out for meals or to grab a coffee. It's only 10 days. You can do it.

The day before you begin, weigh yourself and record your weight. Don't weigh yourself again until the day after you finish the cleanse. Weight fluctuates like the stock market; stepping on the scale all the time, and seeing fluctuations, might frustrate you and distract you from your goal.

STEP 4: FOLLOW THE 10 RULES OF THE CLEANSE

The rules are simple. Refer back to this page if you have any questions while you are on the cleanse.

1. First thing in the morning, drink 2 liters of water to flush out your system and ignite your metabolism.

2. Drink another 8 cups of filtered water throughout the day. You can use some of your quota to make herbal tea, but don't drink anything else—coffee, tea, and alcohol are not allowed. Feel free to squeeze some fresh lemon juice into your water for an infusion of flavor and nutrients.

3. Have 3 smoothies daily, and 1 solid meal for dinner. Every other day, your solid meal should be a salad or a soup. On "salad" or "soup" days, you may have the soup or salad for lunch, and the meal 2 or meal 3 smoothie for dinner.

4. Follow the suggested meal plan (pages 38–39) or feel free to improvise. You can choose a few smoothies you like best and stick to those for the entire 10 days, or you can follow the plan as written. The same goes for the soups and salads, which can be interchanged for lunch or dinner.

5. Eat until you feel full and satisfied—then stop.

6. Don't count calories. Do not weigh or count a thing. If you eat the right detox foods, then you will instinctively know how much to eat and what is right for your body.

7. Don't eat past 8 PM. Food eaten after this time tends to take longer to digest because the body's metabolism slows down toward bedtime. Keep your system clear and working at its peak by avoiding late meals.

8. If you feel tired, sleep. When you rest, your body has a chance to replenish and repair cells.

9. Stay away from the foods I mentioned in Step 2 (pages 35–36).

10. Don't stay on the cleanse longer than 10 days.

THE 10-DAY NEGATIVE CALORIE FOODS CLEANSE MEAL PLAN

DAY 1

MEAL 1 Cucumber-Strawberry Green Smoothie

MEAL 2 Green Goddess Smoothie

MEAL 3 Sangrita Tomato, Orange, and Red Pepper Smoothie

MEAL 4 Seared Tuna Tataki Salad with Citrus, Tofu, and Watercress

DAY 2

MEAL 1 Apple-Lime-Cilantro Protein Smoothie

MEAL 2 Tropical Sunrise Smoothie

MEAL 3 The Virgin Mary Smoothie

MEAL 4 Chicken Soup with Escarole and Leeks

DAY 3

MEAL 1 Spiced Apple Pie Smoothie

MEAL 2 "Dillicious" Green Smoothie

MEAL 3 Spinach, Pineapple, Lime, and Mint Smoothie

MEAL 4 Rocco's Chef Salad

DAY 4

MEAL 1: Strawberry Shortcake Smoothie

MEAL 2: Lemon-Ginger Smoothie

MEAL 3: Almond Vanilla Protein Smoothie

MEAL 4: Mixed Leafy Green Soup "Caldo Verde" with Chickpeas

DAY 5

MEAL 1 Orange Greensicle Smoothie

MEAL 2 Lemon-Ginger Smoothie

MEAL 3 The Virgin Mary Smoothie

MEAL 4 Swiss Chard Turkey Salad with Golden Raisins and Capers

DAY 6

MEAL 1 Blueberry-Basil Smoothie

MEAL 2 Apple-Lime-Cilantro Protein Smoothie

MEAL 3 Spinach, Pineapple, Lime, and Mint Smoothie

MEAL 4 Vegetable Pot-au-Feu

DAY 7

MEAL 1 Citrus-Berry Smash Smoothie

MEAL 2 Green Goddess Smoothie

MEAL 3 Tropical Sunrise Smoothie

MEAL 4 Crabmeat Salad with Apple, Celery, and Leafy Greens

DAY 8

MEAL 1 Cucumber-Strawberry Green Smoothie

MEAL 2 Sangrita Tomato, Orange, and Red Pepper Smoothie

MEAL 3 Spiced Apple Pie Smoothie

MEAL 4 Flank Steak Salad with Horseradish and Apple

DAY 9

MEAL 1   Orange Greensicle Smoothie

MEAL 2   "Dillicious" Green Smoothie

MEAL 3   Spinach, Pineapple, Lime, and Mint Smoothie

MEAL 4   Asian Curry Mussel Soup

DAY 10

MEAL 1   Almond Vanilla Protein Smoothie

MEAL 2   Lemon-Ginger Smoothie

MEAL 3   Strawberry Shortcake Smoothie

MEAL 4   Shrimp and Cucumber Salad with Red Onion and Poblanos

THE SHOPPING LIST

We're going to detox your weekly shopping list, too. As I've stated before—but it's especially important on the cleanse—try to buy organic, fresh, seasonal vegetables and fruits whenever possible. You don't want to cleanse your body . . . only to load it up with pesticides from conventionally grown produce. Switching to organic foods for even a short period of time can have a measurable impact on your health: Researchers at Emory University had participants go on an organic diet for a few days, then a conventional diet for the next few days. When urine samples were taken, they revealed that levels of two common pesticides fell to undetectable levels when the people ate organically, but reverted back to high levels after conventional foods were reintroduced into their diets.

Here is a sample shopping list for the cleanse. I've divided it into two 5-day lists, since you'll have to go shopping at least twice during the 10 days to make sure you have fresh produce on hand. Your shopping list will look a little different if you choose to use fewer smoothies for the cleanse. This list is based on shopping for one person. Naturally, if others in your family are cleansing with you, you'll have to increase the amount of food you purchase.

DAYS 1–5

FRUITS

◊ 1 banana

◊ 6 Granny Smith apples

◊ 2 kiwi fruits

◊ 4–6 lemons

◊ 4 limes

◊ 3 or 4 oranges

◊ 1 carton fresh strawberries

Dried Fruit

◊ One 5-ounce package unsweetened dried cranberries

◊ One 5-ounce package unsweetened golden raisins

VEGETABLES

◊ 1 bunch kale

◊ 1 or 2 bunches spinach

◊ 1 bunch collard greens

◊ 1 bunch mustard greens

◊ 2 bunches escarole

◊ 2 bags romaine hearts

◊ 2 bunches Swiss chard

◊ 1 bag celery

◊ 2 or 3 cucumbers

◊ 1 small leek

- ◇ 1 bunch scallions
- ◇ 1 white onion
- ◇ 1 red onion
- ◇ 1 garlic bulb
- ◇ 1 small red bell pepper
- ◇ 1 small head broccoli
- ◇ 3 or 4 tomatoes
- ◇ 1 carton cherry tomatoes

Fresh Herbs
- ◇ Cilantro
- ◇ Dill
- ◇ Mint
- ◇ Thyme

PROTEINS
- ◇ One 8-ounce package raw almonds
- ◇ One 2-pound container protein powder (such as Rocco's. If not mine, choose a protein powder made from organic egg white powder, dehydrated beef broth, or pea protein. Make sure there is no sugar added to the brand you choose.)
- ◇ One 20-ounce package silken tofu (such as Nasoya Organic)
- ◇ 1 package skinless store-roasted turkey breast, sliced thin
- ◇ 1 dozen eggs
- ◇ Sushi-grade tuna steak
- ◇ 1 to 2 pounds skinless, boneless chicken breasts

FROZEN FOODS
- ◇ One 12-ounce bag frozen no-sugar-added strawberries

CANNED FOODS
- ◇ One 15-ounce can no-salt-added chickpeas (garbanzo beans)
- ◇ One 15-ounce can pineapple chunks, canned in their own juice

SWEETENERS
- ◇ One 4.8-ounce bag monk fruit extract (such as Monk Fruit In The Raw)

SPICES AND FLAVORINGS
- ◇ Fresh ginger
- ◇ Cayenne pepper
- ◇ Organic vanilla extract
- ◇ Almond extract
- ◇ Chipotle chili powder (or other spicy and/or smoky chili)
- ◇ Ground cinnamon
- ◇ Salt, preferably unprocessed Celtic sea salt (see page 178)
- ◇ Black peppercorns, for grinding
- ◇ Smoky paprika

CONDIMENTS
- ◇ Miso paste
- ◇ Raw coconut aminos such as Coconut Secret
- ◇ Red wine vinegar
- ◇ Extra-virgin olive oil
- ◇ 1 jar prepared horseradish
- ◇ 1 jar capers

MISCELLANEOUS
- ◇ One 4-ounce bag acacia fiber (such as Navitas or Renew Life)

- ◊ One 15-ounce jar coconut manna (such as Nutiva Organic)
- ◊ ½ gallon vanilla almond beverage (such as So Delicious)
- ◊ Olive oil cooking spray
- ◊ Two or three 32-ounce cartons unsalted chicken stock (such as Kitchen Basics)
- ◊ 1 package grated Parmigiano-Reggiano cheese

──────── **DAYS 6–10** ────────

FRUITS

- ◊ 1 banana
- ◊ 6–8 Granny Smith apples
- ◊ 2 kiwi fruits
- ◊ 4 lemons
- ◊ 4 limes
- ◊ 3 oranges
- ◊ 1 carton fresh strawberries

Dried Fruit

- ◊ One 5-ounce package unsweetened dried cranberries
- ◊ One 5-ounce package unsweetened golden raisins

VEGETABLES

- ◊ 1 bunch packaged kale
- ◊ 2 bunches packaged spinach
- ◊ 1 bunch collard greens
- ◊ 1 bunch mustard greens
- ◊ 4 heads butter lettuce
- ◊ 1 bag celery (if you don't have any left over from the previous 5 days)
- ◊ 10 cucumbers
- ◊ 1 or 2 Japanese eggplants

- ◊ 1 head cauliflower
- ◊ 3 white onions
- ◊ 1 red onion
- ◊ 4 red bell peppers
- ◊ 1 poblano pepper, or 1 green bell pepper
- ◊ 1 red jalapeño pepper
- ◊ 1 small head broccoli
- ◊ One 8-ounce package cremini mushrooms
- ◊ One 8-ounce package dried shiitake mushrooms
- ◊ 2 cartons cherry tomatoes

Fresh Herbs

- ◊ Basil
- ◊ Cilantro
- ◊ Dill
- ◊ Mint
- ◊ Parsley

PROTEINS

- ◊ One 20-ounce package silken tofu (such as Nasoya Organic)
- ◊ 12 ounces blue crabmeat
- ◊ One 12-ounce flank steak
- ◊ 1 pound peeled steamed shrimp
- ◊ 2 pounds mussels

FROZEN FOODS

- ◊ One 12-ounce bag frozen no-sugar-added blueberries
- ◊ One 12-ounce bag frozen no-sugar-added mixed berries

CANNED FOODS

- ◊ One 15-ounce can pineapple chunks, canned in their own juice

SPICES AND FLAVORINGS

◊ Crab boil spice (such as reduced-sodium Old Bay)

◊ Curry powder

◊ Condiments

◊ 1 jar Dijon mustard

◊ Unrefined coconut oil

MISCELLANEOUS

◊ ½ gallon vanilla almond beverage (such as So Delicious, sweetened naturally with monk fruit)

◊ ½ gallon unsweetened almond milk

◊ 1 carton frozen unsweetened coconut dessert (such as So Delicious)

◊ Two or three 32-ounce cartons vegetable stock

◊ One 6-ounce carton fat-free, no-sugar-added Greek yogurt

HANDLING HUNGER AND CRAVINGS

Hankering for pizza or chocolate cake? The first few days of the cleanse can be tough, but my advice is to hang in there and take it meal by meal. Cravings will not last. By day 3, you'll be fine. You'll begin to experience the positive effects of the cleanse—your sugar and salt cravings will subside, your taste buds will change, and you won't desire stuff you used to want.

Now for some specific tips to guide you on your cleanse:

• Eat mindfully. When you're on the cleanse, try to stretch out your meals. Relax your mind, chew or sip slowly, and really taste the food you're eating and drinking.

• Water your body. Most hunger cravings between meals are signs of dehydration, which can be put to rest with a glass of water. Another strategy is to sip a cup of warm herbal tea. Mint tea is great for warding off sweet cravings.

• Have your morning smoothie. Don't skip your first beverage in the morning, or you might be besieged by cravings throughout the day.

• Supplement with greens. Add a few teaspoons of spirulina, barley grass, wheatgrass, or a combo of green powders to your smoothie or juice. These are superfoods in supplement form that help our cells to thrive, increasing energy and vitality.

• Limit caffeine. If you're still drinking coffee, consider cutting back or easing off it altogether. Caffeine can stimulate stress hormones that heighten hunger. Instead, try a cup of green tea, which still has caffeine but isn't as hard on your system.

• Stop your urge to splurge. Before you cave in, stop and ask yourself: *"Am I really hungry? Or am I mad? Stressed out? Lonely or bored? Tired?"* It's easy to reach for food when you're feeling emotional or overwhelmed. Instead of turning to food, give yourself the mental or physical outlet you really need: Work out, read a book, take a walk, write an e-mail to a friend—anything to get your mind off food and dissipate your emotions. The urge to splurge will pass.

• Sleep. Try to get 7 to 8 hours of shut-eye every night. Poor sleep quality increases your appetite and throws your hunger-controlling hormones out of whack. The net effect is that you want to eat everything in sight.

• Don't get too hungry. Space your smoothies and daily meal out so that you're eating every 3 to 4 hours. Doing so will help control your hunger.

• Stay active. Walk, do some yoga, or engage in some light exercise. Movement stimulates the release of mood-lifting chemicals such as serotonin, endorphins, and dopamine; plus, it reins in your appetite and helps you stay energized. And if you sweat a little, that's good, too, since perspiration is an effective natural detoxifier that releases toxins through the skin.

After the 10-Day Cleanse is over—and you've completed it successfully—check in with yourself: How do you feel, mentally and physically? Doing a cleanse is an opportunity for real, live biofeedback: it gives you a chance to connect with your body and see how it's really feeling. Many people note that they have improved mental clarity, more energy, and better digestion after the cleanse. Did you notice that your stomach felt better after you avoided certain foods? How did you fare without caffeine? Did your skin clear up, or did your daily headache go away?

And, of course, now that you're done, it's time to get on the scale. Depending on your starting weight, you may find that you've lost 10 pounds or more—what a great way to kick off the next phase of the Negative Calorie Diet.

Let's go!

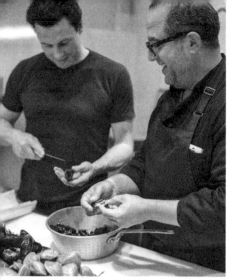
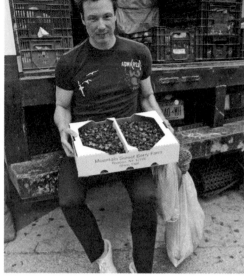
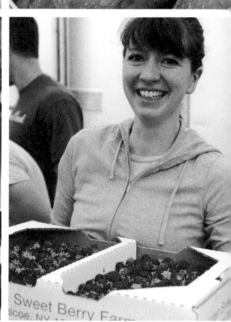
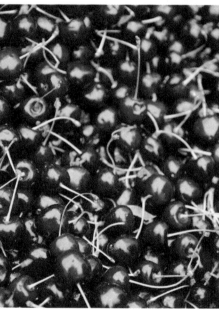
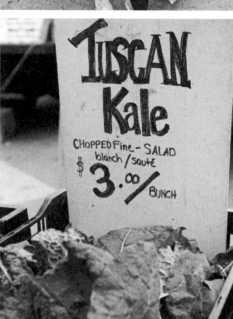

TUSCAN
Kale
CHOPPED Fine - SALAD
blanch/sauté
$ 3.00/BUNCH

Sweet Berry Farm
scoe, NY

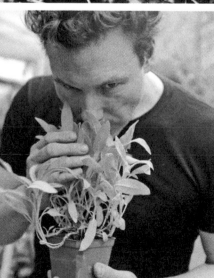
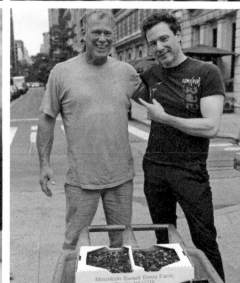

Mountain Sweet Berry Farm
Roscoe, NY 12776

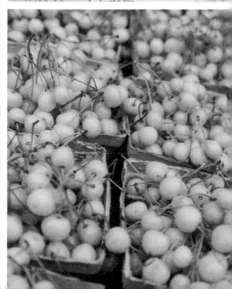

CHAPTER FIVE

THE 20-DAY ALL YOU CAN EAT PLAN

I HOPE your results after the 10-Day Cleanse—sparkling eyes, shiny hair, glowing skin, more energy, and, of course, significant weight loss—have inspired you to start the next phase of this journey: the Negative Calorie Diet.

This diet is different from most diets you've probably tried in the past. Why? Well for one thing, it doesn't eliminate any food groups or macronutrients: it's not anti-fat, low-carb, or high-protein. One great example of the all-inclusiveness of this program is fruit—an entire category of food that is shunned on many diets, because fruit contains sugar and carbs. But as you already know, three of my top 10 Negative Calorie Foods are fruit! Apples, citrus fruit, and berries are not just allowed, but also encouraged.

Another difference between this style of eating and many other diets is that I'm not going to police your portion sizes. When you are eating negative calorie foods, you can enjoy yourself and eat without restriction. It's not about exact measurements or calorie calculations—it's about learning to recognize, and choose, foods for their nutritive and fat-burning potential.

This diet is really a way of life: it is all about balance and nutrition. You'll get the nutrients you need from plenty of fresh fruits and vegetables, energy from carbs, and satiety from healthy protein. The results are truly amazing, and when they are added to the health benefits, such as reduced inflammation and better blood sugar regulation, you have a prescription for a whole new way of living better and slimmer in your world.

Remember, I'm asking you for only 20 days. Think of how quickly 20 days go by . . . not even three weeks! You owe it to yourself to set aside this time to get healthy and feel your best.

PREPARING FOR A NEW, HEALTHIER BODY

You can't go on a trip without first deciding on your destination, mapping out your route, or making reservations. As with most things in life, there's a logical, organized way to begin an eating plan. I encourage you to do the following in order to set yourself up for success:

ASK YOURSELF WHY YOU WANT TO LOSE WEIGHT

There are a lot of reasons to lose weight, but one of the most commonly cited among my clients is cosmetic. Let's face it, we all want to look better, fit into our favorite jeans, and feel confident without having to hide our spare tire. While it's important to acknowledge that our body image ideals have gotten out of hand in this country and not everyone is meant to have a 25-inch waist, there's certainly nothing wrong with wanting to look your best. When you see a slimmed-down you in the mirror, it's a great confidence booster. Visible results are also motivating, reminding you that the changes you are making and the work you are doing are really paying off.

In addition to body confidence, there are a host of other reasons to lose weight, including preventing or alleviating serious health problems such as high blood pressure, type 2 diabetes, heart disease, stroke, gallbladder disease, and even some cancers. Other benefits of weight loss include:

◊ Being able to climb up a flight of stairs without huffing or puffing.
◊ Participating in your kids' activities.
◊ Extending the length and quality of your life.
◊ Improving chronic pain conditions in your joints and back.
◊ Gaining more energy and boosting your mental outlook

At the end of the day, this is your journey; the only person making you stick to your new eating plan is you. It's important to think hard about the reasons that brought you here. Every time your resolve wavers, remember those reasons.

SET YOUR FOCUS ON THE POSITIVE

When your goal is to lose weight, you're obviously focusing on something you *don't* want—extra pounds. But focusing on a negative can be counterproductive, because instead of focusing on where you want to be, you're caught up in thoughts of where you don't want to be. And if you've struggled to lose weight in the past, you may also be coming at your new plan from a negative mind-set, with your perceived shortcomings at the forefront of your mind.

Begin by thinking about what you *want* instead of what you don't want. Ditch negative thinking. Tell yourself: *"I look forward to feeling great and being slim and healthy"* or *"I can't wait to shop for new clothes in 20 days"* rather than *"I'm so fat . . . I look gross today,"* or *"I hate dieting."*

It's also helpful to focus on small steps and short-term goals as you go along. In fact, researchers have shown that incremental, practical goal-setting is the key to weight loss. Psychologists at the Free University of Berlin observed that dieters were more successful if they had an "implementation intention"—*how* they'd achieve weight loss—as opposed to a "goal intention": *what* they'd achieve on their plan. Think about what you can do right now to get what you want. On week one, instead of thinking, *"I'm going to lose 20 pounds,"* shift your focus to: *"I'm going to cook myself a nice dinner tonight with fresh, wholesome foods."*

So try shifting your mind-set in a more positive, practical direction. Remember, what you focus on, you give life to.

PREPARE YOUR FAMILY AND FRIENDS

Before you start your new eating plan, it's a good idea to explain your intention to your family and friends. They may be supportive (I hope so!); heck, they may even want to join you. On the other hand, they might be skeptical. Expect it: there are always going to be those folks who say, "There she goes on *another* diet." Fine! Let them think what they want. Just don't let their negativity throw you off course. This is about you, not them.

Try to take any negative comments in stride and remember that no one knows what's right for your body and your health as well as you do. In Chapter 13, I've got some advice on how to follow this program with and without your family, and how to handle family issues that sometimes arise when one person changes his or her eating habits. The great thing about this plan is that it is so adaptable to family life that your spouse and kids won't ever feel they're on a "diet."

PICK A START DATE

It's important to plan for—and stick to—a start date. No pushing it back to "tomorrow"—once you select a date, circle it in red on your calendar, set an alarm on your phone, even post it on social media so that you're accountable to others. Once you make the commitment, there's no opting out.

When is the best time to start a new eating program? Interestingly, a British poll of 2,000 female dieters found that starting on a Sunday or a Monday offers the best chance for success. Psychologically, you'll be motivated to continue if you start afresh at the beginning of the week. The poll also found that 88 percent of people who started their diet on Sunday were able to keep their weight off.

So pick your start day wisely!

THE ESSENTIALS OF THE 20-DAY DIET

As I've emphasized, the Negative Calorie Diet focuses on a fat-burning, health-supportive 20-day eating plan in which you enjoy 10 negative calorie foods in unlimited quantities. You will also eat a variety of the 10 proteins, along with other foods that are high in fiber and nutrients.

YOU WILL EAT:

◇ 4 meals a day: breakfast, lunch, dinner, and 1 snack
◇ Unlimited amounts of negative calorie foods

YOU'LL LIMIT:

◇ Certain carbohydrates
◇ Dairy foods (Greek yogurt and some Italian cheeses are included in small amounts)

YOU WON'T EAT:

◇ Refined or processed foods
◇ Nonorganic or GMO food
◇ Trans fats
◇ Sugar or alcohol
◇ Soda or any beverages made with sugar or artificial sweeteners
◇ Regular coffee (espresso is allowed)

FRUITS AND VEGETABLES TO INCLUDE IN YOUR MEALS:

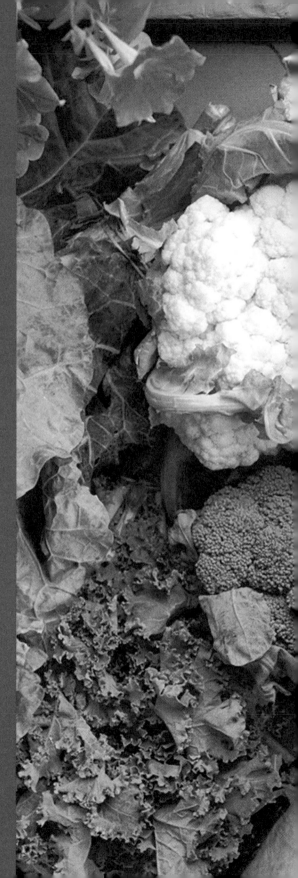

WHOLE VEGETABLES

Arugula
Asparagus
Beet greens
Bok choy
Broccoli
Broccoli rabe
Brussels sprouts
Cabbage, all types
Cauliflower
Celery
Collard greens
Cucumber
Dandelion greens
Eggplant
Endive
Kale
Garlic
Green beans
Jicama
Lettuce, all types
Mushrooms, all types
Mustard greens
Okra
Onions
Parsley
Pea pods
Peppers, all types
Scallions
Spinach
Sprouts (alfalfa, broccoli,
    mung, and so forth)
Swiss chard
Summer squash
Tomatoes, all varieties
Turnip greens
Water chestnuts
Watercress
Yellow beans
Zucchini

WHOLE FRUITS

Apples
Apricot
Bananas
Blackberries
Blueberries
Cherries
Cranberries
Grapefruit
Grapes
Guava
Mango
Melon, all varieties
Nectarine
Orange
Papaya
Passion fruit
Peach
Pear
Persimmon
Pineapple
Plum
Pomegranate
Raspberries
Strawberries
Tangelo
Tangerine
Watermelon

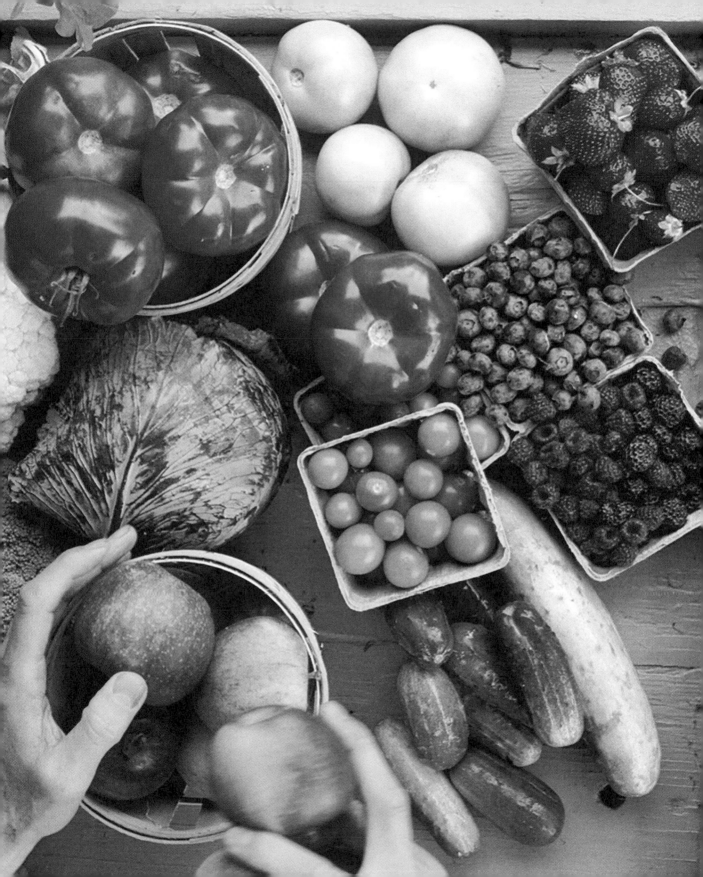

HOW THE NEGATIVE CALORIE DIET WORKS

Every day you will eat three meals and one snack. To give you a sense of how you can put together your meals, I've created a 20-day meal plan with sample menus. The menus incorporate my recipes, which begin on page 68. With the exception of smoothies, all of my recipes are scaled to feed four people—so halve the ingredients, as well as the shopping lists, if you are cooking for two. If you're going solo on the diet, you can cook for two or four and have leftovers for the next day or two, or freeze leftovers for another week.

If you're someone who doesn't like making decisions about what to eat and you're not particularly picky about your food, then I would suggest following these menus to the letter. It will make your life easier by taking the guesswork out of meal planning. If you're someone who prefers to create your own menus, that's fine; this plan gives you the flexibility to do that. What I suggest is that you turn to Part II and read through the recipes; select the ones that most appeal to you, and repeat them for breakfast, lunch, dinner, and snacks as often as you like. If you've found a couple of smoothie recipes from the cleanse that you absolutely love, enjoy them for breakfast every day for the next 20 days. You can also find guidance for planning your own menus on page 60, under "Making the Negative Calorie Diet Your Own."

If you are vegan or vegetarian, you can still follow this eating plan. In fact, a number of my recipes are designed just for you! Anytime you see a meat entrée on the meal plan, simply swap in one of my meatless recipes from Chapter 9. You'll also want to refer to Chapter 12, which addresses the needs of people who want to do a 100-percent plant-based version of the Negative Calorie Diet. I'll explain how to do this, and the benefits of going meat-free.

As you follow the Negative Calorie Diet, feel free to add in other high-fiber, low-starch vegetables, as well as other fresh fruits (see page 48 for ideas). Just keep most starches out of the mix so that the negative calorie foods can work their magic. And don't forget to drink water throughout the day—eight to ten 8-ounce glasses—since water is a true negative calorie nutrient.

I strongly encourage you to get in the kitchen over the next 20 days, and I promise you that the recipes in this book are easy enough for even a novice cook—there are no chef tricks or fancy tools involved. I use my background and training to create flavor in innovative ways—not to overcomplicate things. Remember, cooking your own food gives you control over everything that goes into your body, and this gives you control over your weight. If you like to eat at restaurants, or need to do so for convenience, please check out Chapter 14 on eating out. It will show you how to navigate a restaurant menu while sticking to the Negative Calorie Diet.

To help you on the diet, I've included shopping lists for days 1 to 7, days 8 to 14, and days 15 to 20. They are intended to be used as guidelines only—I wrote these lists for a household of four people, but obviously the amount of food you need to buy will vary according to the number of people you are cooking for, so be sure to scale the amounts of each ingredient accordingly. The lists will also vary based on how closely you want to follow the sample menus. For example, if you have smoothies for breakfast or snacks, rather than my suggested breakfasts, you'll need to customize the shopping lists to include the ingredients you like in your favorite smoothies. As for the spices and condiments listed, you probably have most of these in your pantry already—no need to go out and buy a whole new spice rack!

Although this is a 20-day plan, there's no need to stop at the end of 20 days! Many of my clients find that they enjoy the food so much, and they are experiencing such great results, that they want to stay on the plan indefinitely. You can also go back on the cleanse at any point if you feel that your weight loss has reached a plateau, or if a recent vacation or holiday splurge has set you back. The cleanse will put you on the right track again.

Okay . . . here we go. Time to get cooking!

SUGGESTED MENUS FOR THE 20-DAY NEGATIVE CALORIE DIET

DAY 1

BREAKFAST

Apple and Cinnamon Breakfast "Risotto" with Oat Bran and Almonds, or a Negative Calorie Smoothie

LUNCH

Charred Thai-Style Broccoli Salad with Almonds and Lime

SNACK

Cucumber and Almond Rice Sushi or a Negative Calorie Smoothie

DINNER

Baked Chicken with Sweet-and-Sour Red Cabbage + Crepes Suzette with Oranges and Vanilla Cream

DAY 2

BREAKFAST

Blueberry and Quinoa Porridge with Mint or a Negative Calorie Smoothie

LUNCH

Chicken Soup with Escarole and Leeks

SNACK

Cucumber and Almond Rice Sushi or a Negative Calorie Smoothie

DINNER

Almond-Encrusted Flounder with Chopped Spinach and Clam Broth + Citrus and Mixed Berry Bowl with Whipped Topping

DAY 3

BREAKFAST

Breakfast Citrus Salad with Cucumbers and Basil or a Negative Calorie Smoothie

LUNCH

Crabmeat Salad with Apple, Celery, and Leafy Greens

SNACK

Apple, Cranberry, and Almond Bars or a Negative Calorie Smoothie

DINNER

Eggplant Roll-Ups + Chocolate and Almond Butter Truffles

BREAKFAST

Breakfast Pizza with Mushrooms and Broccoli or a Negative Calorie Smoothie

LUNCH

Leftover Chicken Soup with Escarole and Leeks

SNACK

Apple, Cranberry, and Almond Bars or a Negative Calorie Smoothie

DINNER

Filet of Beef with Braised Kale and Black Olives + Chocolate and Almond Butter Truffles

── DAY 5 ──

BREAKFAST

Kale, Red Onion, and Tomato Frittata or a Negative Calorie Smoothie

LUNCH

Shrimp and Cucumber Salad with Red Onion and Poblanos

SNACK

Cauliflower and Apples with Thai Almond Butter Sauce or a Negative Calorie Smoothie

DINNER

"Pappardelle" of Chicken with Winter Pesto + Chocolate-Dipped Strawberries with Crushed Almonds

── DAY 6 ──

BREAKFAST

Avocado Toast with Spinach and Tomatoes or a Negative Calorie Smoothie

LUNCH

Mixed Leafy Green Soup "Caldo Verde" with Chickpeas

SNACK

Cauliflower and Apples with Thai Almond Butter Sauce or a Negative Calorie Smoothie

DINNER

Flounder "a la Plancha" with Catalonian Eggplant Relish + Chocolate-Dipped Strawberries with Crushed Almonds

── DAY 7 ──

BREAKFAST

Mexican Cauliflower Chili Scramble or a Negative Calorie Smoothie

LUNCH

Shrimp and Cucumber Salad with Red Onion and Poblanos

SNACK

The Grate Salad Bowl with Chia Seed Dressing or a Negative Calorie Smoothie

DINNER

Meatballs with Mushroom and Spinach Gravy + Cocoa-Dusted Almonds

SHOPPING LIST DAYS 1–7
FRUITS

◇ 4 large Gala, Pink Lady, or Empire apples
◇ 3 or 4 large Red Delicious apples
◇ 7 limes
◇ 2 or 3 lemons
◇ 2 avocados
◇ 6 oranges
◇ 2 or 3 grapefruits
◇ 2 cartons fresh blueberries
◇ Several cartons of various types of berries
◇ 1 carton strawberries

Dried Fruit

◊ One 5-ounce package unsweetened dried unsulfured cranberries

◊ One 5-ounce package unsweetened unsulfured golden raisins

VEGETABLES

◊ Several heads escarole

◊ Eight 10-ounce bags spinach

◊ 4 heads butter lettuce

◊ 2 bunches curly kale

◊ 4 bunches Tuscan kale

◊ Four 10-ounce bags mixed leafy greens (kale, collards, and mustard)

◊ 1 garlic bulb

◊ 1 or 2 onions

◊ 1 red onion

◊ 1 large eggplant

◊ 3 large Japanese eggplants

◊ 1 leek

◊ 2–5 heads broccoli

◊ 3 heads cauliflower

◊ 1 or 2 packages cremini mushrooms

◊ 3 or 4 fresh tomatoes

◊ 5 cartons cherry tomatoes

◊ 10 cucumbers

◊ 2 heads red cabbage

◊ 1 package celery sticks

◊ 2 red bell peppers

◊ 1 green bell pepper

◊ 2 poblano peppers, or green bell peppers

◊ 4 carrots

Fresh Herbs

◊ Ginger

◊ Cilantro (several bunches)

◊ Mint

◊ Thyme

◊ Basil

BEEF

◊ Four 3-ounce filets lean beef tenderloin, trimmed of fat

◊ 12 ounces 96% lean ground beef (such as Laura's Lean)

FISH AND SHELLFISH

◊ 2 pounds peeled steamed shrimp

◊ 2 pounds littleneck clams (about 24 clams)

◊ Five 4-ounce fluke or flounder fillets

◊ 12 ounces blue crab crabmeat, picked to remove all shells

POULTRY

◊ Four 4-ounce skinless, boneless chicken cutlets

◊ 8 ounces boneless, skinless chicken thighs

◊ 12 ounces skinless, boneless chicken breasts

EGGS

◊ 3 dozen eggs

CEREALS AND GRAINS

◊ One 12-ounce package oat bran

◊ One 16-ounce package red quinoa

◊ One 24-ounce box rolled oats

◊ 208 grams (about 7.4 ounces) frozen gluten-free pizza dough (such as Gillian's)

◊ 1 loaf gluten-free bread (such as Canyon)

◊ 6-ounce package puffed brown rice (such as Arrowhead Mills)

CANNED FOODS

◇ One 15-ounce can cannellini beans (such as Eden)

◇ One 2¼-ounce can sliced black olives

◇ One 15-ounce can chickpeas (garbanzo beans)

◇ Two 15-ounce cans no-salt-added crushed tomatoes

SWEETENERS

◇ One 4.8-ounce bag monk fruit extract (such as Monk Fruit In The Raw)

◇ One 12-ounce bottle raw coconut nectar (such as Coconut Secret)

◇ Three 3-ounce no-sugar-added naturally sweetened dark chocolate bars (such as Lily's)

OILS AND VINEGARS

◇ Coconut oil

◇ Extra-virgin olive oil

◇ Olive oil cooking spray

◇ Rice wine vinegar

◇ Apple cider vinegar

SPICES AND FLAVORINGS

◇ Black peppercorns

◇ Cinnamon

◇ Salt, preferably unprocessed Celtic sea salt (see sidebar, page 178)

◇ Chopped caraway seeds

◇ Vanilla extract

◇ 1 vanilla bean

◇ Crushed red pepper flakes

◇ Crab boil spice (such as reduced-sodium Old Bay)

◇ Cayenne pepper

◇ Whole fennel seeds

◇ Paprika

◇ Smoked paprika

◇ Ground coriander

◇ Cumin

◇ Chili powder

◇ Garlic powder

◇ Arrowroot

◇ One 8-ounce canister unsweetened organic cocoa powder

CONDIMENTS AND SAUCES

◇ Hot sauce (such as Tabasco)

◇ Green hot sauce (such as Tabasco)

◇ Thai fish sauce (such as Thai Kitchen)

◇ Coconut aminos

◇ Wasabi powder

◇ Dijon mustard

◇ One 26.46-ounce package fat-free, salt-free marinara sauce (such as Pomi)

◇ Thai red curry paste (such as Thai Kitchen)

DAIRY AND NONDAIRY FOODS

◇ Parmigiano-Reggiano cheese

◇ Pecorino Romano cheese

◇ ½ gallon unsweetened vanilla almond milk

◇ One 6-ounce carton fat-free Greek yogurt

◇ ½ gallon unsweetened coconut milk

MISCELLANEOUS

◇ Two or three 8-ounce packages raw almonds

◇ One 8-ounce package slivered almonds

◇ One 12-ounce bag ground chia seeds

◇ One 10- or 50-quantity package nori (seaweed wraps)

◇ One 12-ounce canister psyllium husk flakes

◇ One 8-ounce bag egg white powder (such as Deb El)

◇ Several 32-ounce cartons unsalted chicken stock (such as Kitchen Basics)

◇ Several 32-ounce cartons unsalted beef stock (such as Kitchen Basics)

◇ One 8-ounce package gelatin powder

◇ One 1.69-ounce package freeze-dried apple chips (such as Bare Fruit Simply Cinnamon)

◇ One 12-ounce jar raw almond butter

DAY 8

BREAKFAST

Breakfast Bowl with Quinoa and Berries or a Negative Calorie Smoothie

LUNCH

Leftover Mixed Leafy Green Soup "Caldo Verde" with Chickpeas

SNACK

The Grate Salad Bowl with Chia Seed Dressing or a Negative Calorie Smoothie

DINNER

Shiitake and Bok Choy Stir-Fry + Cocoa-Dusted Almonds

DAY 9

BREAKFAST

Spinach and Mushroom Omelet or a Negative Calorie Smoothie

LUNCH

Flank Steak Salad with Horseradish and Apple

SNACK

Eggplant and Almond Dip with Celery or a Negative Calorie Smoothie

DINNER

Shrimp and Cabbage Hot Pot with Chile Peppers + Instant Almond Cake with Mixed Berries

DAY 10

BREAKFAST

Apple and Cinnamon Breakfast "Risotto" with Oat Bran and Almonds or a Negative Calorie Smoothie

LUNCH

Mushroom Bouillon with Leeks, Tofu, and Wasabi

SNACK

Eggplant and Almond Dip with Celery or a Negative Calorie Smoothie

DINNER

Beef-Stuffed Cabbage with Pepper and Tomato Goulash + Instant Almond Cake with Mixed Berries

DAY 11

BREAKFAST

Blueberry and Quinoa Porridge with Mint or a Negative Calorie Smoothie

LUNCH

Leafy Green Salad with Creamy Almond Dressing and Radishes

SNACK

Peanutty Apple Slices or a Negative Calorie Smoothie

DINNER

Spinach Pesto Pasta with Tomatoes + Chocolate and Almond Butter Truffles

BREAKFAST

Breakfast Citrus Salad with Cucumbers and Basil or a Negative Calorie Smoothie

LUNCH

Leftover Mushroom Bouillon with Leeks, Tofu, and Wasabi

SNACK

Peanutty Apple Slices or a Negative Calorie Smoothie

DINNER

Grilled Shrimp with Marinated Cucumbers, Kale, and Cauliflower + Chocolate and Almond Butter Truffles

---

 DAY 13

BREAKFAST

Breakfast Pizza with Mushrooms and Broccoli or a Negative Calorie Smoothie

LUNCH

Rocco's Chef Salad

SNACK

No-Sugar-Added Organic Cranberry Sauce with crackers or a Negative Calorie Smoothie

DINNER

Beef-Stuffed Cabbage with Pepper and Tomato Goulash + Chocolate-Dipped Strawberries with Crushed Almonds

---

 DAY 14

BREAKFAST

Kale, Red Onion, and Tomato Frittata or a Negative Calorie Smoothie

LUNCH

Asian Curry Mussel Soup

SNACK

No-Sugar-Added Organic Cranberry Sauce with whole-grain crackers or a Negative Calorie Smoothie

DINNER

Sliced Pepper Steak with Swiss Chard and Mushrooms + Chocolate-Dipped Strawberries with Crushed Almonds

SHOPPING LIST DAYS 8–14

FRUITS

◇ 4 large Gala, Pink Lady, or Empire apples

◇ 5 apples

◇ 1 Granny Smith apple

◇ 2 or 3 lemons

◇ 3 or 4 oranges

◇ 2 or 3 grapefruits

◇ 2 cartons fresh blueberries

◇ Several cartons of various types of berries

◇ 1 cup fresh cranberries

◇ 1 carton strawberries

VEGETABLES

◇ One 17.6-ounce bag spinach

◇ 1 large bunch mustard greens

◇ 6 heads butter lettuce

◇ One 20-ounce bag washed spinach

◇ 2 heads romaine lettuce, cleaned

◇ 4 or 5 bunches of kale

◇ 1 head napa cabbage

◇ 2 heads savoy cabbage

◇ 1 bunch Swiss chard

◇ 4 large radishes

◇ 1 garlic bulb

◇ 2 large onions

- ◇ 1 bunch scallions
- ◇ 3 shallots
- ◇ 2 medium Italian eggplants
- ◇ 1 large Japanese eggplant
- ◇ 1 bunch leeks
- ◇ 2 heads broccoli
- ◇ 2 heads cauliflower
- ◇ One 10-ounce package shiitake mushrooms
- ◇ 1½ pounds cremini mushrooms
- ◇ 1½ pounds sliced mixed mushrooms
- ◇ 3 large tomatoes
- ◇ 3 or 4 cartons cherry tomatoes
- ◇ 7–9 cucumbers
- ◇ 1 head red cabbage
- ◇ 7 or 8 red bell peppers
- ◇ 4 carrots
- ◇ One 12-ounce package bean sprouts
- ◇ I large head bok choy

Fresh Herbs

- ◇ Cilantro (several bunches)
- ◇ Mint
- ◇ Basil

BEEF

- ◇ One 12-ounce flank steak, trimmed of all visible fat
- ◇ One 16-ounce flank steak, trimmed of all visible fat
- ◇ 32 ounces 96% lean ground beef (such as Laura's Lean)

FISH AND SHELLFISH

- ◇ 16 ounces peeled, cleaned, and deveined shrimp
- ◇ 2 pounds mussels

POULTRY

- ◇ 8 ounces skinless store-roasted turkey breast, sliced thin

EGGS

- ◇ 3 dozen eggs

VEGETABLE PROTEIN

- ◇ One 20-ounce package medium-firm tofu

CEREALS AND GRAINS

- ◇ One 16-ounce package quinoa
- ◇ 208 grams (about 7.4 ounces) frozen gluten-free pizza dough (such as Gillian's)
- ◇ One 4.5-ounce package unsalted brown rice thins (such as Suzie's Thin Cakes)

CANNED FOODS

- ◇ Two 15-ounce cans garbanzo beans (chickpeas)
- ◇ One 15-ounce can no-salt-added tomato puree

SWEETENERS

- ◇ Three 3-ounce no-sugar-added naturally sweetened dark chocolate bars (such as Lily's)

VINEGAR

- ◇ Sherry vinegar

SPICES AND FLAVORINGS

- ◇ Baharat spice blend
- ◇ Curry powder
- ◇ Almond extract

CONDIMENTS AND SAUCES

◊ 1 jar prepared horseradish

◊ 1 jar chili garlic sauce

◊ 1 bottle reduced-sodium, gluten-free soy sauce

DAIRY AND NONDAIRY FOODS

◊ ½ gallon unsweetened vanilla almond milk

MISCELLANEOUS

◊ 2 tablespoons hemp hearts

◊ Two or three 8-ounce packages raw almonds

◊ One 16-ounce bag almond meal/flour

◊ One 6.5-ounce jar peanut butter powder

◊ One 3.5-ounce jar caper berries

◊ One 1-ounce package citrus pectin (such as Pomona)

◊ One 16-ounce jar pickled cherry peppers

◊ Several 32-ounce cartons unsalted chicken Stock (such as Kitchen Basics)

◊ Four 6-ounce noncoated paper cups

DAY 15

BREAKFAST

Avocado Toast with Spinach and Tomatoes or a Negative Calorie Smoothie

LUNCH

Seared Tuna Tataki Salad with Citrus, Tofu, and Watercress

SNACK

Red Ants on a Log or a Negative Calorie Smoothie

DINNER

Chicken with Mustard Greens, Quinoa, and Oranges + Cocoa-Dusted Almonds

---

DAY 16

BREAKFAST

Mexican Cauliflower Chili Scramble or a Negative Calorie Smoothie

LUNCH

Leftover Asian Curry Mussel Soup

SNACK

Red Ants on a Log or a Negative Calorie Smoothie

DINNER

Meatballs with Mushroom and Spinach Gravy + Cocoa-Dusted Almonds

---

DAY 17

BREAKFAST

Breakfast Bowl with Quinoa and Berries or a Negative Calorie Smoothie

LUNCH

Shaved Brussels Sprouts with Warm Toasted Garlic, Almond, and Lemon Dressing

SNACK

Apple, Cranberry, and Almond Bars or a Negative Calorie Smoothie

DINNER

Shrimp with Mustard Greens, Mushrooms, and Miso + Crepes Suzette with Oranges and Vanilla Cream

---

DAY 18

BREAKFAST

Spinach and Mushroom Omelet or a Negative Calorie Smoothie

LUNCH

Chicken Soup with Escarole and Leeks

Apple, Cranberry, and Almond Bars or a
Negative Calorie Smoothie

DINNER

Spinach Pesto Pasta with Tomatoes + Citrus and
Mixed Berry Bowl with Whipped Topping

———— DAY 19 ————

BREAKFAST

Mexican Cauliflower Chili Scramble or a
Negative Calorie Smoothie

LUNCH

Swiss Chard Turkey Salad with Golden Raisins
and Capers

SNACK

The Grate Salad Bowl with Chia Seed Dressing or
a Negative Calorie Smoothie

DINNER

Shiitake and Bok Choy Stir-Fry + Instant Almond
Cake with Mixed Berries

———— DAY 20 ————

BREAKFAST

Breakfast Bowl with Quinoa and Berries or a
Negative Calorie Smoothie

LUNCH

Chicken Soup with Escarole and Leeks

SNACK

The Grate Salad Bowl with Chia Seed Dressing or
a Negative Calorie Smoothie

DINNER

Flounder "a la Plancha" with Catalonian Eggplant
Relish + Instant Almond Cake with Mixed Berries

SHOPPING LIST DAYS 15–20

FRUITS

◇ 3 avocados
◇ 2 apples
◇ 4–6 lemons
◇ 10–12 oranges
◇ 6–8 cartons of various types of berries

Dried Fruits

◇ One 5-ounce package dried unsweetened
  cranberries
◇ One 1.69-ounce package freeze-dried apple
  chips (such as Bare Fruit Simply Cinnamon)

VEGETABLES

◇ 16 cups spinach
◇ 4 quarts tightly packed, cleaned spinach
  (17.6 ounces)
◇ One 20-ounce bag washed spinach
◇ 16 cups mustard greens
◇ 12 cups cleaned and chopped escarole
◇ 6 cups Swiss chard
◇ 1–3 onions
◇ 1 red onion
◇ 1 bunch scallions
◇ 1 package celery sticks
◇ 3 pints Brussels sprouts
◇ 2 or 3 shallots
◇ 3 large Japanese eggplants
◇ 1 bunch leeks
◇ 3 heads broccoli
◇ 4 heads cauliflower
◇ 1½ pounds cremini mushrooms
◇ 1½ pounds sliced mixed mushrooms
◇ ¾ pound mushrooms, any type
◇ 1 large tomato

- ◇ 3 cartons cherry tomatoes
- ◇ 2 heads red cabbage
- ◇ 2 or 3 red bell peppers
- ◇ 8 carrots
- ◇ One 12-ounce package bean sprouts
- ◇ 1 large head bok choy

Fresh Herbs
- ◇ Parsley
- ◇ Thyme
- ◇ Basil

BEEF
- ◇ 12 ounces 96% lean ground beef (such as Laura's Lean)

FISH AND SHELLFISH
- ◇ One 12-ounce sushi-grade tuna steak
- ◇ 1 pound cleaned, shelled, and deveined shrimp
- ◇ Four 4-ounce fillets fluke or flounder

POULTRY
- ◇ Four 4-ounce boneless, skinless chicken cutlets
- ◇ 8 ounces boneless, skinless chicken thighs
- ◇ 6 ounces store-roasted skinless turkey breast

EGGS
- ◇ 4 dozen eggs

VEGETABLE PROTEIN
- ◇ One 20-ounce package medium-firm tofu

CANNED FOODS
- ◇ Three 15-ounce cans no-salt-added crushed tomatoes

SPICES AND FLAVORINGS
- ◇ Mustard seeds
- ◇ 2 vanilla beans
- ◇ Reduced-sodium seafood boil seasoning (such as reduced-sodium Old Bay)

CONDIMENTS AND SAUCES
- ◇ Miso paste

DAIRY AND NONDAIRY FOODS
- ◇ ½ gallon unsweetened vanilla almond milk
- ◇ Parmigiano-Reggiano cheese
- ◇ One 6-ounce carton fat-free Greek yogurt

MISCELLANEOUS
- ◇ One or two 8-ounce packages raw almonds
- ◇ Several 32-ounce containers unsalted beef stock (such as Kitchen Basics)
- ◇ One or two 32-ounce containers unsalted chicken stock (such as Kitchen Basics)
- ◇ Four to eight 6-ounce noncoated paper cups

MAKING THE NEGATIVE CALORIE DIET YOUR OWN

In this chapter, I've provided you with a meal-by-meal plan for a full 20 days, using every one of my recipes. With those recipes, the plan is quite varied, and you'll eat the full range of negative calorie foods. I've made liberal use of these foods. The more of them you pack away, the less likely you are to pack on pounds!

You have the option of following the 20-day plan exactly as I've written it, or varying it according to your time, schedule, and food preferences.

Let me show you how to do that, by walking you through "a day in the life of the Negative Calorie Diet."

BREAKFAST

For starters, don't skip breakfast. It's well established that people who eat breakfast lose more weight and have fewer hunger pangs that people who skip it. A typical breakfast on the Negative Calorie Diet can include any of the following choices:

- A Negative Calorie Smoothie.
- Several scrambled egg whites, plus one or two negative calorie fruits on the side. Scramble your eggs with spinach, mushrooms, and/or tomatoes for an extra fat-burning boost.
- A small bowl of oatmeal, topped with berries.
- One of my breakfast recipes.

LUNCH

At lunchtime, have a salad—a generous bed of leafy greens, chopped tomatoes, chopped celery, sliced cucumbers, or other negative calorie vegetables, topped with chicken, shrimp or other shellfish, turkey, tuna, or beef. Drizzle with olive oil, plus some vinegar and maybe a fat-burning spice or two, and you've just made yourself the perfect negative calorie salad. Other lunch options include:

- A tomato stuffed with crabmeat, shrimp, or tuna, along with a negative calorie fruit for dessert, if you wish.
- Some leftover beef or chicken with a side of cooked greens or cruciferous vegetables or both.
- One of my soup or salad recipes.
- Leftovers from one of my entrée recipes.

DINNER

Dinner is a cinch, too. Match up a protein such as grilled chicken with a cooked negative calorie vegetable and a soup or salad, and you've whipped up a meal that will promote weight loss. You don't

SETTING UP YOUR KITCHEN

I promised you there would be no crazy equipment involved in making my recipes, and I stand by that. However, I do want to make sure we are on the same page as to what qualifies as out-of-the-ordinary equipment (we chefs tend to get carried away when purchasing gear). This is a list of all the "specialty" items you will need to make the recipes in this book.

- Blender—The smoothie recipes were made with a standard domestic blender. If you are ready for an upgrade, however, I suggest Vitamix or Blendtec. The NutriBullet is not as powerful as these two, but it will also work and it is extremely convenient.

- Microplane rasp grater/zester—A few of the recipes call for freshly grated Parmigiano-Reggiano or Pecorino Romano. You cannot beat the surface coverage of cheese when grated with a Microplane. It is also hands down the best option for citrus zests.

- Nonstick skillet and grill pan—Look for nontoxic, eco-friendly, nonstick pans that do not contain coatings made from polytetrafluoroethylene (PTFE) and perfluorooctanoic acid (PFOA). Ecolution is one brand that makes some great, safe options.

even have to limit your vegetable choices to only those in the negative calorie category. You can include other low-calorie; high-fiber veggies, too (see the list on page 48). Just make sure you have at least two negative calorie foods at main meals. Don't forget to include one of my negative calorie desserts, too! Some dinner ideas:

- Any of the 10 fat-burning proteins paired up with two or more the of 10 negative calorie foods.
- A soup or salad from my recipes.
- Any one of my entrée recipes, plus one of my desserts if you wish.
- Leftover entrée recipe from the night before.
- Go meatless: Enjoy one of the plant-based entrées.

SNACKING

The Negative Calorie Diet is a four-meal-a-day plan, and one of those meals is a snack. You can choose to have your snack at mid-morning or mid-afternoon, whenever you feel hungrier. The snack foods I recommend are negative calorie fruits such as apples, citrus fruits, or berries, or any negative calorie veggie. Pair these with some almonds, and you'll fill yourself up with fiber and good fats. That means you'll feel satiated all morning or afternoon, and you won't be ravenous at lunch or dinner. Some other snack ideas include:

- Leftover negative calorie soup.
- A negative calorie smoothie.
- Celery with almond butter.
- Any of my negative calorie snacks.

A CONFIGURATION OF EATING

There is a simple configuration of eating on this diet. The meals are combinations of negative calorie foods, lean proteins, and healthy fats. So when you plan your own meals, keep this configuration in mind: two or more negative calorie foods + 1 lean protein + a small amount of fat such as extra-virgin olive oil or avocado. And remember, there's no talking about calorie counts, fat grams, carb counts, or serving sizes. When you're eating negative calorie foods, you don't need to analyze every bite that goes into your mouth.

By the time you're well into the 20 days, you'll have a feel for what to eat and how to put your meals together. You'll be familiar with the metabolic principles of negative calorie foods and how they work to help you lose body fat.

In the next chapters, you'll find the recipes for the cleanse and the diet. Each one is simple and easy to prepare. As you follow both the cleanse and the diet, you can select your favorite recipes and smoothies and rearrange them in any way you like, repeating your favorites as often as you want.

Most of the ingredients used in my recipes can be found at your local grocery store, though there are a few specialty ingredients that may require a trip to the health food store or ethnic grocer. They are also widely available online—I've listed recommended brands for anything out of the ordinary. Also, except for my smoothies, all recipes will yield four servings. Even if you're cooking for one or two, I suggest making the full recipe so that you have leftovers on hand for quick meals.

Even if you haven't spent much time in the kitchen, there is no better time to step up to the dinner plate. I swear my recipes are foolproof—you can't go wrong!

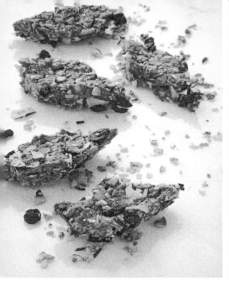
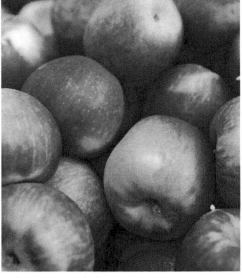
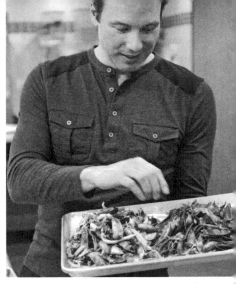
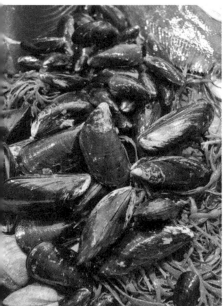
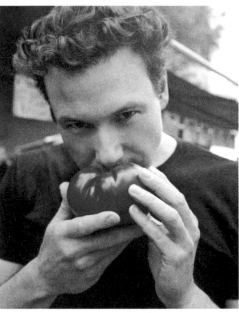
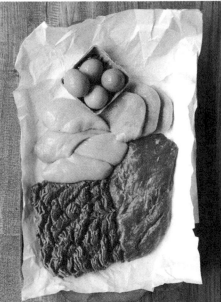
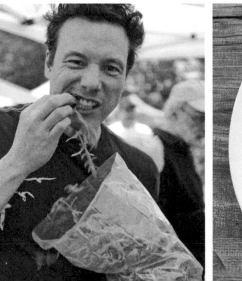
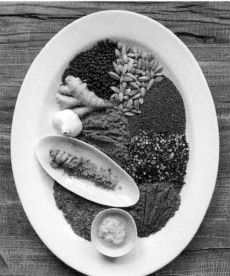
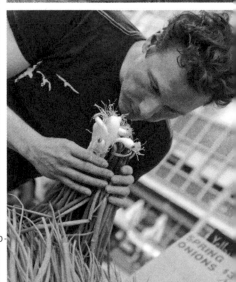

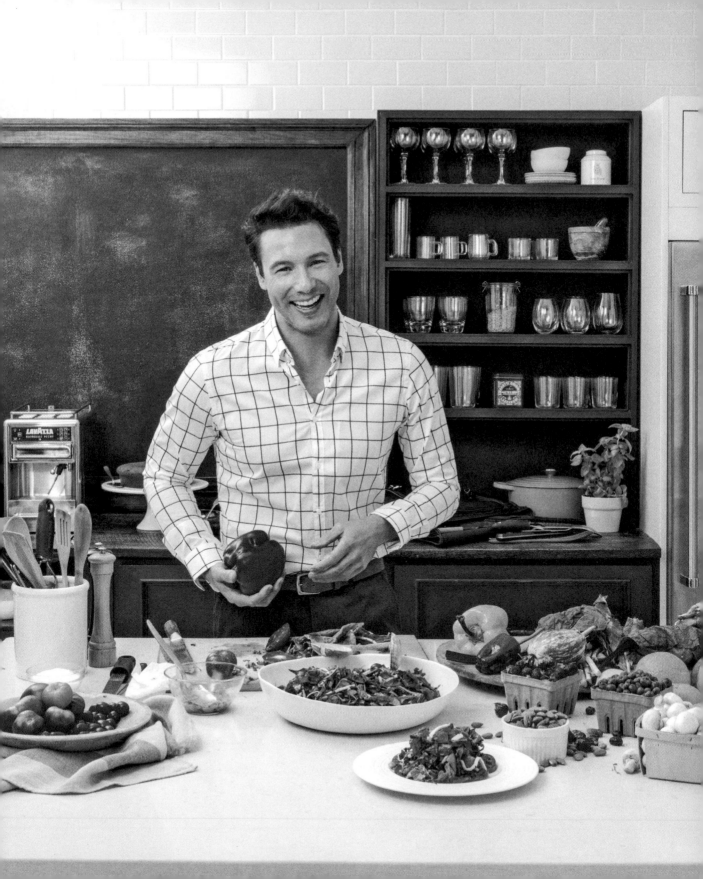

PART II

THE NEGATIVE CALORIE RECIPES

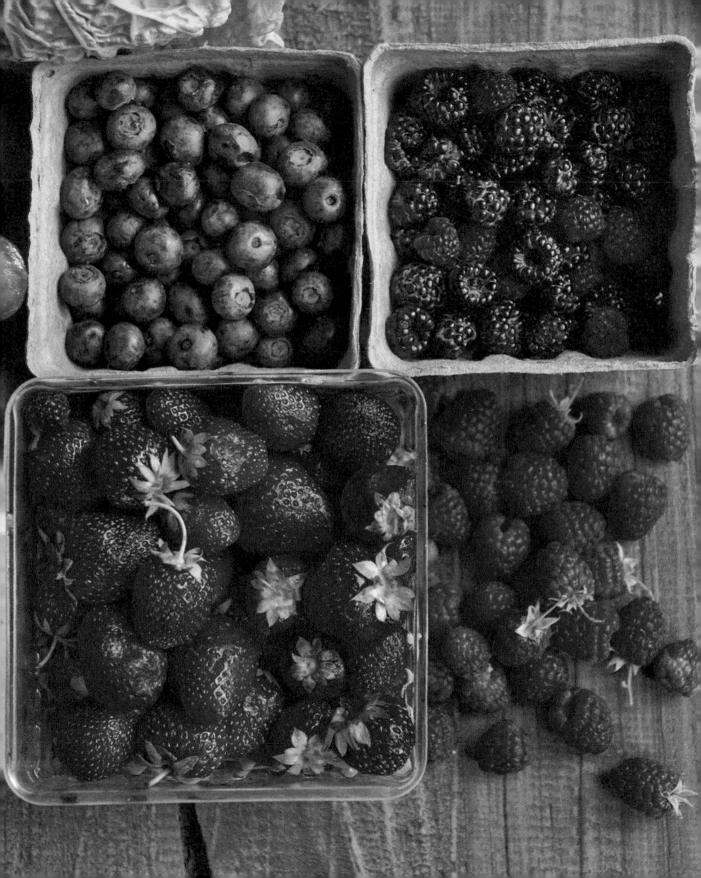

CHAPTER SIX

SMOOTHIES

Cucumber-Strawberry Green Smoothie 68

Spinach, Pineapple, Lime, and Mint Smoothie 70

Apple-Lime-Cilantro Protein Smoothie 72

Green Goddess Smoothie 74

Tropical Sunrise Smoothie 76

"Dillicious" Green Smoothie 78

Lemon-Ginger Smoothie 80

Orange Greensicle Smoothie 82

Sangrita Tomato, Orange, and Red Pepper Smoothie 84

The Virgin Mary Smoothie 86

Strawberry Shortcake Smoothie 88

Almond Vanilla Protein Smoothie 90

Spiced Apple Pie Smoothie 92

Blueberry-Basil Smoothie 94

Citrus-Berry Smash Smoothie 96

CUCUMBER-STRAWBERRY GREEN SMOOTHIE

MAKES 1 SMOOTHIE
PREP TIME: 5 MINUTES
PROCESSING TIME: 3 MINUTES

I salute the inventor of the smoothie, whoever that person may be. What other beverage so admirably multitasks, working as a meal, a snack, a postexercise replenisher, or even a dessert? This refreshing green smoothie is packed with vitamins and minerals. It is perfect for breakfast on the go, or even a quick lunch—just be sure to include the protein powder to keep you full until dinner!

PER SERVING

253 calories
3.5g fat
28.5g protein
31g carbohydrates
9g fiber
411mg sodium

INGREDIENTS

½ cup water

1 packet monk fruit extract (such as Monk Fruit In The Raw)

5 raw almonds

1 tablespoon pure acacia fiber (such as Renew Life)

1 cup kale leaves, tough ribs removed, firmly packed

½ cup chopped cucumber

Heaping ¼ cup frozen no-sugar-added strawberries

¼ cup sliced banana

1 scoop protein powder (such as Rocco's)

½ cup crushed ice, or small cubes of ice

METHOD

1. Put the water, monk fruit extract, almonds, and acacia fiber in a blender and blend until smooth. Add the kale, cucumbers, strawberries, and banana and blend until smooth.

2. Add the protein powder and the ice and continue to blend until smooth. Serve immediately.

TIP

When you have a seriously ripe banana that's on its last legs, don't toss it out. Wrap it in aluminum foil and freeze it. You'll have an instant healthy add-in for your smoothies, and you won't need any ice. Frozen bananas give smoothies a thick, indulgent consistency—kind of like a healthy milk shake!

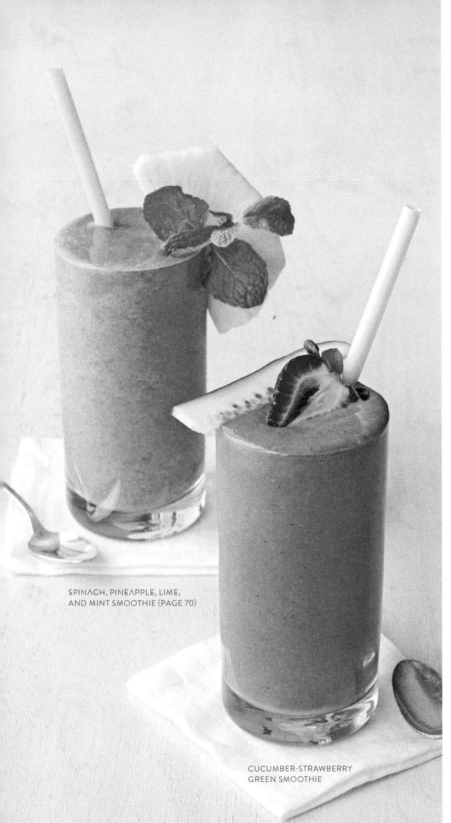

SPINACH, PINEAPPLE, LIME, AND MINT SMOOTHIE (PAGE 70)

CUCUMBER-STRAWBERRY GREEN SMOOTHIE

ACACIA FIBER

A relatively new fiber supplement on the market is acacia fiber, made from the gum of the acacia tree. It comes in powder form and can be easily added to smoothies or cereals. Although new to the United States, acacia fiber has been used as a natural medicine since ancient days; Egyptians used it to embalm mummies!

I consider acacia a negative calorie supplement because the body can't digest it, and it helps to usher excess calories, sugar, and fat from your body. Acacia fiber also helps you feel full and satisfied—another negative calorie benefit.

If you have digestive troubles, such as irritable bowel syndrome (IBS), acacia is a great natural treatment option. You can purchase this versatile fiber in health food stores—I recommend the brand Renew Life—and some grocery stores.

SPINACH, PINEAPPLE, LIME, AND MINT SMOOTHIE

MAKES 1 SMOOTHIE
PREP TIME: 5 MINUTES
PROCESSING TIME: 3 MINUTES

I love the taste of fresh mint—it reminds me of summer. Mint also has a whole host of medicinal qualities: it has been shown to soothe migraines, indigestion, stomach upset, irritable bowel syndrome, and muscle pain. And its scent can even energize your workout. In one study, athletes ran faster and completed more push-ups after sniffing some mint!

PER SERVING

250 calories
0.5g fat
27g protein
39g carbohydrates
10.5g fiber
425mg sodium

INGREDIENTS

¼ cup water

1 tablespoon pure acacia fiber (such as Renew Life)

½ cup Granny Smith apple chunks

1 cup fresh or frozen pineapple chunks

1 cup spinach, firmly packed

⅓ cup fresh mint leaves, firmly packed

1 teaspoon freshly squeezed lime juice

⅛ teaspoon lime zest

1 scoop protein powder (such as Rocco's)

½ cup crushed ice, or small cubes of ice

METHOD

1. Put the water, fiber, apple, pineapple, spinach, mint, lime juice, and lime zest in a blender and blend until smooth.

2. Add the protein powder and the ice and blend until smooth. Serve in a tall glass.

PROTEIN POWDER—WHAT TO LOOK FOR

There are so many protein powders on the market these days that it can be confusing to decide what to buy. Let me help you cut through that confusion. When looking for a protein powder I have a few considerations:

Total protein percentage: The most important thing to remember in selecting a protein powder for weight management is that you should get one with the highest amount of protein per serving: 90 percent protein or above is best but anything over 80 percent will do. To calculate, simply look at the label and divide the amount of protein by the serving size (in grams). So, for example, if a 30-gram serving contains 25 grams of protein, the powder is 83 percent protein.

Flavor: Each variety of protein powder has a different flavor and, unfortunately, that tends to vary from brand to brand. I like egg white powder because it generally has the most neutral taste, though for certain shakes, I will combine it with chocolate-flavored brown rice protein simply because it tastes better.

Texture: Some protein powders can be gritty. Egg white powder has a silky sheen and gives shakes a light texture. Pea protein tends to have a heavier texture, so it is best used in fruit smoothies. Brown rice protein has a very small grit to it, so it is best used in conjunction with other powders or in a smoothie with a fruit or vegetable base.

Protein Source: The source of protein you choose will most likely be based on your personal preferences or dietary restrictions. For example, vegans and vegetarians will want to stick to a plant-based protein, while meat eaters can choose any variety they'd like. Here's a quick breakdown of my top three favorite types of powdered protein:

- **Egg white protein.** Among protein powders, this one is absorbed the best by the body and is an excellent source of protein. Generally, 1 serving contains 30 grams of protein, 0.5 gram of carbohydrate, 0 grams of fat, and only 100 calories.
- **Yellow pea protein.** Pea protein is a plant-based protein. It packs between 15 and 30 grams of protein per serving, plus 2 grams of carbohydrate, 2 grams of fat, and 140 calories. The only drawback is that pea protein powder tends to be a little "sludgy" when blended into smoothies.
- **Soy protein isolate.** Unless you're intolerant of or allergic to soy, this is a worthy choice. Per serving, it contains 30 grams of protein, 16 grams of carbohydrate, 3 grams of fat, and 216 calories.

All of these protein powders can be wonderfully useful in other cooking applications besides making smoothies or shakes, such as aeration, binding, or emulsification. Just be sure to choose "raw" protein powder so its protein properties are 100 percent pure and intact.

APPLE-LIME-CILANTRO PROTEIN SMOOTHIE

MAKES 1 SMOOTHIE
PREP TIME: 5 MINUTES
PROCESSING TIME: 3 MINUTES

Ever see those weight lifter guys at the gym drinking their protein smoothies and wonder what it's all about? The truth is, they're onto something: consuming a combination of carbs and protein post-workout has been shown to accelerate the action of hormones involved in muscle-building and fat-burning. So drink up after you work out! Your muscles will thank you.

PER SERVING

238 calories
0g fat
26g protein
34g carbohydrates
10.5g fiber
410mg sodium

INGREDIENTS

½ cup water

1½ cups Granny Smith apples, chopped

1 tablespoon pure acacia fiber (such as Renew Life)

Small pinch of cayenne pepper (optional)

1 cup spinach

1 tablespoon freshly squeezed lime juice

⅛ teaspoon lime zest

1 cup fresh cilantro leaves, firmly packed

1 scoop protein powder (such as Rocco's)

½ cup crushed ice, or small cubes of ice

METHOD

1. Put the water, apples, and fiber in a blender and blend until smooth.

2. Add the cayenne, if using, spinach, lime juice, lime zest, and cilantro and blend until smooth.

3. Add the protein powder and the ice and blend until smooth. Serve immediately.

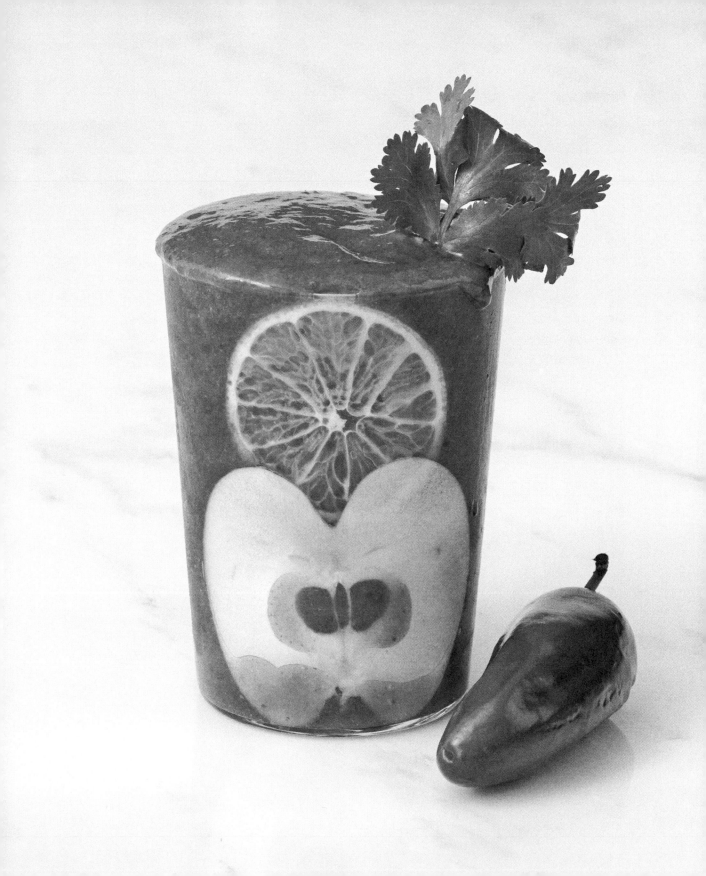

GREEN GODDESS SMOOTHIE

MAKES 1 SMOOTHIE
PREP TIME: 5 MINUTES
PROCESSING TIME: 3 MINUTES

If you scanned the list of ingredients here and got scared when you saw "broccoli," never fear: the kiwi sweetens this smoothie quite a bit, and fresh ginger adds a hit of spice—you'll never know you're "drinking" broccoli! This smoothie is a great way to knock back four negative calorie foods in one drink.

PER SERVING

224 calories
1g fat
28.25g protein
29.5g carbohydrates
10.25g fiber
433mg sodium

INGREDIENTS

½ cup water

1 tablespoon pure acacia fiber (such as Renew Life)

1 teaspoon chopped peeled fresh ginger

1 cup broccoli florets

¼ cup celery, chopped (about one 5-inch stalk)

1 ripe kiwi, peeled

½ teaspoon lemon juice

1 scoop protein powder (such as Rocco's)

½ cup crushed ice, or small cubes of ice

METHOD

1. Put the water, fiber, and ginger in a blender and blend until smooth.

2. Add the broccoli, celery, kiwi, and lemon juice and blend until smooth.

3. Add the protein powder and the ice and blend until smooth. Serve immediately.

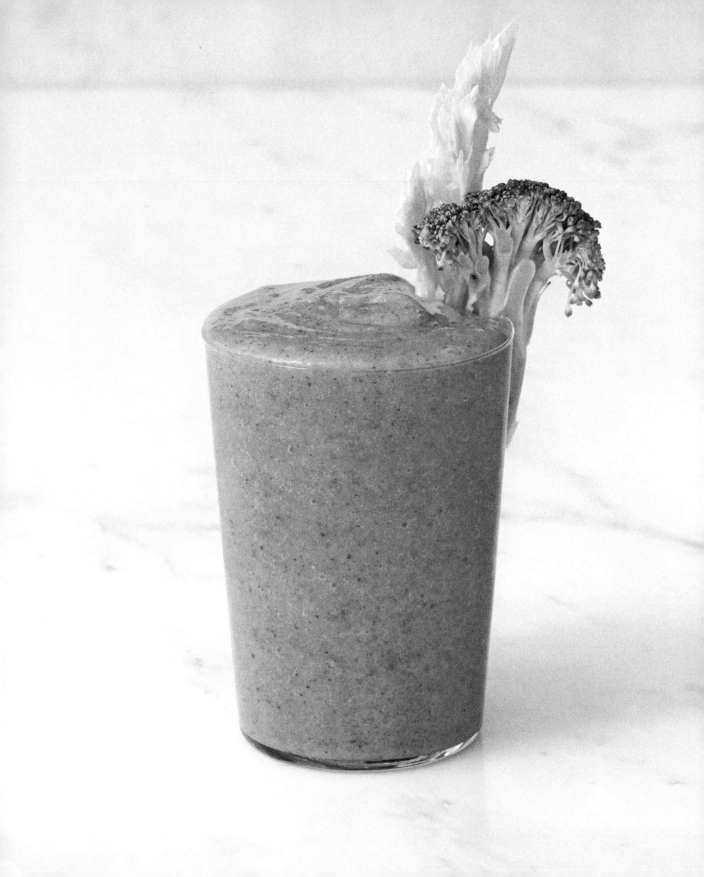

TROPICAL SUNRISE SMOOTHIE

MAKES 1 SMOOTHIE
PREP TIME: 5 MINUTES
PROCESSING TIME: 3 MINUTES

I love to make this decadent-tasting smoothie for breakfast. The combination of coconut, lime, and kiwi tastes like something you would enjoy with your feet in the sand, and brings a little island relaxation to your morning. Throw in a cup of collards (or any other leafy green you have on hand) for some phytonutrients and negative calorie cucumber for good measure, and you're off to a sunny start!

PER SERVING

253 calories

5g fat

27g protein

27.5g carbohydrates

10g fiber

393mg sodium

INGREDIENTS

½ cup water

½ teaspoon vanilla extract

1 tablespoon pure acacia fiber (such as Renew Life)

1½ teaspoons coconut manna (such as Nutiva Organic)

1 cup collard greens, firmly packed

1 cup chopped cucumber

1 kiwi, peeled

⅛ teaspoon lime zest

1 tablespoon freshly squeezed lime juice

1 scoop protein powder (such as Rocco's)

½ cup crushed ice, or small cubes of ice

METHOD

1. Put the water, vanilla extract, fiber, coconut manna, collards, cucumber, kiwi, lime zest, and lime juice in a blender and blend until smooth.

2. Add the protein powder and the ice and blend until smooth. Serve immediately.

TIP

Try cold-steeping a bag of chamomile tea in the water before making this smoothie.

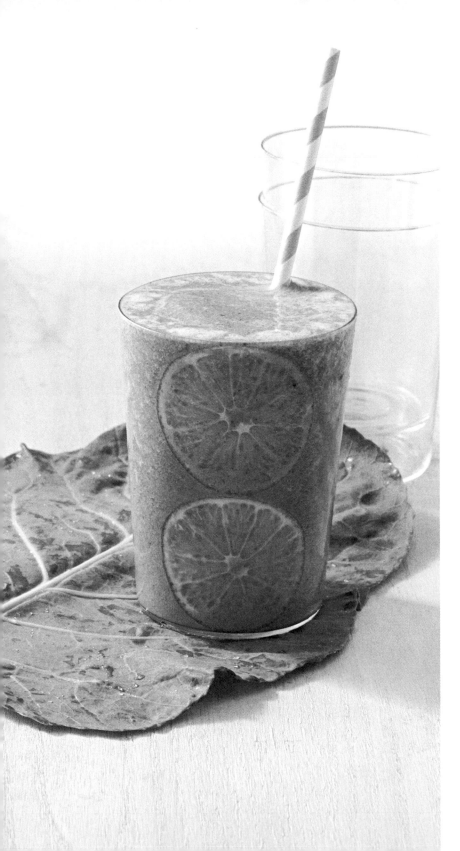

COCONUT MANNA

Coconut manna is to coconut what peanut butter is to peanuts or what almond butter is to almonds. It is ground coconut mixed with coconut oil to form a creamy, buttery spread.

Like other forms of coconut, it's high in medium-chain triglycerides (MCTs), a class of fats that are easily absorbed by the body, help reduce body fat, and improve insulin sensitivity.

Although coconut manna is high in saturated fat, it helps lower total and LDL cholesterol, while raising HDL ("good" cholesterol) levels. And like coconut oil, coconut manna is also rich in lauric acid, a compound that fights bacteria and germs. Coconut manna also has anti-inflammatory properties,

Coconut manna is highly versatile. You can cook with it or use it as a spread to replace butter, peanut butter, or mayonnaise. It tends to become solid at room temperature, so you have to dip the jar in warm water to soften it for spreading.

"DILLICIOUS" GREEN SMOOTHIE

MAKES 1 SMOOTHIE
PREP TIME: 5 MINUTES
PROCESSING TIME: 3 MINUTES

Vitamin C, calcium, fiber, and negative calorie ingredients—this morning smoothie will start your day with a good dose of each. I've added a little fresh dill to give it a tangy, herbaceous flavor. Dill is also beneficial for the digestive system. The silken tofu gives the smoothie a creamy texture, not to mention a blast of protein, but you can substitute almond milk if you prefer.

PER SERVING

230 calories
2.5g fat
31.25g protein
22g carbohydrates
7g fiber
414mg sodium

INGREDIENTS

½ cup water

1 tablespoon pure acacia fiber (such as Renew Life)

1 cup kale leaves, tough ribs removed, firmly packed

½ cup chopped Granny Smith apple

1 cup chopped cucumber

⅛ package silken tofu (such as Nasoya Organic), or ½ cup of almond milk

½ cup chopped fresh dill

1 tablespoon freshly squeezed lemon juice

1 scoop protein powder (such as Rocco's)

½ cup crushed ice, or small cubes of ice

METHOD

1. Put the water, fiber, kale, granny smith apple, and cucumber in a blender and blend until smooth.

2. Add the tofu, dill, and lemon juice and blend until smooth.

3. Add the protein powder and the ice and blend until smooth. Serve in a tall glass.

TIP

Add one-fourth of an avocado to this recipe for a smoother texture, extra fiber, and a dose of heart-healthy, monounsaturated fat.

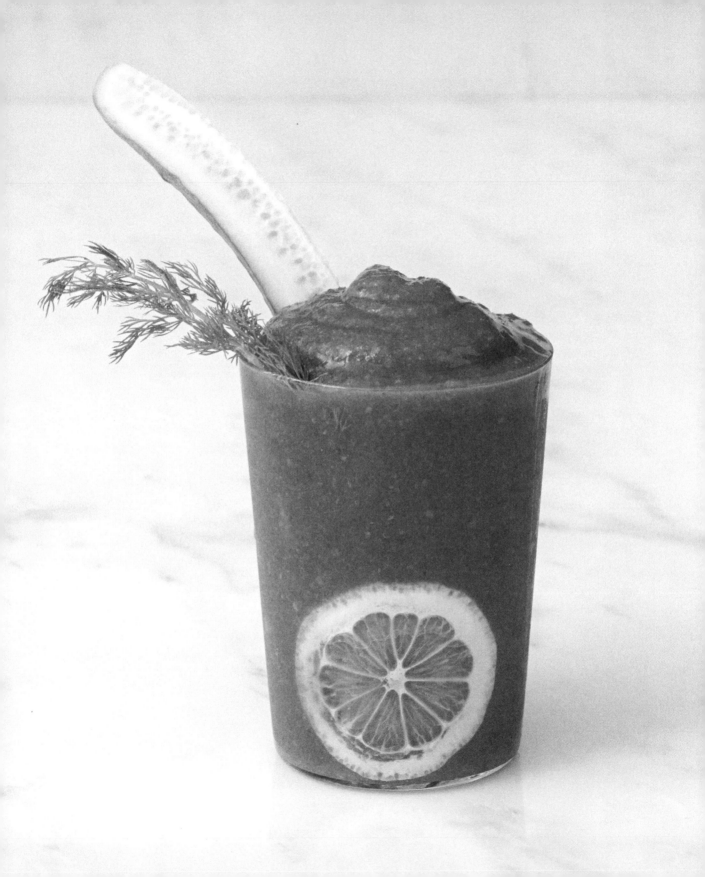

LEMON-GINGER SMOOTHIE

MAKES 1 SMOOTHIE
PREP TIME: 5 MINUTES
PROCESSING TIME: 3 MINUTES

I love this smoothie. It has a light, clean, simple flavor, and it is packed with vitamins and nutrients. The sweetness of the apple is balanced by the addition of freshly squeezed lemon juice. Add some celery and kale for a punch of green goodness and some grated fresh ginger for a little bite—delicious!

PER SERVING

270 calories
1g fat
27g protein
44g carbohydrates
11g fiber
425mg sodium

INGREDIENTS

½ cup water

1 tablespoon pure acacia fiber (such as Renew Life)

⅛ teaspoon cinnamon

¾ teaspoon chopped peeled fresh ginger

1½ cups chopped apple

1 cup kale leaves, tough ribs removed, firmly packed

One 5-inch stalk celery, chopped

1 tablespoon freshly squeezed lemon juice

1 scoop protein powder (such as Rocco's)

½ cup crushed ice, or small cubes of ice

METHOD

1. Put the water, fiber, cinnamon, ginger, apple, kale, celery, and lemon juice in a blender and blend until smooth.

2. Add the protein powder and the ice and blend until smooth. Serve in a tall glass.

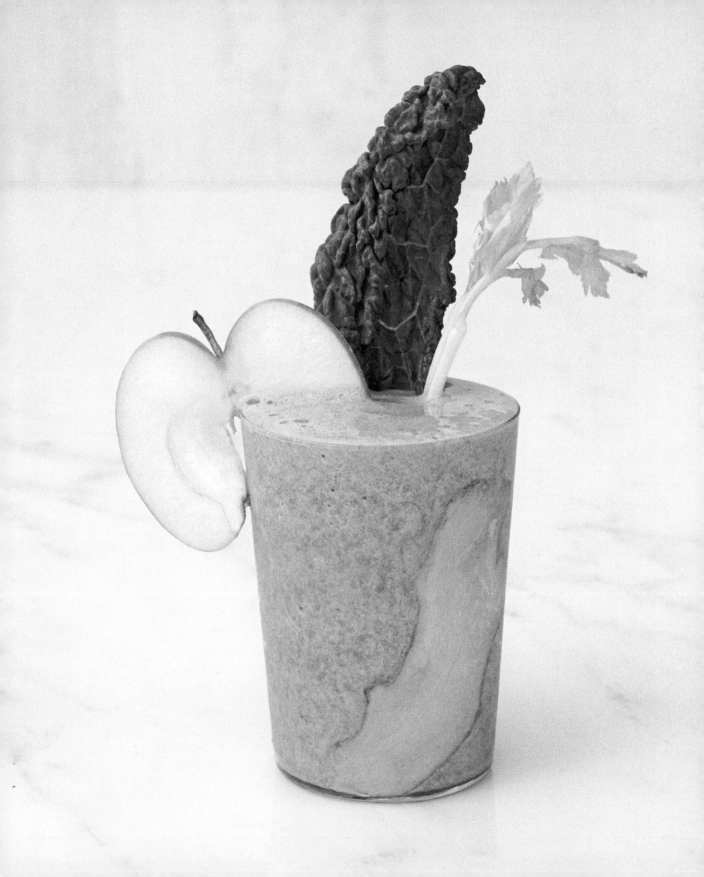

ORANGE GREENSICLE SMOOTHIE

MAKES 1 SMOOTHIE
PREP TIME: 5 MINUTES
PROCESSING TIME: 3 MINUTES

Even though green drinks are packed with nutrients and offer detoxifying and alkalizing vitamins and antioxidants, a lot of people are afraid they'll taste too . . . well, "green." Not so with this creamy smoothie, which contains vanilla almond milk and fresh oranges . . . it tastes like dessert!

PER SERVING

247 calories
2.5g fat
32g protein
28g carbohydrates
9.5g fiber
450mg sodium

INGREDIENTS

¾ cup unsweetened vanilla almond milk, or homemade almond milk (see page 91)

1 tablespoon pure acacia fiber (such as Renew Life)

2 cups spinach

⅛ teaspoon orange zest

¾ cup orange segments

1 teaspoon vanilla extract

1 scoop protein powder (such as Rocco's)

½ cup crushed ice, or small cubes of ice

METHOD

1. Put the almond milk, fiber, spinach, orange zest, orange segments, and vanilla in a blender and blend until smooth.

2. Add the protein powder and the ice and blend until smooth. Serve in a tall glass.

TIP

Add 1½ teaspoons coconut manna for extra creaminess.

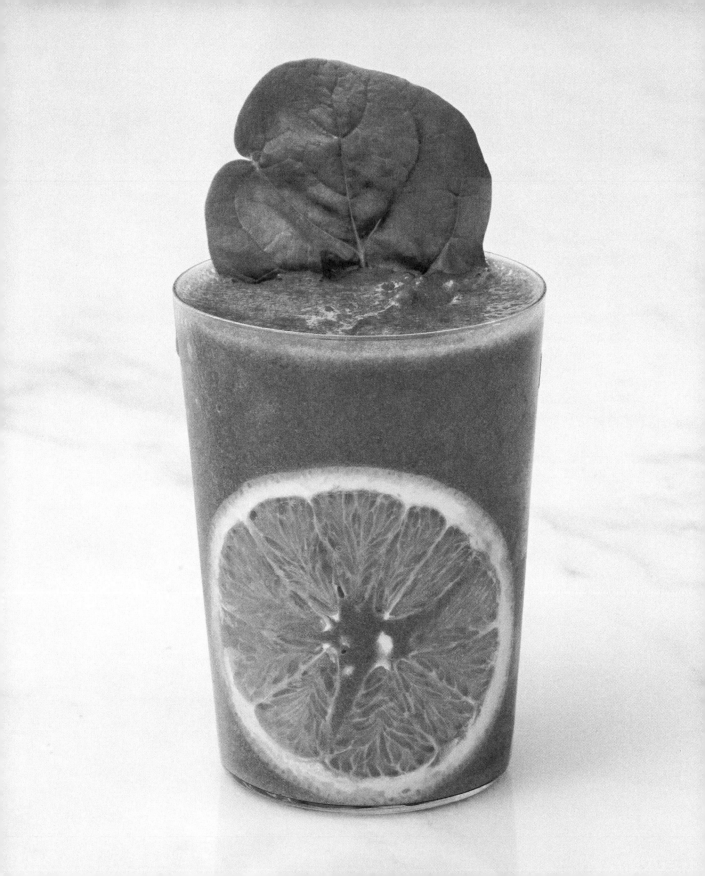

SANGRITA TOMATO, ORANGE, AND RED PEPPER SMOOTHIE

MAKES 1 SMOOTHIE
PREP TIME: 5 MINUTES
PROCESSING TIME: 3 MINUTES

I was inspired by the traditional Mexican *sangrita* to create this tangy, refreshing drink. Originally, the sangrita was concocted to quench the fire of tequila shots. You'd drink the sangrita alternately with tequila to cool your palate. I'm not advising the tequila, but the pure spicy flavor of this smoothie is delicious all on its own.

PER SERVING

245 calories
0.5g fat
28g protein
39.5g carbohydrates
12g fiber
390mg sodium

INGREDIENTS

1 cup chopped fresh tomatoes

1 tablespoon pure acacia fiber (such as Renew Life)

¾ cup peeled orange segments

½ cup chopped red bell pepper

1 tablespoon plus 1 teaspoon freshly squeezed lime juice

⅛ teaspoon ancho chili powder (or other spicy and/or smoky chili)

1 scoop protein powder (such as Rocco's)

½ cup crushed ice, or small cubes of ice

METHOD

1. Put the tomatoes, fiber, orange segments, bell pepper, lime juice, and chili powder in a blender and blend until smooth.

2. Add the protein powder and the ice and blend until smooth. Serve in a tall glass.

TIPS

1. Give this a dash or two of your favorite hot sauce if you like.

2. Add a splash of bitters to this for a real authentic boozy brunch flavor.

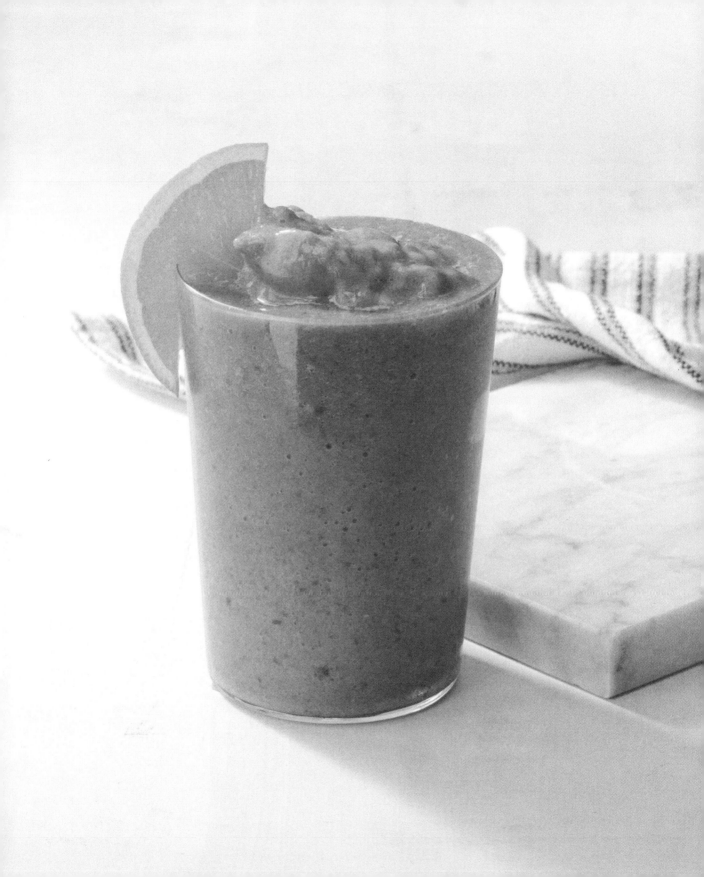

THE VIRGIN MARY SMOOTHIE

MAKES 1 SMOOTHIE
PREP TIME: 5 MINUTES
PROCESSING TIME: 3 MINUTES

When I'm creating smoothie recipes, I like to experiment with different flavor combinations, but sometimes I also get inspired by the classics. This mixture of tomato, celery, and horseradish reminds me of a Bloody Mary—but with energy-boosting protein instead of empty-calorie alcohol!

PER SERVING

203 calories
0.5g fat
7g protein
26.5g carbohydrates
10g fiber
450mg sodium

INGREDIENTS

¼ cup water

1 tablespoon pure acacia fiber (such as Renew Life)

1½ cups chopped fresh tomatoes

½ cup chopped celery

1 teaspoon prepared horseradish

1 tablespoon freshly squeezed lemon juice

2 frozen unsweetened strawberries

1 scoop protein powder (such as Rocco's)

½ cup crushed ice, or small cubes of ice

Freshly ground black pepper

METHOD

1. Put the water, fiber, tomatoes, celery, horseradish, lemon juice, and strawberries in a blender and blend until smooth.

2. Add the protein powder and the ice and blend until smooth. Serve in a tall glass with some freshly ground black pepper on top.

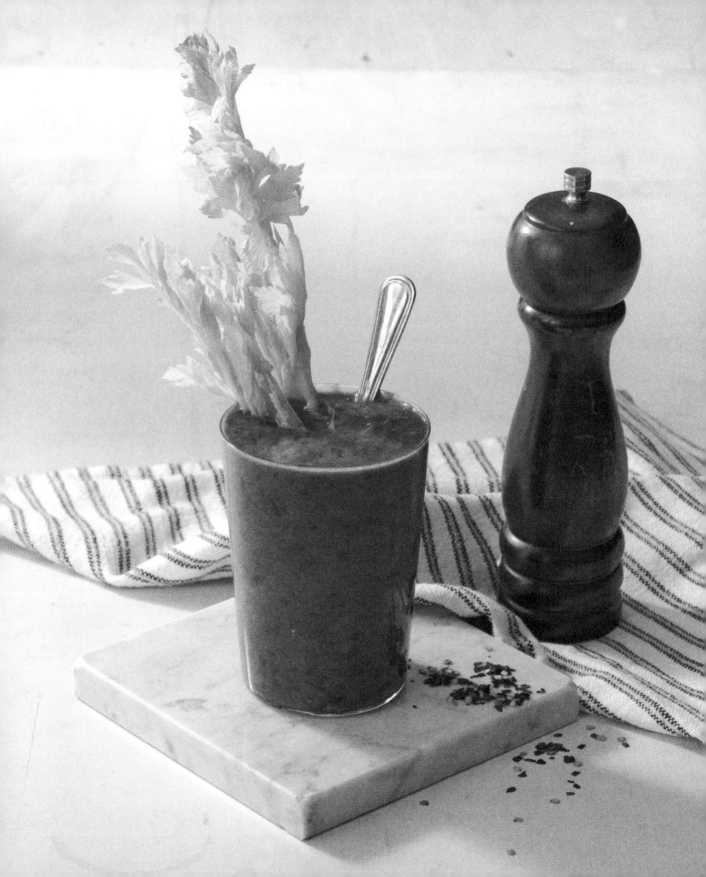

STRAWBERRY SHORTCAKE SMOOTHIE

MAKES 1 SMOOTHIE
PREP TIME: 5 MINUTES
PROCESSING TIME: 3 MINUTES

One of the best ways to taste-test a smoothie is with your children. If your kids approve, it must be good! This dessert-like smoothie is a great way to sneak some nutrition into their day.

PER SERVING

247 calories
2.5g fat
30.5g protein
27.5g carbohydrates
9.5g fiber
450mg sodium

INGREDIENTS

1 cup unsweetened vanilla almond milk, or homemade almond milk (page 91)

1 tablespoon pure acacia fiber (such as Renew Life)

1½ cups fresh strawberries

1½ teaspoons vanilla extract

1 packet monk fruit extract (such as Monk Fruit In The Raw)

1 teaspoon freshly squeezed lemon juice

1 scoop protein powder (such as Rocco's)

½ cup crushed ice, or small cubes of ice

METHOD

1. Put the almond milk, fiber, strawberries, vanilla extract, monk fruit extract, and lemon juice in a blender and blend until smooth.

2. Add the protein powder and the ice and blend until smooth. Serve in a tall glass.

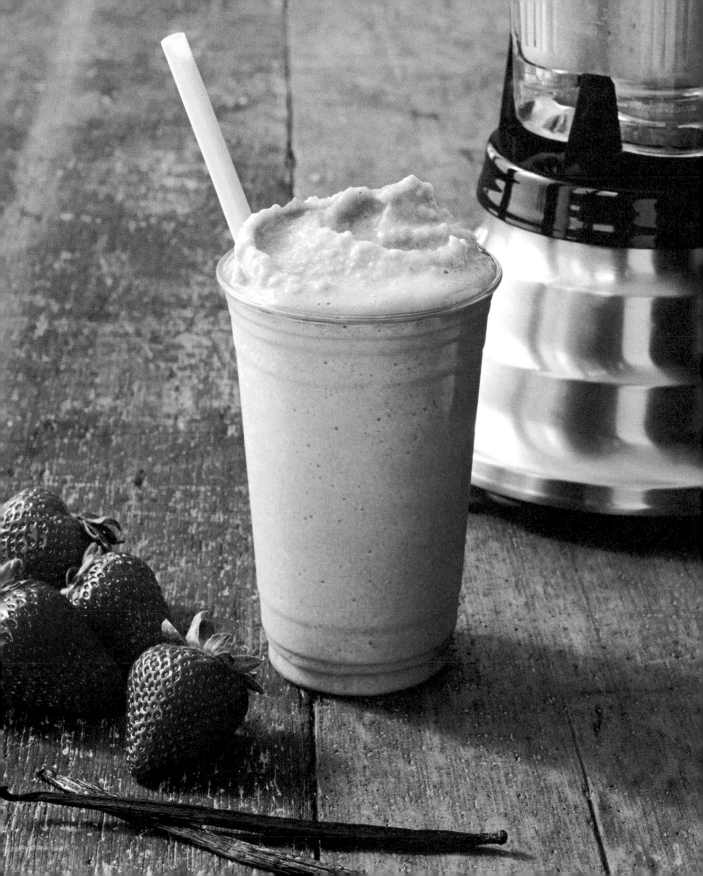

ALMOND VANILLA PROTEIN SMOOTHIE

MAKES 1 SMOOTHIE
PREP TIME: 2 MINUTES
PROCESSING TIME: 3 MINUTES

Want a sweet, creamy smoothie that will fill you up and provide a punch of protein? This recipe falls right in line with that craving. Toast the almonds in advance so you can throw it together in minutes for a quick breakfast beverage or post-workout pick-me-up.

PER SERVING

269 calories
10.5g fat
30.5g protein
18.5g carbohydrates
9.5g fiber
400mg sodium

INGREDIENTS

2 tablespoons almonds

1 cup unsweetened vanilla almond milk, or homemade almond milk (page 91)

½ cup water

1 tablespoon pure acacia fiber (such as Renew Life)

¼ teaspoon almond extract

1 teaspoon vanilla extract

2 packets monk fruit extract (such as Monk Fruit In The Raw)

1 scoop protein powder (such as Rocco's)

½ cup crushed ice, or small cubes of ice

METHOD

1. Preheat the oven to 400°F.

2. Place the almonds in a small skillet or on a rimmed baking sheet and toast in the oven until a deep golden brown, 3 to 4 minutes.

3. Put the almond milk, water, fiber, toasted almonds, almond and vanilla extracts, and monk fruit extract in a blender, and blend until smooth.

4. Add the protein powder and ice and blend until smooth. Serve in a tall glass.

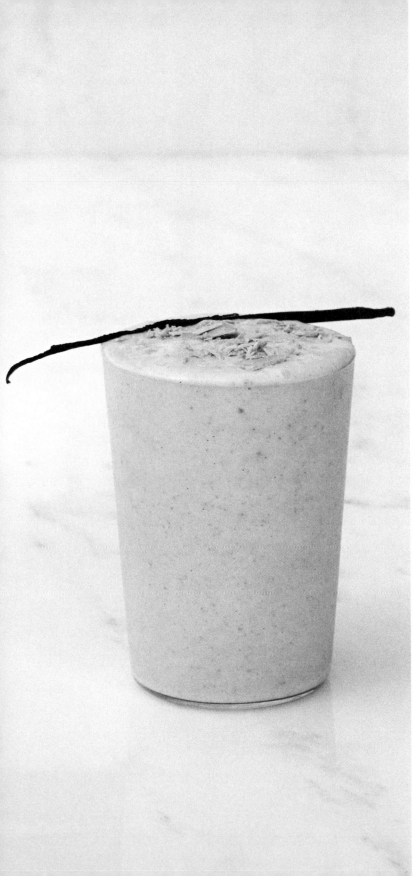

HOMEMADE ALMOND MILK

It's easy to make your own almond milk at home—and you'll find that it's even creamier and more delicious than the packaged almond milk at the grocery store. Be sure to give yourself about twenty-four hours to make it—you'll want to let the almonds soak overnight and then again after blending. Aside from the soaking time, it takes just minutes to make.

Yield: 3 cups

INGREDIENTS

1 cup shelled, skin-on raw almonds
3 cups cold water, plus additional water to cover almonds
1 pinch salt

METHOD

1. Place the almonds in a container, cover with water, add the salt, and let soak overnight.
2. Drain and rinse the almonds, then put them in a blender with 3 cups of cold water and blend until smooth. Place the mixture back in the container, cover, and let stand in the refrigerator for 12 hours.
3. Using a fine-mesh sieve or layers of cheesecloth, strain the milk into a bottle or another container with a lid. Use immediately, or store for up to 2 days in a tightly covered container in the refrigerator.

TIPS

1. Try adding 1 pack of monk fruit extract for sweeter milk.
2. Scrape the contents of one vanilla bean into your mixture before you blend it to make your own amazing vanilla almond milk.

SPICED APPLE PIE SMOOTHIE

MAKES 1 SMOOTHIE
PREP TIME: 5 MINUTES
PROCESSING TIME: 3 MINUTES

Yes, this liquid meal tastes like Mom's apple pie, but you can take comfort in knowing that it provides a serving of negative calorie foods and spices, plus protein and fiber. Enjoy!

PER SERVING

274 calories
2.5g fat
30g protein
36g carbohydrates
9.5g fiber
450mg sodium

INGREDIENTS

1 cup unsweetened vanilla almond milk, or homemade almond milk (page 91)

1 tablespoon pure acacia fiber (such as Renew Life)

1 cup roughly chopped apple

1 teaspoon vanilla extract

2 packets monk fruit extract (such as Monk Fruit In The Raw)

1 teaspoon ground cinnamon

1 scoop protein powder (such as Rocco's)

½ cup crushed ice, or small cubes of ice

METHOD

1. Put the almond milk, fiber, apple, vanilla, monk fruit extract, and cinnamon in a blender and blend until smooth.

2. Add the protein powder and ice, and blend until smooth. Serve in a tall glass.

TIP

Add a teaspoon of raw coconut nectar if you want it a little bit sweeter.

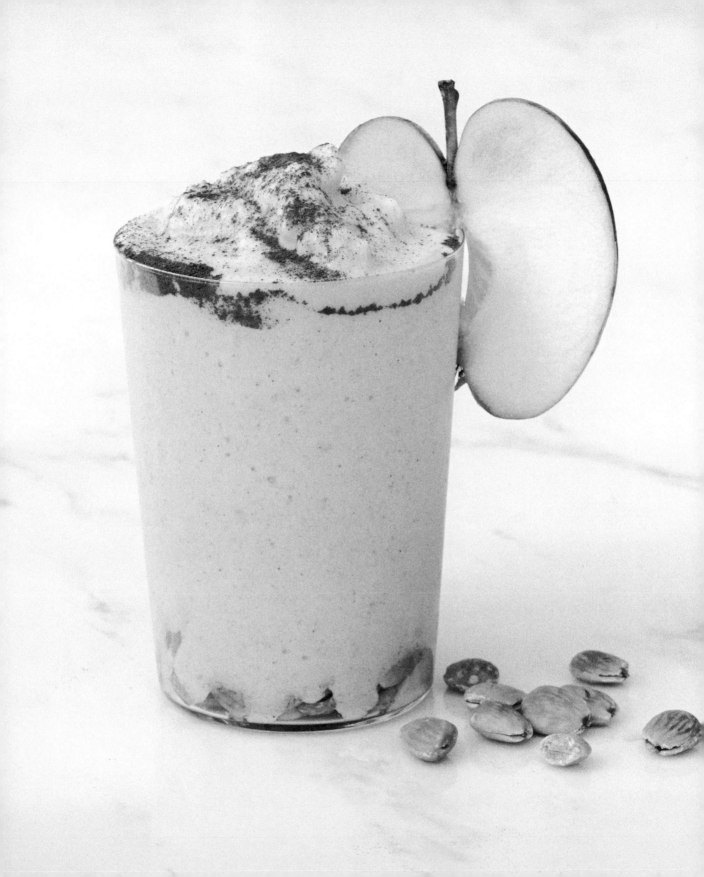

BLUEBERRY-BASIL SMOOTHIE

MAKES 1 SMOOTHIE
PREP TIME: 2 MINUTES
PROCESSING TIME: 3 MINUTES

Everyone loves blueberries, and blueberries love us right back: they have one of the highest antioxidant values of any fruit. Here, I've paired this superstar berry with basil, an herb packed with vitamin K, calcium, and its own team of antioxidants. The result is a jazzed-up smoothie destined to become one of your favorites.

PER SERVING

256 calories
2.5g fat
30g protein
31.5g carbohydrates
9g fiber
450mg sodium

INGREDIENTS

½ cup unsweetened vanilla almond milk, or homemade almond milk (page 91)

1 tablespoon pure acacia fiber (such as Renew Life)

1 cup blueberries, fresh or frozen

¼ teaspoon vanilla extract

2 packets monk fruit extract (such as Monk Fruit In The Raw)

¼ cup fresh basil leaves, firmly packed

1 scoop protein powder (such as Rocco's)

½ cup crushed ice, or small cubes of ice

METHOD

1. Put the almond milk, fiber, blueberries, vanilla extract, monk fruit extract, and basil in a blender and blend until smooth.

2. Add the protein powder and the ice and blend until smooth. Serve immediately.

TIP

Add a teaspoon of raw coconut nectar if you want it a little sweeter.

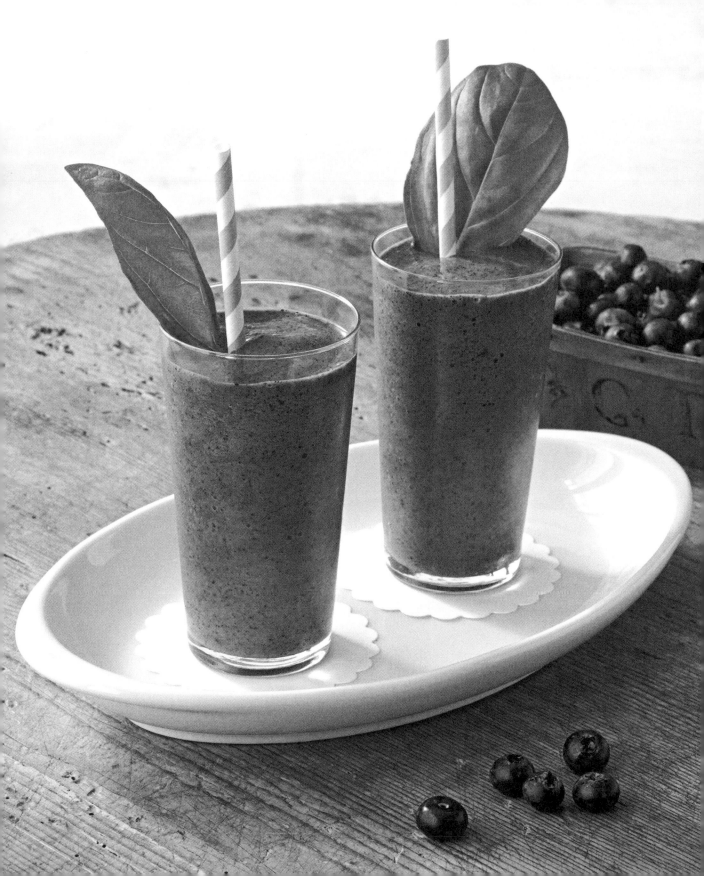

CITRUS-BERRY SMASH SMOOTHIE

MAKES 1 SMOOTHIE
PREP TIME: 5 MINUTES
PROCESSING TIME: 3 MINUTES

I never know whether to have this smoothie for breakfast or for dessert. What I do know is that it's loaded with vitamin C and packed with flavor. The vanilla coconut dessert adds a creamy richness that makes this smoothie especially filling and satisfying.

PER SERVING

250 calories
4.5g fat
26g protein
34g carbohydrates
12.5g fiber
400mg sodium

INGREDIENTS

¼ cup water

½ tablespoon pure acacia fiber (such as Renew Life)

½ cup peeled orange segments

½ cup mixed berries, fresh or frozen

1 teaspoon vanilla extract

1 packet monk fruit extract (such as Monk Fruit In The Raw)

6 fresh mint leaves

¼ cup frozen unsweetened vanilla coconut dessert (such as So Delicious)

1 scoop protein powder (such as Rocco's)

1 cup crushed ice, or small cubes of ice

METHOD

1. Put the water, fiber, orange segments, berries, vanilla extract, monk fruit extract, and mint in a blender and blend until smooth.

2. Add the frozen dessert, protein powder, and ice and blend until smooth. Serve in a tall glass.

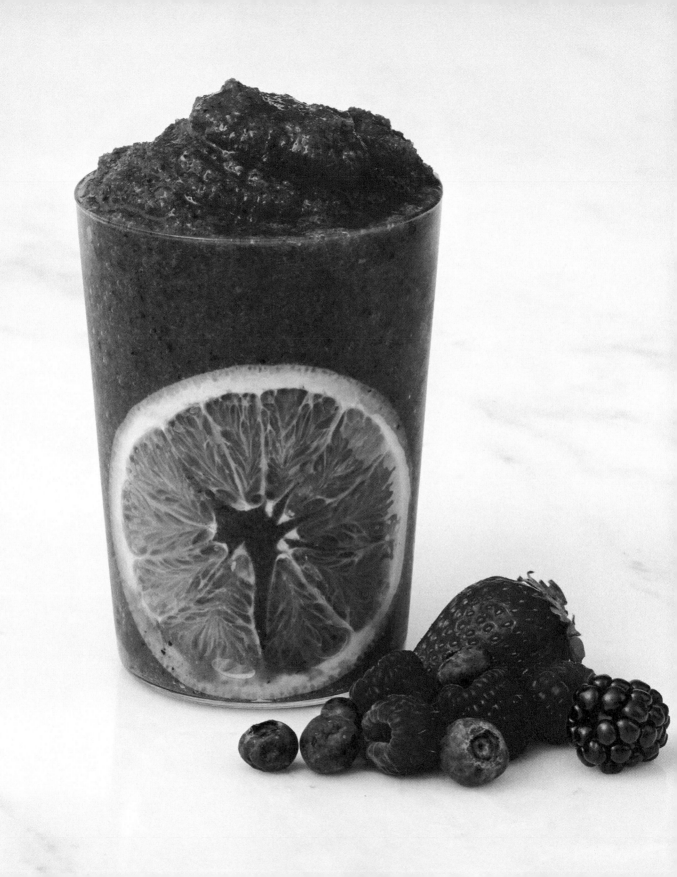

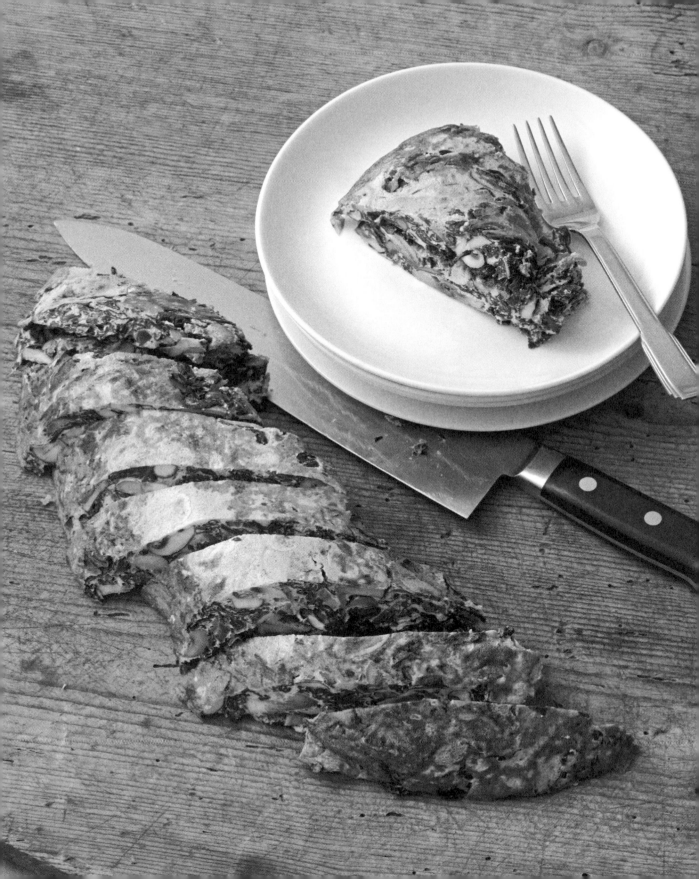

CHAPTER SEVEN

BREAKFAST

Apple and Cinnamon Breakfast "Risotto" with Oat Bran and Almonds 100

Blueberry and Quinoa Porridge with Mint 102

Breakfast Citrus Salad with Cucumbers and Basil 104

Breakfast Pizza with Mushrooms and Broccoli 106

Kale, Red Onion, and Tomato Frittata 108

Avocado Toast with Spinach and Tomatoes 110

Mexican Cauliflower Chili Scramble 112

Breakfast Bowl with Quinoa and Berries 114

Spinach and Mushroom Omelet 116

APPLE AND CINNAMON BREAKFAST "RISOTTO" WITH OAT BRAN AND ALMONDS

MAKES 4 SERVINGS
PREP TIME: 10 MINUTES
COOK TIME: 10 MINUTES

Everyone knows breakfast is the most important meal of the day. Mom, Grandmother, and our doctors have all told us so. Still, breakfast is the most skipped meal in America—30 percent of us go without it. When I was a busy restaurant chef, I ranked among that group. Then it hit me like a ton of bacon: I was missing out on a *meal*! As a food lover, I got back into the swing of things, and I now know that eating breakfast has helped me maintain my weight loss. This hearty and filling breakfast should help you get back into the breakfast groove, too.

PER SERVING

137 calories
4.5g fat
3g protein
23.25g carbohydrates
5g fiber
81.5mg sodium

INGREDIENTS

4 large Gala, Pink Lady, or Empire apples

1 teaspoon unrefined coconut oil

1 teaspoon ground cinnamon

2 cups unsweetened vanilla almond milk, or homemade almond milk (page 91)

¼ cup oat bran (such as Bob's Red Mill)

2 packets monk fruit extract (such as Monk Fruit In The Raw)

10 almonds, toasted and chopped

METHOD

1. Wash the apples and cut them into very small dice, or chop them into small pieces, about ¼-inch dice. Melt the coconut oil in a large nonstick skillet over medium-high heat. Add the apples and cinnamon and cook until softened, 2 to 3 minutes.

2. Remove the apples from the heat. Add the almond milk and stir in the oat bran and monk fruit extract. Place the mixture back on medium heat and bring to a simmer, stirring. Cook until the mixture is thick and creamy, about 1 minute.

3. Divide the mixture equally among four small bowls and sprinkle each evenly with toasted almonds.

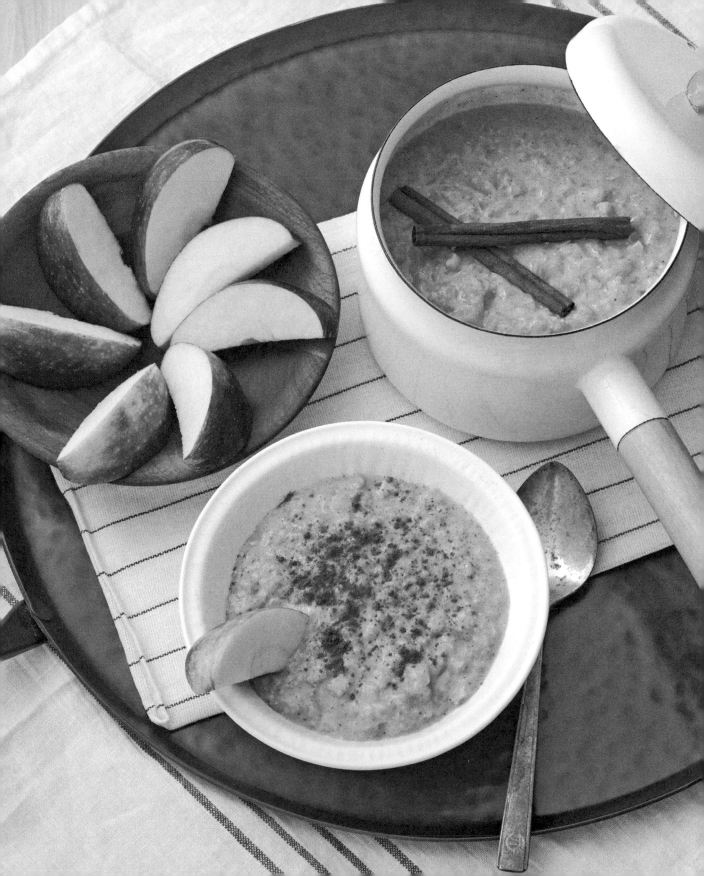

BLUEBERRY AND QUINOA PORRIDGE WITH MINT

MAKES 4 SERVINGS
PREP TIME: 5 MINUTES
COOK TIME: 10 MINUTES

When you prepare this dish for your family or friends, expect to hear a lot of "oohs," "aahs," and "yummys" from everyone . . . followed by more than a few "How do you say the name of it again?" I'm hot on quinoa (pronounced KEEN-wah) because it packs lots of protein, fiber, and flavor, especially when paired with blueberries and mint.

PER SERVING

135 calories
2.75g fat
4g protein
24.25g carbohydrates
3.25g fiber
90mg sodium

INGREDIENTS

½ cup red quinoa

2 cups unsweetened almond milk, or homemade almond milk (page 91)

1 teaspoon vanilla extract

⅛ teaspoon salt

2 packets monk fruit extract (such as Monk Fruit In The Raw)

2 cups fresh washed blueberries

8 leaves fresh mint, lightly chopped

METHOD

1. Place the quinoa in a fine strainer and rinse it well under cold running water. Shake off any excess water. Transfer the quinoa to a blender with the almond milk, vanilla extract, salt, and monk fruit extract. Blend on high to break up the quinoa into smaller pieces, about 30 seconds.

2. Pour the mixture into a wide-bottomed saucepan and place over medium-high heat. Cook the mixture until simmering, whisking constantly to prevent lumps. Once the mixture has simmered, add half of the blueberries and mix to warm them through, letting them break apart slightly.

3. Divide the mixture equally among four bowls. Sprinkle the remaining blueberries equally over each bowl and top with the mint.

TIP

Look for quinoa flakes on the shelves of your supermarket; then you can skip the blending step.

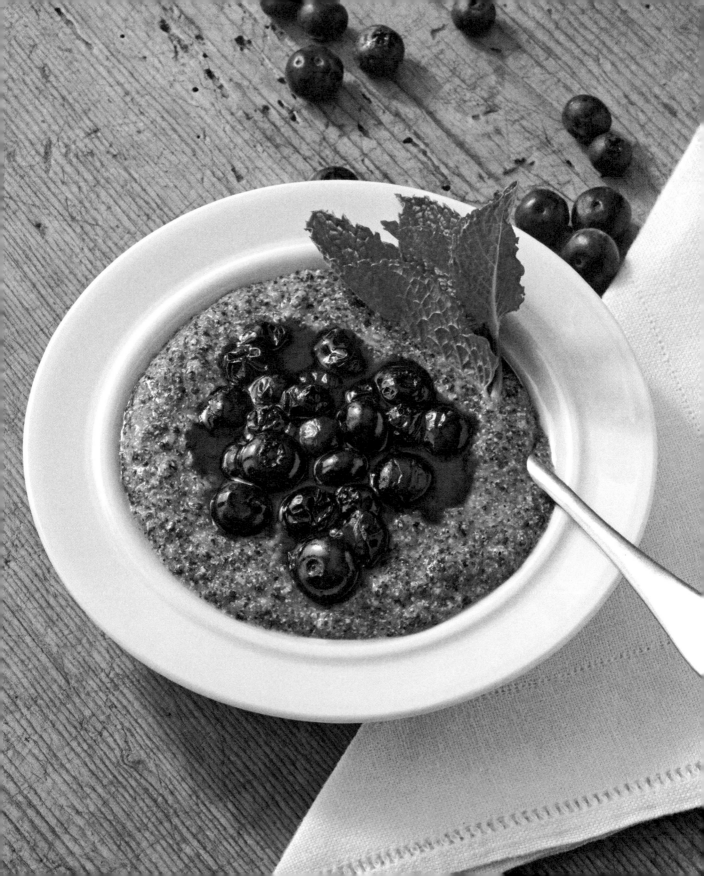

BREAKFAST CITRUS SALAD WITH CUCUMBERS AND BASIL

MAKES 4 SERVINGS
PREP TIME: 10 MINUTES

Salad—it's what's for breakfast. That's right, especially when you want to start your day off with a blast of negative calorie foods, like oranges, grapefruit, and cucumber. Remember, grapefruit contains a special fat-burning chemical; oranges are endowed with fat-burning vitamin C; and cucumber is a detox vegetable that flushes toxins from your body.

PER SERVING

134 calories
0.5g fat
3g protein
33.4g carbohydrates
6.25g fiber
1.5mg sodium

INGREDIENTS

4 cups orange segments
2 cups grapefruit segments
3 cups cucumber slices
½ cup fresh basil, firmly packed

METHOD

Combine all the ingredients in a large bowl and toss them gently together. Spoon the salad into four bowls, dividing it equally.

TIPS

1. Try adding 1 teaspoon of minced jalapeño to the salad for a great kick. You can skip your coffee!
2. Add 1 diced avocado to this recipe for an extra dose of healthy fat and fiber.

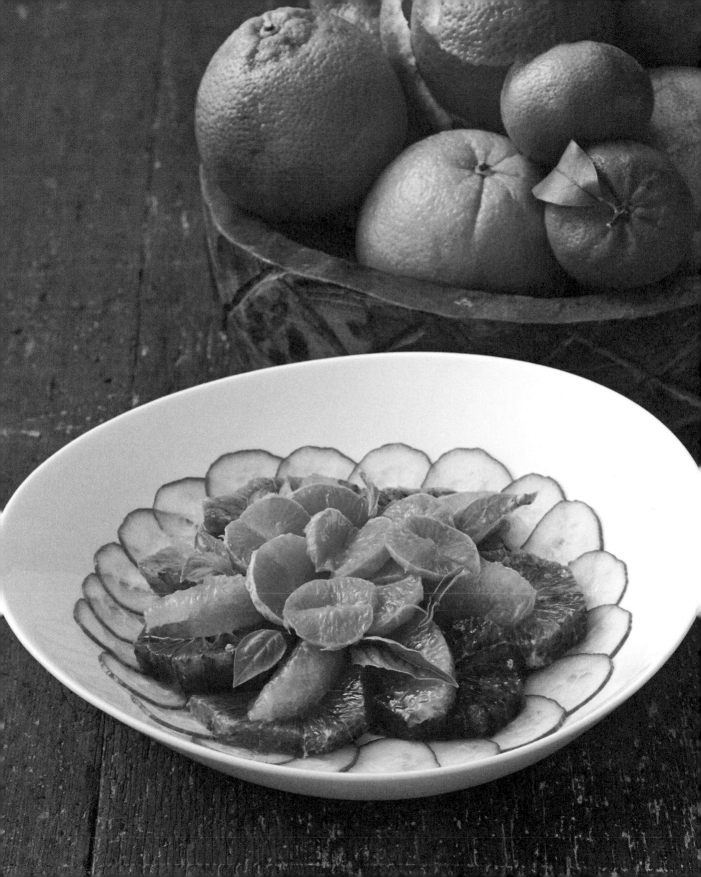

BREAKFAST PIZZA WITH MUSHROOMS AND BROCCOLI

MAKES 4 SERVINGS
PREP TIME: 5 MINUTES
COOK TIME: 15 MINUTES

I spend a great deal of time talking about everything I love to eat, and pizza is at the top of the list. I love pizza anytime, any way. With this negative calorie food–loaded recipe, I now officially declare pizza a "breakfast food."

PER SERVING

209 calories
5.6g fat
10.25g protein
35g carbohydrates
4g fiber
266mg sodium

INGREDIENTS

208 grams (about 7.4 ounces) frozen gluten-free pizza dough (such as Gillian's), defrosted but chilled

Olive oil cooking spray

2 patties no-nitrate chicken breakfast sausage (such as Applegate), broken into bite-size pieces

4 cups chopped broccoli

2 teaspoons chopped garlic

2 cups sliced mushrooms

½ cup fresh basil leaves, torn into small bite-size pieces

2 cups chopped fresh tomatoes

Salt

Crushed red pepper flakes

METHOD

1. Preheat the oven to 400°F.
2. Roll out the dough between two sheets of plastic wrap to a thickness of ¼ inch. Remove the top sheet and flip the dough onto a large baking sheet. Transfer to the oven and bake until the dough is set, 3 to 5 minutes. Remove from the oven and set aside. Leave the oven on.
3. Barely coat a large nonstick skillet with cooking spray and place over medium-high heat. Add the sausage and cook until lightly browned, then transfer to a bowl. Add the broccoli to the skillet and cook until tender, about 2 minutes; transfer to the bowl. Add the garlic to the skillet and cook until golden, about 1 minute; add the mushrooms and cook until softened. Transfer

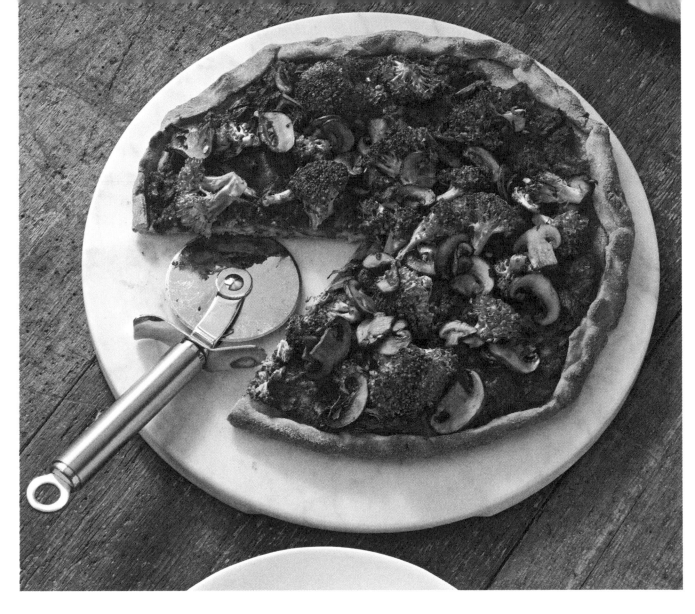

to the bowl. Add the basil and half the chopped tomatoes to the skillet. Simmer until the tomatoes have thickened. Return the broccoli, sausage, and mushrooms to the skillet to warm. Season with salt and red pepper flakes.

4. Spread the sauce mixture over the pizza dough and return it to the oven. Bake until the edges of the pizza are brown. Remove from the oven and top with the remaining tomatoes. Serve immediately.

KALE, RED ONION, AND TOMATO FRITTATA

MAKES 4 SERVINGS
PREP TIME: 10 MINUTES
COOK TIME: 15 MINUTES

You like omelets, right? Well, a frittata is essentially the same thing, but easier to make than an omelet. Here, you'll be mixing three delicious veggies into the egg whites for a hearty, high-protein breakfast that will keep you energized all morning.

Put 1 cup of torn fresh basil leaves in the skillet when adding the onions, for more flavor.

PER SERVING

147 calories
2.5g fat
16g protein
18.3g carbohydrates
3.5g fiber
225mg sodium

INGREDIENTS

8 cups washed kale, tough ribs removed, chopped into 1-inch pieces
2 tablespoons water
12 large egg whites, or 1 pint of liquid egg whites
1 teaspoon extra-virgin olive oil
1 teaspoon chopped fennel seeds
1 tablespoon minced garlic
Crushed red pepper flakes
½ cup thinly sliced red onion
1 cup cherry tomatoes, halved
Salt

METHOD

1. Preheat the oven to 350°F.
2. Place the kale in a microwave-safe dish with 2 tablespoons of water, cover with parchment paper, and cook on high until tender, 3 to 5 minutes. Drain excess water, and reserve.
3. Whisk the egg whites in a mixing bowl and set aside. Pour the olive oil into a large nonstick skillet, place over medium-high heat, add the fennel seeds and garlic, and cook until the garlic is golden brown, about 1 minute. Add the red pepper flakes and onion.
4. Reduce the heat to medium and cook the onion until soft, 3 to 4 minutes. Add the tomatoes and kale, season, and cook until the mixture is hot. Add the egg whites and mix well. Once the egg whites are almost set, transfer the skillet to the oven and bake until the eggs are cooked through, about 2 minutes. Remove the skillet and serve immediately.

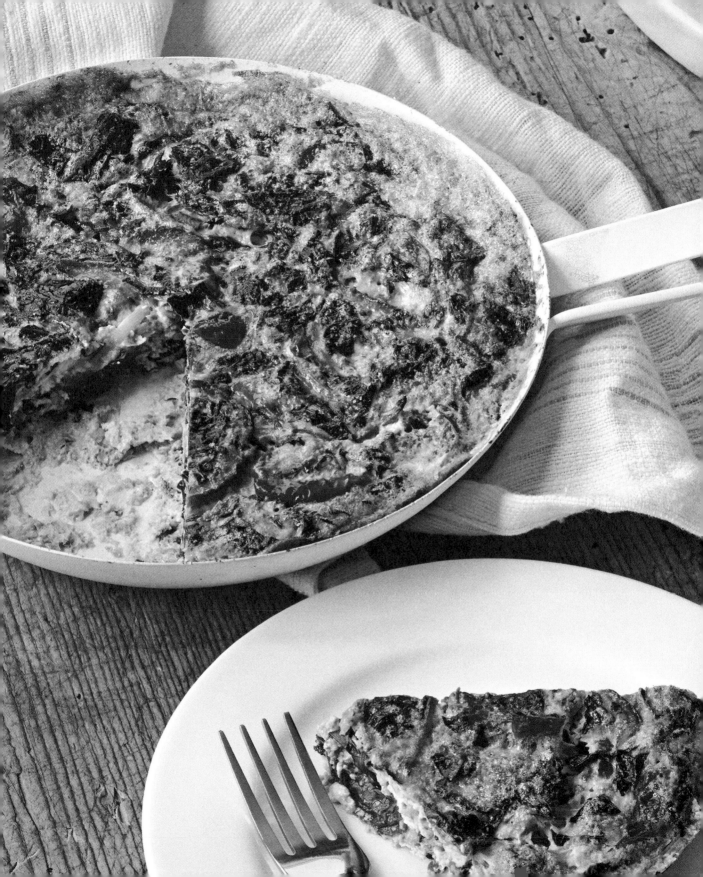

AVOCADO TOAST WITH SPINACH AND TOMATOES

MAKES 4 SERVINGS
PREP TIME: 10 MINUTES
COOK TIME: 10 MINUTES

From food blogs to Instagram posts, avocado toast is enjoying its moment in the food-trend sun, with countless varieties and photos that make your mouth water. A brunch favorite among the healthy set, it's even made its way onto restaurant and café menus in New York City! My version incorporates negative calorie vegetables and eggs for a complete and satisfying meal.

PER SERVING

180 calories
8.5g fat
10g protein
19g carbohydrates
5g fiber
200mg sodium

INGREDIENTS

8 cups spinach

Salt

Green hot sauce (such as Tabasco)

4 slices natural gluten-free bread (such as Canyon)

½ ripe avocado, mashed with a fork

4 thick (½-inch) slices ripe tomato

Freshly ground black pepper

4 medium eggs, poached

METHOD

1. Heat a large nonstick skillet over medium-high heat. Put in the spinach and cook until wilted. Transfer the spinach to a colander and press out as much of the water as possible. Put the drained spinach in a mixing bowl and season with salt and green hot sauce.

2. Toast the bread in the toaster. Season the avocado with salt. Once the toast is done, spread the avocado evenly over each piece of toast and place a slice of tomato on top. Season the tomatoes with salt and pepper and top each slice with an even amount of the spinach mixture.

3. Place each piece of toast on a plate, top with a poached egg, and serve.

TIP

Hot sauce not hot enough for you? Try adding 1 teaspoon of minced jalapeño to the avocado mash for an extra kick.

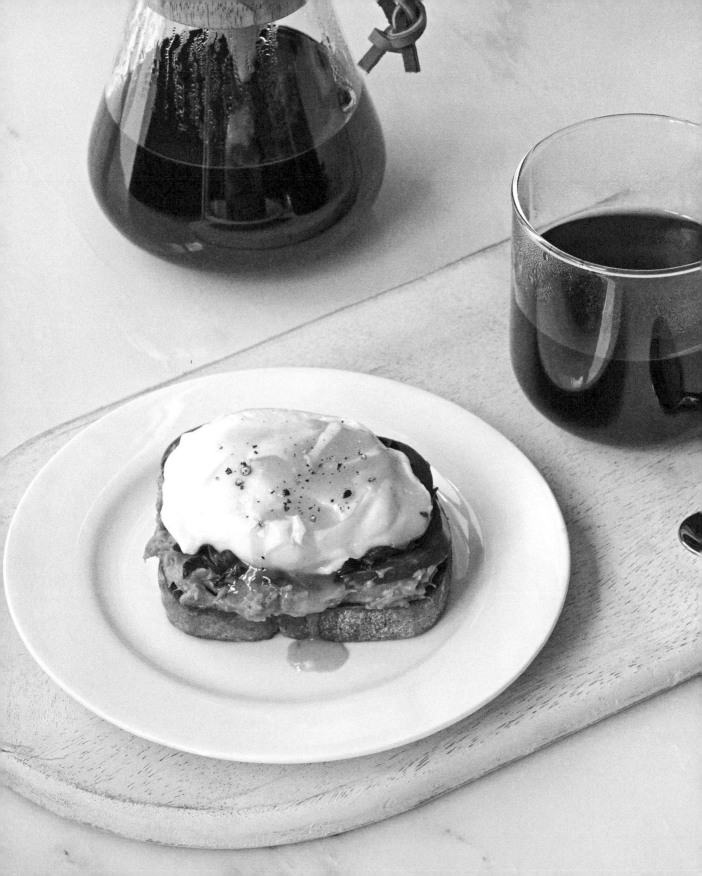

MEXICAN CAULIFLOWER CHILI SCRAMBLE

MAKES 4 SERVINGS
PREP TIME: 10 MINUTES
COOK TIME: 10 MINUTES

I love to go out for breakfast, especially when I can enjoy a great Tex-Mex breakfast buffet. But I tend to stuff myself silly at buffets, so I've learned to create my own guilt-free all-you-can-eat breakfast buffet at home. Here is one of my favorite at-home breakfasts.

Feel free to use a variety of dried chili powders to personalize this dish to your taste. I love adding a little ancho chili powder!

PER SERVING

184 calories
5.5g fat
15.5g protein
17g carbohydrates
7g fiber
207mg sodium

INGREDIENTS

Olive oil cooking spray

½ head cauliflower, grated on the large side of a box grater (about 3 cups yield)

2 tablespoons minced onion

½ cup small-diced red bell pepper (about 1 medium pepper)

¼ teaspoon ground cumin

1 teaspoon chili powder

½ teaspoon garlic powder

1 cup crushed tomatoes

Salt

Crushed red pepper flakes

1 cup very small broccoli florets

12 large egg whites, or 1 pint of liquid egg whites

1 avocado, cut into bite-size chunks

METHOD

1. Lightly coat a large nonstick skillet with cooking spray and place over medium-high heat. Add the cauliflower and cook until browned; transfer to a bowl. Add the onion, bell pepper, cumin, chili powder, and garlic powder to the skillet and cook until the onion and bell pepper have softened, 2 to 3 minutes. Add the tomatoes and cook until the mixture is soft and thick. Add the cauliflower, season with salt and red pepper flakes, and stir to combine. Transfer the vegetable "chili" to a bowl.

2. Wipe the skillet clean, lightly coat again with cooking spray, and place over medium-high heat. Add the broccoli and cook until

tender, 1 to 2 minutes. Add the egg whites and cook, scrambling them, about 2 minutes. Season.

3. Spoon the eggs and cauliflower chili onto four plates; top with avocado and serve.

BREAKFAST BOWL WITH QUINOA AND BERRIES

MAKES 4 SERVINGS
PREP TIME: 5 MINUTES

Breakfast bowls are the new green juice: they've become an in-demand menu item for the post-yoga, post–spin class set, despite some eyebrow-raising prices for what boils down to a pretty simple breakfast. Why spend all of that money on something you can easily make at home? This hearty, gluten-free bowl takes just minutes to throw together and is absolutely delicious.

PER SERVING

142 calories

6g fat

5g protein

19.75g carbohydrates

7g fiber

2mg sodium

INGREDIENTS

4 cups mixed berries (raspberries, strawberries, blueberries, blackberries)

2 tablespoons hemp hearts (available in the natural section of most supermarkets in a variety of brands)

20 whole almonds, toasted and chopped

¼ cup cooked quinoa

METHOD

Divide the berries equally among four bowls. Place the remaining ingredients in another bowl, and toss to combine. Sprinkle the mixture over each of the four bowls and serve.

TIP

Add 1½ heaping tablespoons of fat-free Greek yogurt to this dish for more protein.

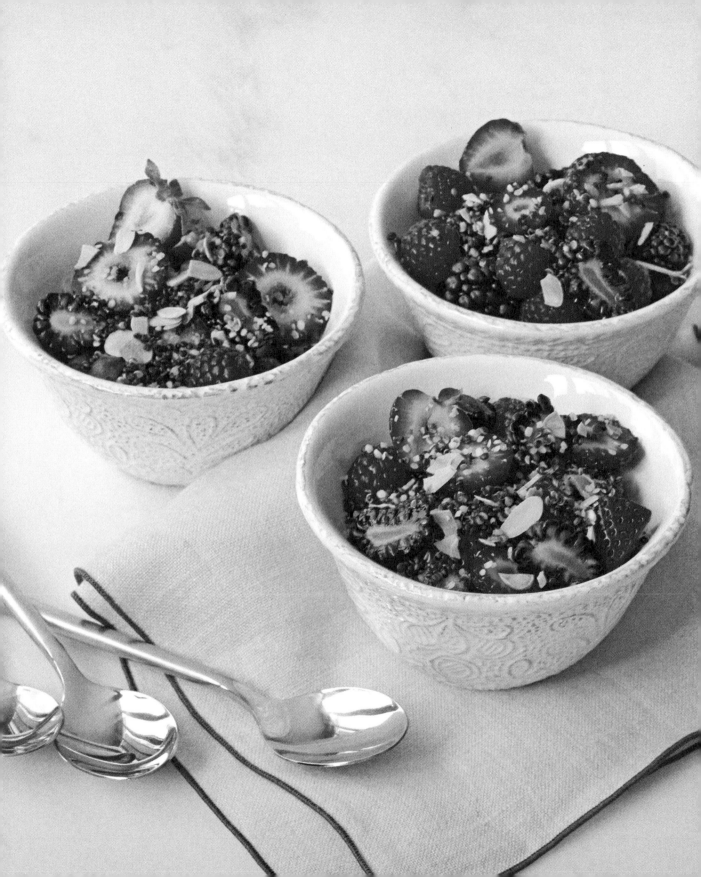

SPINACH AND MUSHROOM OMELET

MAKES 4 SERVINGS
PREP TIME: 10 MINUTES
COOK TIME: 15 MINUTES

Most of us are on a mission to get more vegetables into our diets. One of the easiest ways I've found to do that—besides smoothies—is by adding superstar leafy greens into egg recipes, such as omelets. Not only are greens negative calorie foods; they're also excellent sources of vitamin A, vitamin C, and other nutrients, including calcium, iron, and fiber.

Feel free to top your dish with a dash of hot sauce or a sprinkle of Parmigiano-Reggiano for extra flavor.

PER SERVING

108 calories
2g fat
16g protein
9g carbohydrates
3g fiber
263mg sodium

INGREDIENTS

12 large egg whites, or 1 pint liquid egg whites

1 teaspoon extra-virgin olive oil

4 cups sliced cremini mushrooms

Salt

2 tablespoons finely chopped shallots

Crushed red pepper flakes

One 16-ounce package tightly packed, cleaned spinach

METHOD

1. Preheat the oven to 350°F.
2. In a mixing bowl, whisk the egg whites until foamy; set aside. Pour the olive oil into a large nonstick, oven-safe skillet and place over medium-high heat. Once the oil has begun to show wisps of smoke, add the mushrooms. Cook the mushrooms until browned and softened. Season with salt, remove from the skillet, and reserve on a plate.
3. Add the shallots and a pinch of red pepper flakes to the skillet and cook until soft, about 2 minutes. Add the spinach and cook until wilted and soft and all the water has evaporated, 3 to 4 minutes. Push the spinach with the back of a spatula to release excess water and discard the liquid.
4. Return the mushrooms to the skillet. Taste and adjust the seasoning as needed and pour in the egg whites. Cook, stirring, until the egg whites have almost set. Transfer the skillet to the oven to finish the cooking, about 2 minutes. Fold the omelet in half; cut into 4 equal pieces and place a piece on each of four plates.

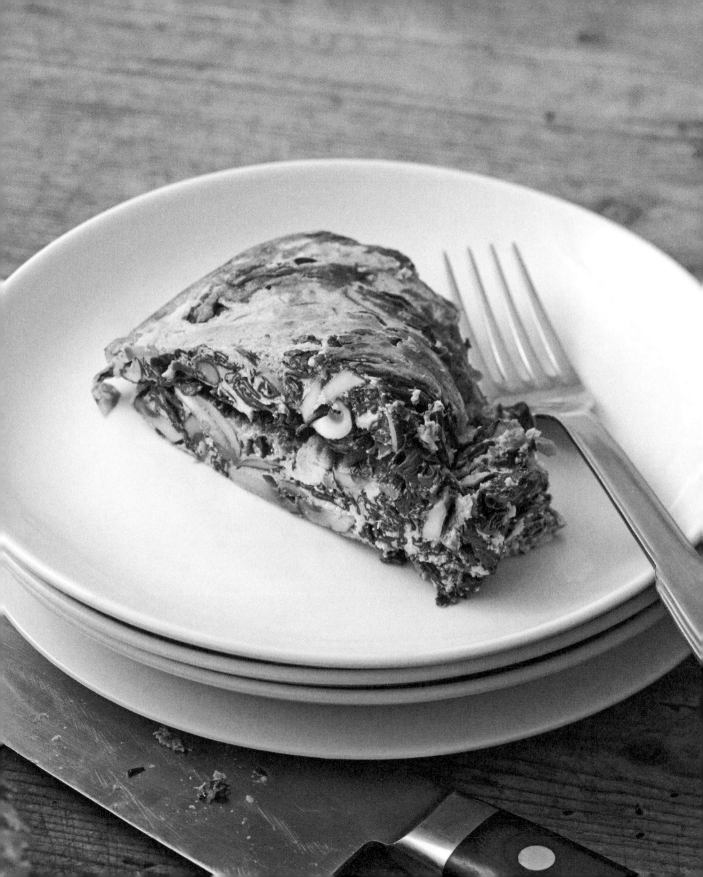

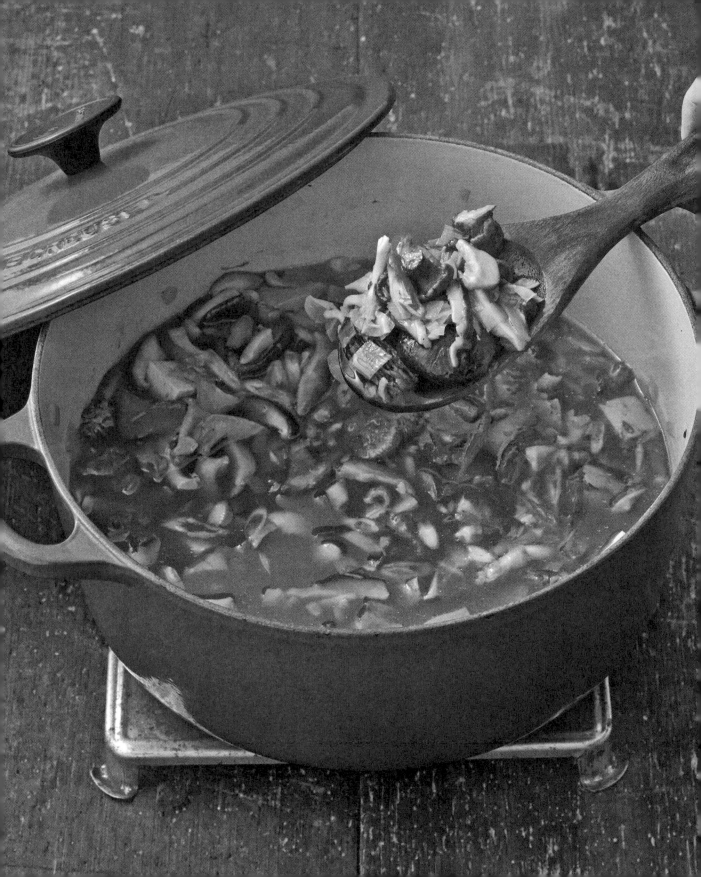

CHAPTER EIGHT

SOUPS AND SALADS

Charred Thai-Style Broccoli Salad with Almonds and Lime   120

Crabmeat Salad with Apple, Celery, and Leafy Greens   122

Chicken Soup with Escarole and Leeks   124

Shrimp and Cucumber Salad with Red Onion and Poblanos   126

Flank Steak Salad with Horseradish and Apple   128

Mixed Leafy Green Soup "Caldo Verde" with Chickpeas   130

Rocco's Chef Salad   132

Seared Tuna Tataki Salad with Citrus, Tofu, and Watercress   134

Asian Curry Mussel Soup   136

Shaved Brussels Sprouts with Warm Toasted Garlic, Almond, and Lemon Dressing   138

Strawberry and Spinach Salad with Almonds and Basil   140

Swiss Chard Turkey Salad with Golden Raisins and Capers   142

The Grate Salad Bowl with Chia Seed Dressing   144

Mushroom Bouillon with Leeks, Tofu, and Wasabi   146

Leafy Green Salad with Creamy Almond Dressing and Radishes   148

CHARRED THAI-STYLE BROCCOLI SALAD WITH ALMONDS AND LIME

MAKES 4 SERVINGS
PREP TIME: 5 MINUTES
COOK TIME: 10 MINUTES

There's no culinary rule that says salads must contain lettuce. You can create a salad with any vegetable (fruit, too) and heap it up on your plate. This salad starts with a base of broccoli, a negative calorie food brimming with vitamins, minerals, and antioxidants.

For an extra dose of protein, add 3 ounces of steamed shrimp per serving.

PER SERVING

97 calories
5g fat
5g protein
7g carbohydrates
4g fiber
266mg sodium

INGREDIENTS

¼ cup almonds, toasted and chopped

2 teaspoons grated peeled fresh ginger

1 teaspoon grated garlic

2 teaspoons grated onion

1 tablespoon plus 1 teaspoon golden monk fruit extract (such as Lakanto)

¼ teaspoon grated lime zest

3 tablespoons freshly squeezed lime juice

2 teaspoons Thai fish sauce (such as Thai Kitchen)

Hot sauce

Olive oil cooking spray

8 cups broccoli florets

1 cup fresh cilantro, torn into 2-inch pieces

4 lime wedges, for serving

Hot sauce, for serving

METHOD

1. Preheat the oven to 350°F.
2. For the dressing: Combine the almonds, ginger, garlic, onion, monk fruit extract, lime zest and juice, and fish sauce in a large mixing bowl and mix well. Add hot sauce to taste and set aside.
3. Lightly coat a large oven-safe skillet with cooking spray and place over high heat. Once it gets extremely hot, add the broccoli florets and allow them to char on one side. Stir, and allow the other sides to char. Transfer the broccoli to the oven, and cook it until it is just tender, about 5 minutes.

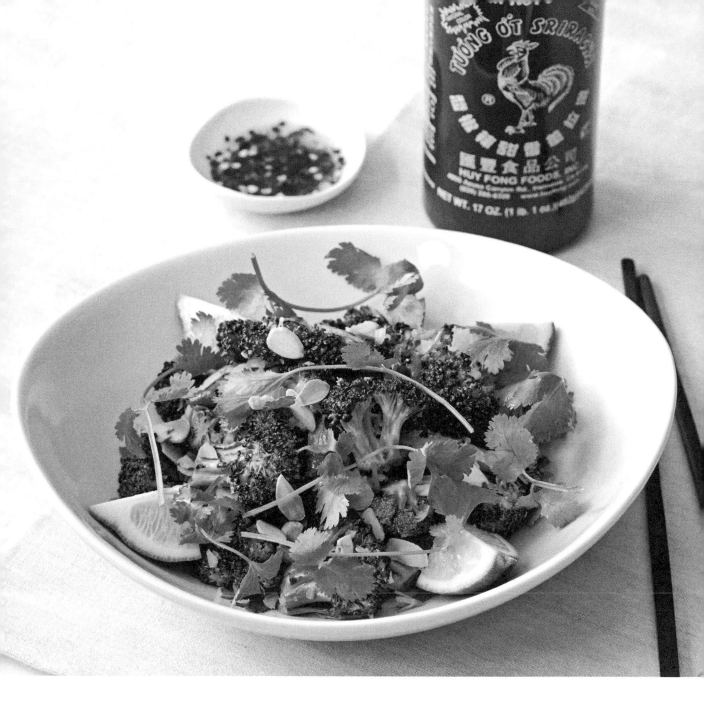

4. Remove broccoli from oven and add it and the cilantro to the mixing bowl. Toss with dressing and spoon into four salad bowls. Serve with lime wedges and hot sauce.

CRABMEAT SALAD WITH APPLE, CELERY, AND LEAFY GREENS

MAKES 4 SERVINGS
PREP TIME: 10 MINUTES

I love seafood salads like this one because they can be easily packed and transported to work or school, but the calories won't travel to your waistline. In this salad—unlike traditional seafood salads that are drowning in mayo—I've used Greek yogurt to create the rich, creamy texture we all know and love. Be sure to splurge for real crabmeat—not the imitation stuff, which is full of chemicals.

PER SERVING

129 calories
2g fat
21g protein
27g carbohydrates
2.5g fiber
291mg sodium

INGREDIENTS

¼ cup fat-free Greek yogurt (such as Fage 0%)

1 tablespoon freshly squeezed lemon juice

1 teaspoon Dijon mustard

⅛ teaspoon crab boil spice (such as reduced-sodium Old Bay)

½ cup thinly sliced celery

12 ounces fresh crabmeat, such as blue crab, picked to remove all shells

Salt

Cayenne pepper

4 heads butter lettuce, outer leaves removed, heads cut in half

½ cup sliced apple

METHOD

1. Put the yogurt, lemon juice, mustard, and crab boil spice into a medium mixing bowl and toss well. Add the celery and fold in the crabmeat without breaking it up too much. Taste and adjust the seasoning with salt and cayenne.

2. Arrange the lettuce halves on four plates. Spoon the crabmeat salad over the lettuce, dividing it equally. Scatter the apple slices over the tops.

TIP

Try putting in some fresh chopped dill and/or chives for an added layer of flavor.

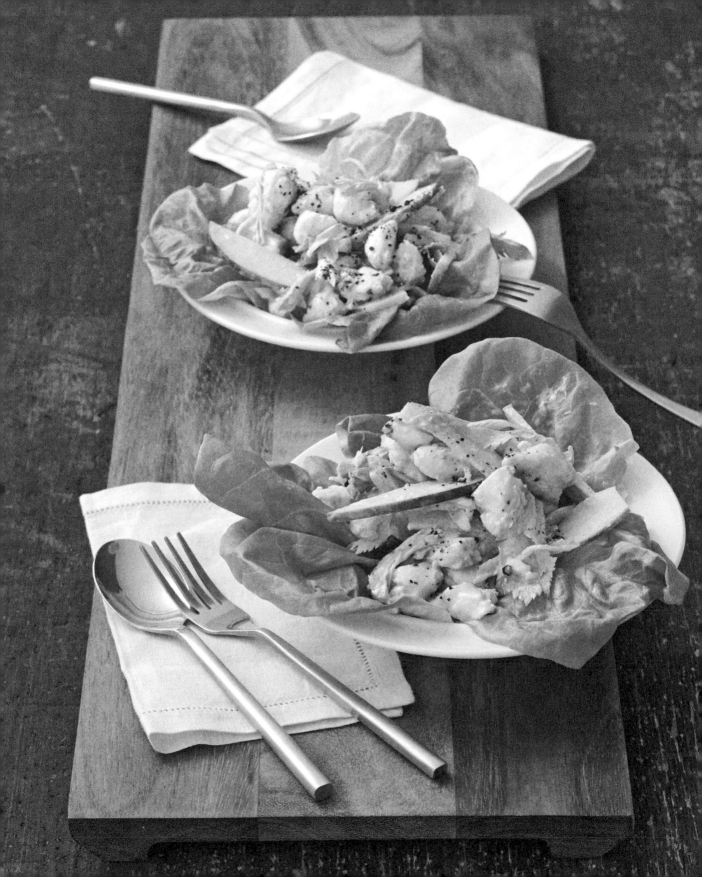

CHICKEN SOUP WITH ESCAROLE AND LEEKS

MAKES 4 SERVINGS
PREP TIME: 10 MINUTES
COOK TIME: 30 MINUTES

Most people don't know escarole from escargot, but that's okay. Just know that escarole is a delicious leafy green vegetable that's high in vitamin C. Leeks, which resemble large scallions, have a slightly oniony flavor. Here, I've used both in a main-meal soup that is filling and nutritious.

Try sprinkling a little smoked paprika over the soup before adding the cheese—it will give a sweet, smoky, slightly spicy flavor.

PER SERVING

163 calories
4.5g fat
21g protein
9.7g carbohydrates
4g fiber
353mg sodium

INGREDIENTS

Olive oil cooking spray

8 ounces boneless, skinless chicken thighs, cut into 1-inch pieces

Salt

Freshly ground black pepper

1 cup well-washed, chopped leeks

12 cups well-washed, chopped escarole

8 cups unsalted chicken stock (such as Kitchen Basics)

2 teaspoons fresh thyme

1 ounce Parmigiano-Reggiano cheese, finely grated on a Microplane grater

METHOD

1. Lightly coat a large pot with olive oil cooking spray and place over medium-high heat. Season the chicken with salt and pepper. Once the oil is hot, add the chicken and brown well on one side. Add the leeks and escarole to the pot and cook, stirring occasionally, until the vegetables have wilted but not browned, 2 to 3 minutes.

2. Add the chicken stock to the pot, cover, and bring to a simmer. Cook until the vegetables are soft and the chicken is tender, about 20 minutes.

3. Add the fresh thyme to the soup. Taste and adjust the seasoning. Ladle the soup into four soup bowls, dividing it equally. Sprinkle with cheese and serve.

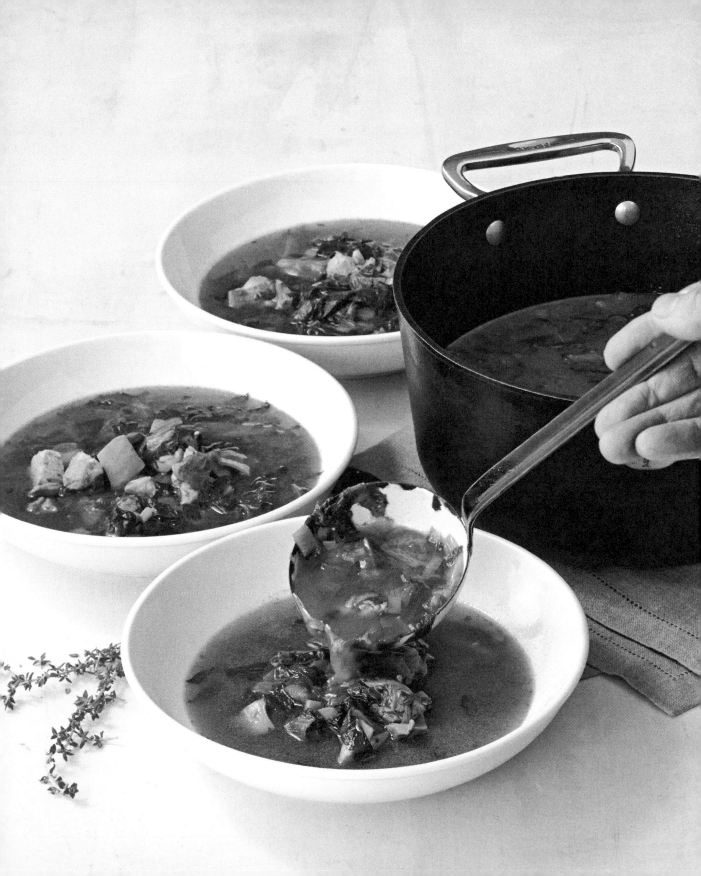

SHRIMP AND CUCUMBER SALAD WITH RED ONION AND POBLANOS

MAKES 4 SERVINGS
PREP TIME: 5 MINUTES
COOK TIME: 10 MINUTES

Daydreaming about a trip to the beach and indulging in some seafood? Then this simple yet flavorful seafood salad will satisfy your craving, and make sure you're in swimsuit shape when you do hit the beach!

PER SERVING

168 calories
1.5g fat
26g protein
13.25g carbohydrates
2.5g fiber
264mg sodium

INGREDIENTS

¾ cup thinly sliced red onion

¼ teaspoon grated lime zest

¼ cup freshly squeezed lime juice

Salt

½ cup thinly sliced poblano peppers

6 cups sliced cucumber

2 cups cherry tomatoes, halved

1 pound peeled steamed shrimp, cut into bite-size pieces

1 cup fresh cilantro, torn into 2-inch pieces

4 lime wedges, for serving

METHOD

1. Place the onion in a coffee mug, and add the lime zest and juice. Season with salt and stir. Let stand for 5 minutes.

2. Combine the peppers, cucumber, tomatoes, shrimp, and cilantro in a medium mixing bowl. Add the onion-lime mixture and toss to coat everything evenly. Taste and season with salt, if needed. Serve with the lime wedges.

TIP

Top with some diced avocado for added nutrients and flavor.

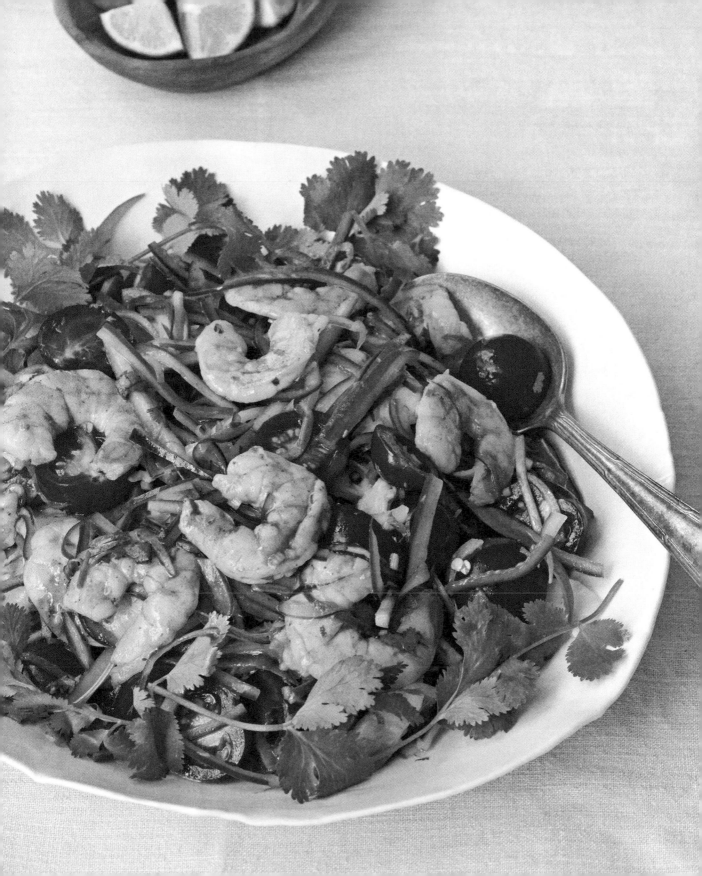

FLANK STEAK SALAD WITH HORSERADISH AND APPLE

MAKES 4 SERVINGS
PREP TIME: 5 MINUTES
COOK TIME: 10 MINUTES

Salads are more satisfying than people think they are—all of those veggies contain fiber and water, which fill you up. Add a healthy protein like flank steak, and you have a complete meal that is not only super satiating, but downright delicious.

PER SERVING

251 calories
6.5g fat
29g protein
21g carbohydrates
6g fiber
400mg sodium

INGREDIENTS

Olive oil cooking spray

One 12-ounce flank steak, trimmed of all visible fat

Salt

Freshly ground black pepper

½ cup sliced onion

12 cremini mushrooms, sliced

2 tablespoons water

8 cups chopped mustard greens

1 large Granny Smith apple, cut into bite-size chunks

¼ cup coconut aminos (such as Coconut Secret)

3 teaspoons prepared horseradish

4 lemon wedges, for serving

METHOD

1. Preheat the oven to 350°F.

2. Lightly coat a large grill pan with cooking spray and place over high heat. Season the steak with salt and pepper and place it in the hot pan. Cook until browned, about 2 minutes. Flip the steak and add the onion and mushrooms to the skillet. Finish in the oven and cook until the steak is warmed through, 3 to 5 minutes. Remove the steak from the pan and let it rest.

3. Add the water to the pan and cook over medium heat until the onion and mushrooms are coated with the sauce. Transfer them to a mixing bowl with the mustard greens, apple, and coconut aminos. Toss to coat; season with more salt and horseradish.

4. Serve steak, sliced, over salad. Garnish with lemon.

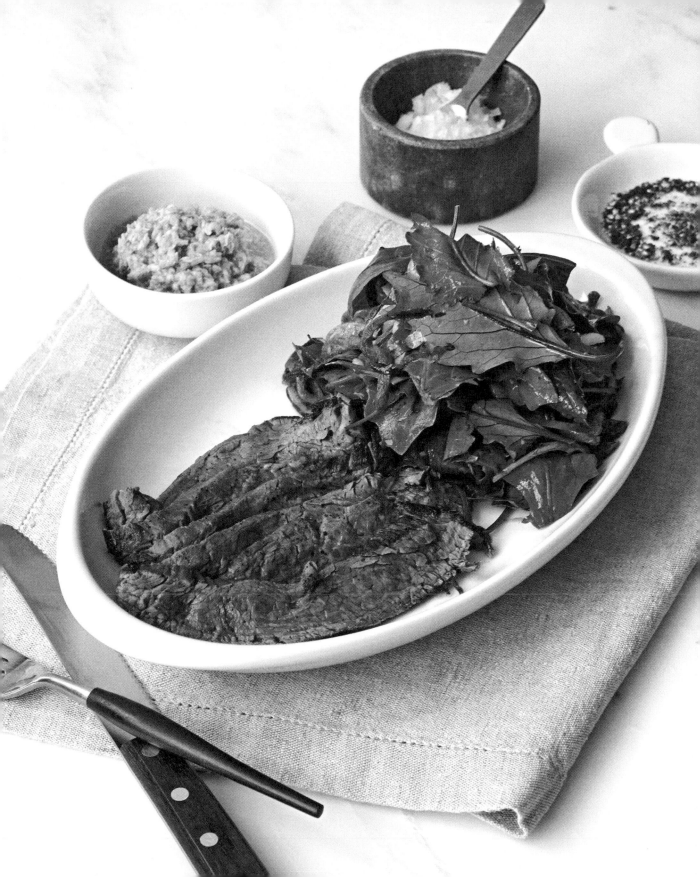

MIXED LEAFY GREEN SOUP "CALDO VERDE" WITH CHICKPEAS

MAKES 4 SERVINGS
PREP TIME: 5 MINUTES
COOK TIME: 20 MINUTES

Caldo verde means "green broth" in Portuguese, and it is Portugal's unofficial national dish. This beautiful green soup is technically a hot smoothie, since its many nutritious greens are pureed together in a blender. Chickpeas are an important ingredient here, too. Fiber- and protein-rich, they've been shown in studies to help people lose weight.

For added protein, top with 4 ounces of shredded chicken or add 2 dozen clams to the broth.

PER SERVING

151 calories
2.5g fat
12.5g protein
25.5g carbohydrates
7g fiber
251mg sodium

INGREDIENTS

1½ teaspoons olive oil

1 tablespoon plus 1 teaspoon chopped garlic

1 cup small-diced onions

1 teaspoon smoked paprika

8 cups mixed leafy greens (kale, collards, and mustard)

1 cup no-salt-added chickpeas (garbanzo beans)

1 quart unsalted chicken stock (such as Kitchen Basics)

Salt

Freshly ground black pepper

METHOD

1. Pour the olive oil into a large pot, and place over medium-high heat. Add the garlic and cook until golden brown, about 2 minutes. Add the onions and paprika; lower the heat to medium; and cook, covered, until tender, 2 to 3 minutes.

2. Put the greens into a blender and blend until pureed (you may use a little water to help, or use the wand tool that comes with some blenders to force the greens to blend without water). Pour this mixture into the pot, increase the heat to high, and cook until the water has evaporated from the greens.

3. Pour two-thirds of the chickpeas into the blender with 1 cup of the stock and blend until smooth. Add the pureed chickpeas to the pot with the remaining chicken stock and chickpeas and bring to a simmer. Cook covered until the greens are tender and the soup has thickened, about 10 minutes. Season with salt and pepper. Ladle the soup into four bowls and serve.

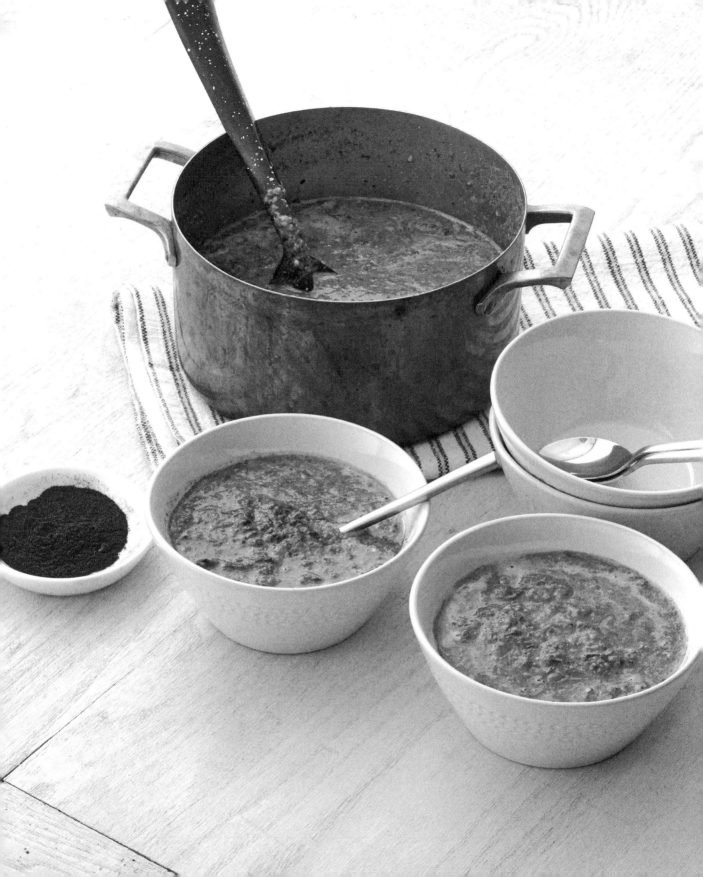

ROCCO'S CHEF SALAD

MAKES 4 SERVINGS
PREP TIME: 10 MINUTES

Traditionally, "chef salads" were mixed by the chef at the diner's table—which is perhaps where the name came from. There's no documentary evidence tying the origin of "chef salad" to any particular chef, however. That being so, I slapped my name on this one because it's my creation! It's healthy and flavorful and will more than satisfy your appetite.

PER SERVING

183 calories
7g fat
22g protein
9g carbohydrates
3.5g fiber
71mg sodium

INGREDIENTS

½ cup unsweetened dried cranberries, roughly chopped

¼ cup plus 2 tablespoons red wine vinegar

Salt

Freshly ground black pepper

1 tablespoon extra-virgin olive oil

8 cups chopped romaine lettuce

1 cup cherry tomatoes, halved

2 cups cucumber slices

2 large hard-boiled eggs, peeled and roughly chopped

8 ounces skinless store-roasted turkey breast, sliced thin

METHOD

1. For the dressing: Put half the cranberries in a blender with the vinegar and blend to a chunky puree. Pour this puree into a bowl and season it with salt and pepper. Stir in the olive oil and set aside.

2. Place the lettuce, tomatoes, and cucumber in a large mixing bowl. Toss with the dressing and season with salt and pepper. Spoon the salad into four salad bowls, dividing it equally, and top each one with the eggs and turkey.

TIPS

1. Some diced avocado is great on this salad if you have it handy.

2. Add 1 teaspoon of Dijon mustard to the dressing if you like it spicy!

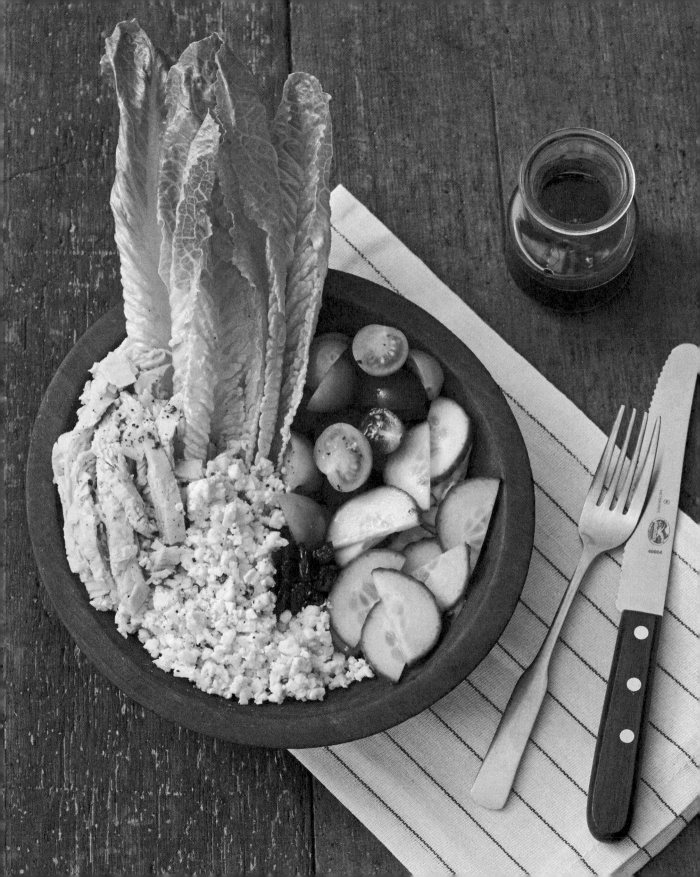

SEARED TUNA TATAKI SALAD WITH CITRUS, TOFU, AND WATERCRESS

MAKES 4 SERVINGS
PREP TIME: 10 MINUTES
COOK TIME: 10 MINUTES

Salads have been around since the ancient Greeks and Romans; they're not a modern-day "diet" food. Salads get their name from the Latin word for salt: *sal*. This was chosen because in ancient times, salt was often used in the dressing. I don't have any big hang-ups about using a little salt in my salads. Miso is a salty paste made from fermented soybeans—it's a great way to add flavor to Asian-inspired dishes like this one.

PER SERVING

201 calories
3g fat
27.5g protein
16.5g carbohydrates
3.5g fiber
418mg sodium

INGREDIENTS

Olive oil cooking spray

One 12-ounce sushi-grade tuna steak

Salt

Freshly ground black pepper

⅛ block of medium-firm tofu (sprouted if available), cut into bite-size chunks

2 tablespoons plus 2 teaspoons raw coconut aminos

1 tablespoon miso paste

¼ cup thinly sliced scallions

1 teaspoon finely grated orange zest

2 cups orange segments (about 4 oranges)

8 cups watercress, large tough stems removed

METHOD

1. Lightly coat a cast-iron skillet or grill pan with cooking spray. Place the skillet over medium-high heat. Season the tuna with salt and pepper. Once the pan is extremely hot, add the tuna and sear on all sides until blackened, about 1 minute per side. Remove from the skillet and let rest on a wire rack.

2. Place the tofu in a mixing bowl with the coconut aminos, miso, and scallions and toss gently to coat. Season with salt. Add the orange zest and segments to the bowl and mix gently to combine. Fold in the watercress.

3. Arrange the salad on four plates, dividing it equally. Cut the tuna into thin slices and place over each salad. Drizzle any remaining sauce from the bowl over the sliced tuna.

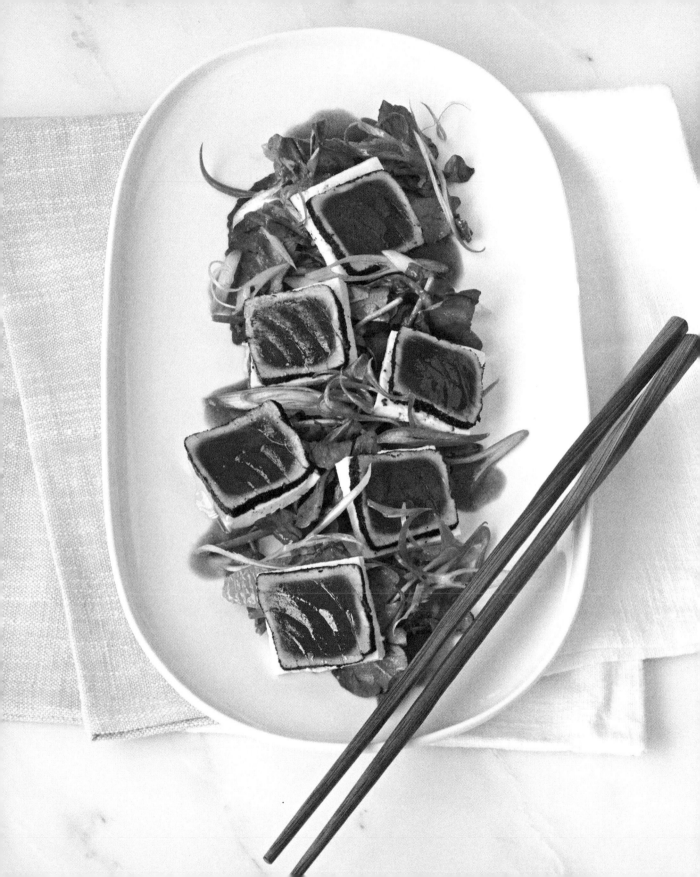

ASIAN CURRY MUSSEL SOUP

MAKES 4 SERVINGS
PREP TIME: 5 MINUTES
COOK TIME: 15 MINUTES

Here's a soup that can be rightly categorized as fusion cuisine. It blends mussel soup, traditionally a Mediterranean dish, with Asian influences to create a uniquely flavorful meal. Note that the recipe calls for a Japanese eggplant. Slender and softer in comparison with the Italian eggplant, this piece of heaven is actually a fruit related to berries. Its unique flavor makes it worth seeking out for this recipe.

PER SERVING

184 calories
7g fat
16.5g protein
9.7g carbohydrates
4g fiber
390mg sodium

INGREDIENTS

1½ teaspoons unrefined coconut oil

2 cups ½-inch-thick sliced rounds Japanese eggplant

1 tablespoon curry powder (I prefer to use mild curry; add more to adjust heat level)

1 tablespoon chopped peeled fresh ginger

2 teaspoons chopped garlic

¾ cup sliced onions

2 cups sliced red bell peppers

1 quart unsweetened almond milk, or homemade almond milk (page 91)

2 pounds mussels, soaked, scrubbed, beards removed (about 48 mussels)

1 cup torn fresh cilantro, for garnish

4 lime wedges, for serving

METHOD

1. Put the oil in a large pot and place over medium-high heat. Add the eggplant and cook until browned. Push the eggplant to the side of the pot and add the curry powder, ginger, garlic, onions, and bell peppers and cook until softened, about 2 minutes.

2. Add the almond milk and bring to a simmer. Add the cleaned mussels, discarding any that are cracked or open; cover the pot; and bring to a simmer. Cook until the mussels have opened, about 3 minutes; discard any that do not open.

3. Divide the mussels equally among four deep soup bowls. Ladle some of the broth into each bowl. Garnish with the cilantro and serve with lime wedges.

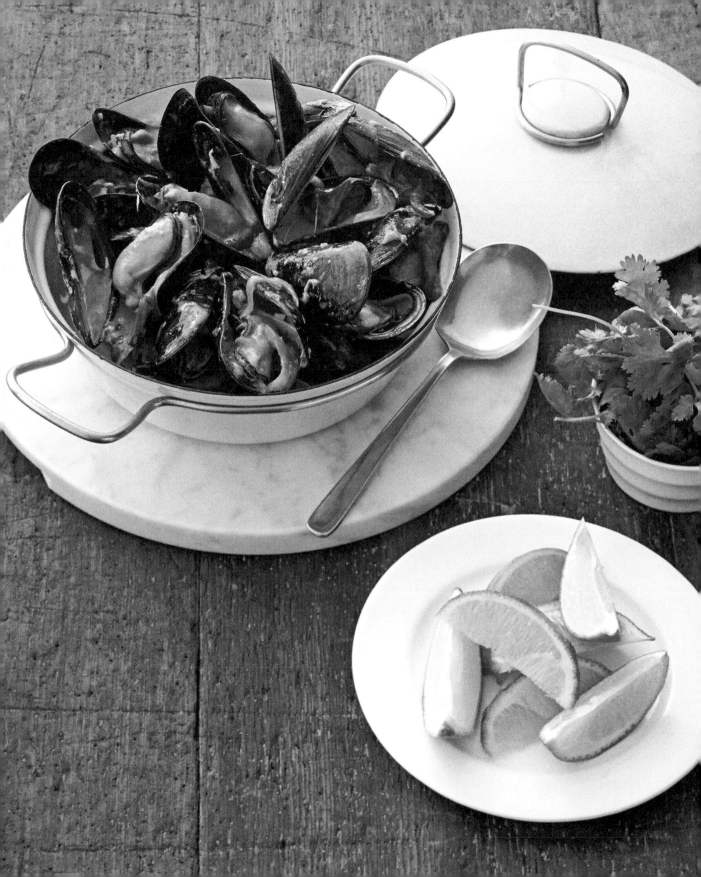

SHAVED BRUSSELS SPROUTS WITH WARM TOASTED GARLIC, ALMOND, AND LEMON DRESSING

MAKES 4 SERVINGS
PREP TIME: 10 MINUTES
COOK TIME: 10 MINUTES

The Brussels sprout is a true nutritional hero, complete with cancer-fighting compounds. I love to pair it with another cancer-fighter, garlic. Shaving the Brussels sprouts creates a hearty yet delicate texture and raw Brussels have a slightly different, lighter flavor compared with cooked Brussels. They make a great salad base for grilled or roasted proteins like chicken or shrimp.

PER SERVING

155 calories
7.5g fat
8.75g protein
17.5g carbohydrates
6.25g fiber
100mg sodium

INGREDIENTS

3 pints Brussels sprouts, shaved thinly with a mandoline, the large side of a box grater, or a sharp knife (this should yield 8 cups)

1½ teaspoons extra-virgin olive oil

5 teaspoons freshly minced garlic

¼ cup toasted almonds, finely chopped

Crushed red pepper flakes

⅛ teaspoon ground cinnamon

½ cup chopped fresh flat-leaf parsley

½ cup freshly squeezed lemon juice

Salt

1 ounce Parmigiano-Reggiano cheese, finely grated on a Microplane grater

METHOD

1. Place the shaved Brussels sprouts in a large mixing bowl and set aside.

2. Place a nonstick skillet over medium-high heat; put in the olive oil and the garlic. Cook the garlic until deep golden brown. Remove from the heat and add the almonds, red pepper flakes, cinnamon, and parsley. Return to the heat and sauté for 10 seconds.

3. Remove the skillet from the heat, add the lemon juice, and season with salt. Transfer the hot mixture to the bowl with the Brussels sprouts and toss well. Add three-quarters of the cheese. Toss again, taste, and adjust the seasoning. Spoon the sprouts into four salad bowls, dividing them equally. Top each dish with the remaining cheese.

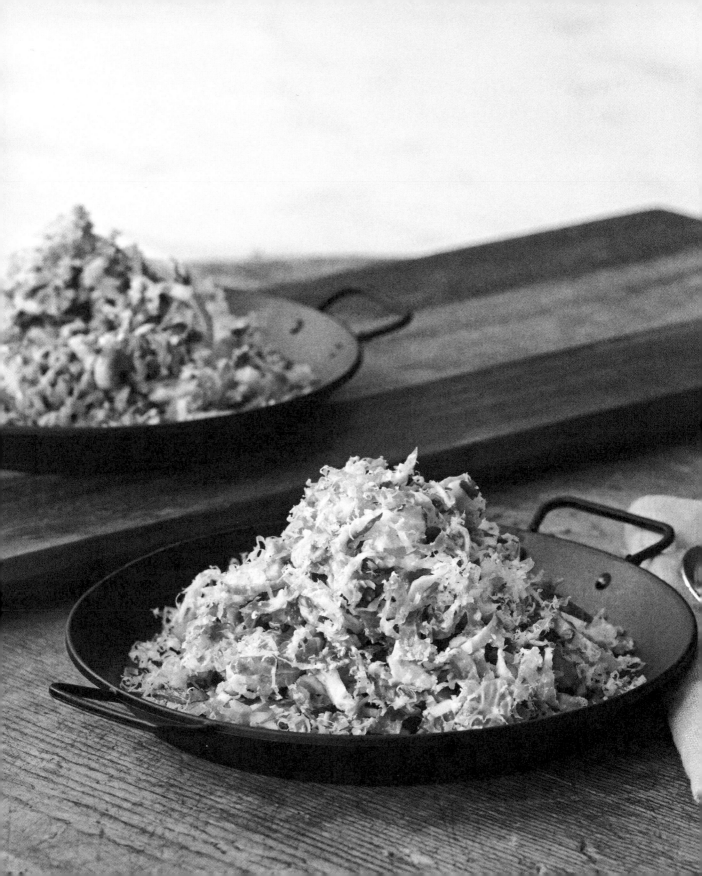

STRAWBERRY AND SPINACH SALAD WITH ALMONDS AND BASIL

MAKES 4 SERVINGS
PREP TIME: 10 MINUTES

Strawberries are my go-to fruit. There are so many ways to enjoy them, from sprinkling them on cereal or yogurt to blending them into smoothies to tossing them into salads. Strawberries and spinach pair especially well, and create a vibrant, beautiful salad.

PER SERVING

116 calories
6g fat
4.5g protein
10.25g carbohydrates
4.5g fiber
51mg sodium

INGREDIENTS

¼ cup lightly toasted almonds, chopped

¼ cup balsamic vinegar

Salt

Freshly ground black pepper

2 cups strawberries, halved or quartered

1 Belgian endive, sliced into thin strips

8 cups washed baby spinach

½ cup fresh basil leaves, torn into bite-size pieces

1 teaspoon extra-virgin olive oil

METHOD

1. In a medium bowl, mix half the almonds with the vinegar and season with salt and pepper. Add the berries and toss gently to coat evenly.

2. Combine the endive, spinach, and basil in a large bowl. Add the olive oil and toss to coat evenly. Season with salt and pepper.

3. Arrange the leafy greens on four salad plates and spoon the strawberries on and around the greens, dividing the greens and berries equally.

TIP

Serve this salad with grilled chicken for a fantastic dinner.

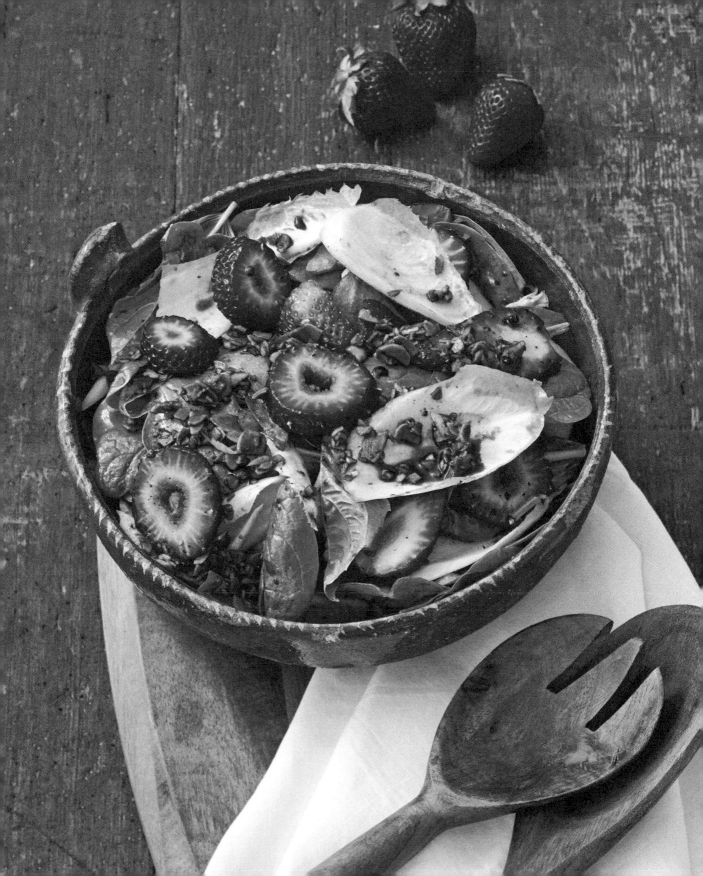

SWISS CHARD TURKEY SALAD
WITH GOLDEN RAISINS AND CAPERS

MAKES 4 SERVINGS
PREP TIME: 5 MINUTES
COOK TIME: 5 MINUTES

If you haven't met Swiss chard yet, let me introduce you. This leafy green is actually a member of the beet family, and has a taste similar to beet leaves and spinach. Swiss chard has a long résumé of health benefits too numerous to list here, but here's one important benefit: a cup of this delightful green supplies over half of your daily requirement of fat-burning, immunity-boosting vitamin C. Okay, you've been formally acquainted—now get cooking with Swiss chard!

PER SERVING

158 calories
5g fat
16g protein
14g carbohydrates
2.75g fiber
315mg sodium

INGREDIENTS

¼ cup chopped golden raisins

2 tablespoons water

2 tablespoons freshly squeezed lemon juice

2 tablespoons chopped capers, plus 1 teaspoon caper brine

¼ cup toasted almonds

Freshly ground black pepper

⅓ cup sliced red onion

1 cup cherry tomatoes

6 cups chopped Swiss chard, stems cut very thin

1 teaspoon extra-virgin olive oil

6 ounces store-roasted skinless turkey breast, shredded

METHOD

1. Combine the raisins in a microwave-safe bowl with the 2 tablespoons water. Cook on high until simmering, 1½ to 2 minutes. Remove from the microwave and let stand for 2 minutes.

2. Put the lemon juice, capers, and almonds in a small bowl and season with black pepper. Add the raisins, their soaking liquid, the onion, and the tomatoes and mix well.

3. In a large bowl, combine the Swiss chard, olive oil, and turkey and toss well. Add the mixture from the small bowl and toss together to combine. Spoon the salad onto four salad plates, dividing it equally, and serve.

TIP

Add 1 chopped avocado to this recipe for some delicious and healthy fat.

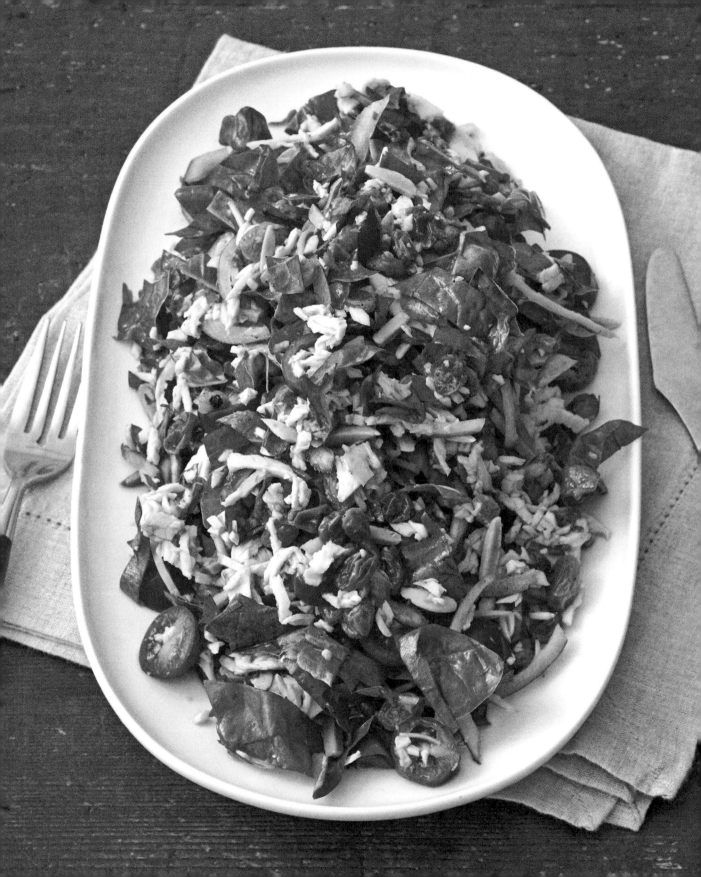

THE GRATE SALAD BOWL WITH CHIA SEED DRESSING

MAKES 4 SERVINGS
PREP TIME: 10 MINUTES

Here's one of the ultimate negative calorie salads, with apple, broccoli, cauliflower, and cabbage. The dressing is made with chia seeds, which have a mild, slightly nutty flavor. These tiny dynamos of nutrition are rich in fiber and protein, and offer a host of health benefits—plus, they fill you up quickly. All the way around, this salad is a negative calorie winner.

PER SERVING

83 calories
1.5g fat
2.5g protein
17g carbohydrates
5g fiber
111mg sodium

INGREDIENTS

1 apple, grated (to yield ⅓ cup)

1 tablespoon chia seeds

2 tablespoons freshly squeezed lemon juice

1 tablespoon apple cider vinegar

2 teaspoons Dijon mustard

Salt

Freshly ground black pepper

½ head broccoli, grated (to yield 1 cup)

⅓ head cauliflower, grated (to yield 1 cup)

½ head red cabbage, grated (to yield 1 cup)

4 carrots, peeled and grated (to yield 1 cup)

METHOD

1. Put the grated apple into a bowl with the chia seeds and let stand for 5 minutes, until thickened. Add the lemon juice, vinegar, and mustard, and season with salt and pepper. Set aside.

2. Mix together the remaining ingredients in a large mixing bowl. Add the chia dressing, and toss to coat evenly. Taste and season with additional salt and pepper, if needed.

TIPS

1. Add 3 ounces of your favorite diced lean protein to this salad for a killer lunch.

2. Add 1 tablespoon of coconut aminos to the dressing for a deeper, richer flavor.

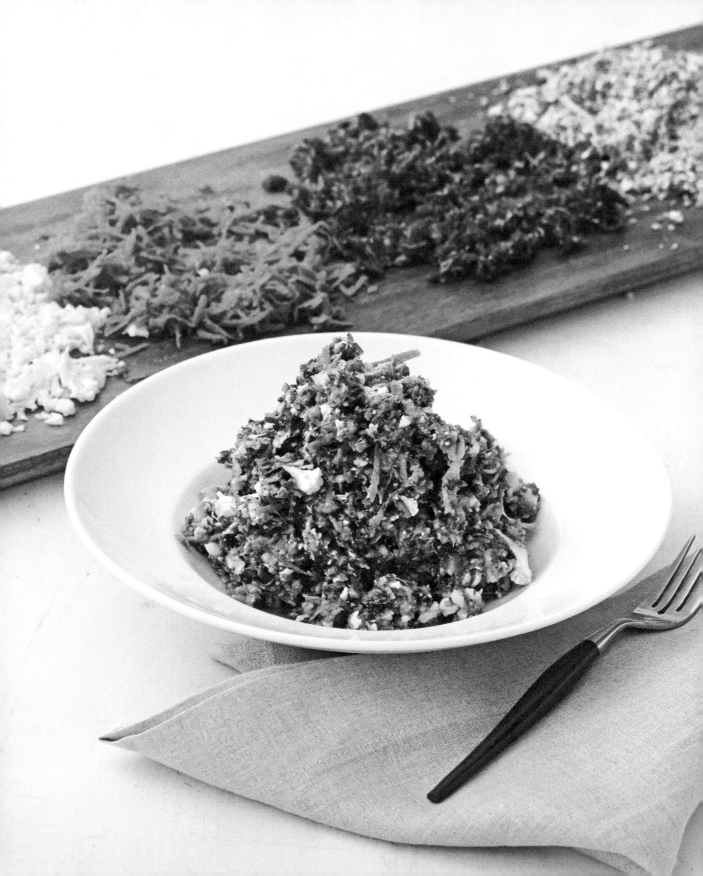

MUSHROOM BOUILLON WITH LEEKS, TOFU, AND WASABI

MAKES 4 SERVINGS
PREP TIME: 10 MINUTES
COOK TIME: 25 MINUTES

Here's a light, flavor-packed Asian-inspired soup with the heavy-hitting, fat-burning power of mushrooms and wasabi, a hot mustard-like condiment that is much more than just a sushi sidekick. Wasabi can also fight tooth decay, and will clear your sinuses like nobody's business. How's that for multitasking?

PER SERVING

101 calories
2g fat
11g protein
11.25g carbohydrates
2g fiber
500mg sodium

INGREDIENTS

2 teaspoons wasabi powder
2 teaspoons water
Olive oil cooking spray
1 cup well-washed thinly sliced leeks
8 cups sliced mixed mushrooms (use wild varieties if possible!)
5 cups unsalted, fat-free chicken stock
2 tablespoons reduced-sodium, gluten-free soy sauce
¼ block medium-firm tofu, drained and cut into bite-size pieces
¼ cup chopped scallions

METHOD

1. In a very small bowl, mix the wasabi with the water to make a thick paste. Invert the bowl, let stand, then form the mixture into 4 equal balls.

2. Lightly coat a large pot with cooking spray and place over medium-high heat. Add the leeks and cook until softened, about 2 minutes. Add the mushrooms and cook, stirring occasionally, until they begin to soften, about 2 minutes. Add the chicken stock and bring to a simmer. Turn off the heat, cover the pot, and let stand for 15 minutes.

3. Add the soy sauce to the soup. Place the tofu in four soup bowls, dividing it equally. Ladle the soup into each bowl over the tofu and serve with scallions and wasabi on the side.

TIPS

1. This soup is also a great base for roasted fish.

2. Add a cup of spinach to each bowl as you ladle out the soup—it will wilt quickly and incorporate well.

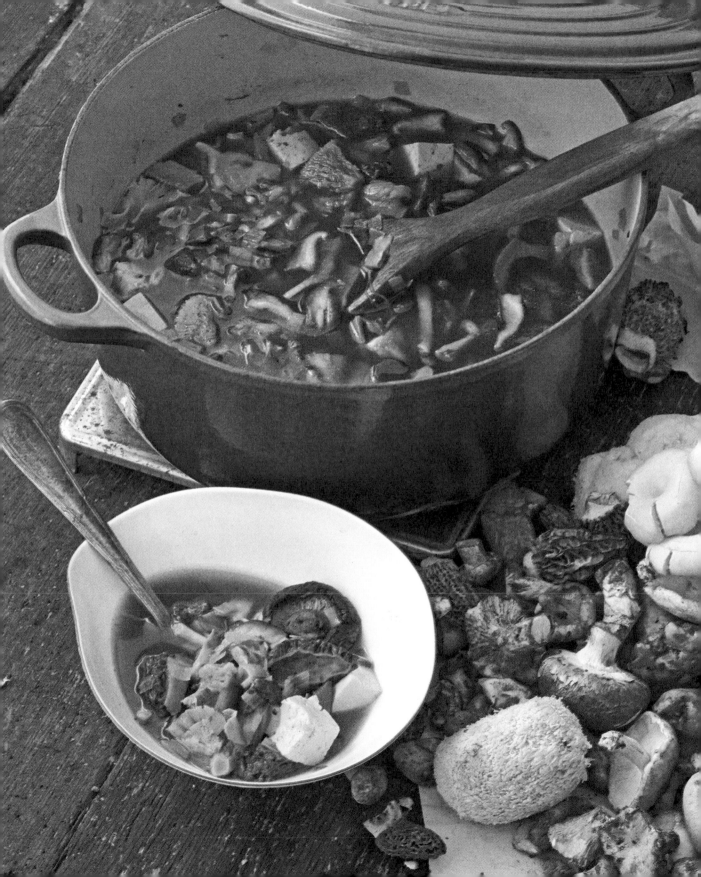

LEAFY GREEN SALAD WITH CREAMY ALMOND DRESSING AND RADISHES

MAKES 4 SERVINGS
PREP TIME: 5 MINUTES
COOK TIME: 10 MINUTES

When you green up your diet, you're getting not only negative calorie benefits but also powerful doses of vitamins A and C, plus calcium, iron, fiber, and disease-fighting nutrients. This creamy, lightly almond-flavored dressing pairs perfectly with delicate butter lettuce and pungent, crunchy radishes.

PER SERVING

136 calories
10g fat
6g protein
9g carbohydrates
4.25g fiber
20mg sodium

INGREDIENTS

⅓ cup almonds, lightly toasted and chopped

1 cup water

3 tablespoons sherry vinegar

1 tablespoon extra-virgin olive oil

Salt

Freshly ground black pepper

⅛ teaspoon almond extract

6 heads butter lettuce, outer leaves removed, heads cut in half

4 large radishes, sliced thinly

METHOD

1. Place ¼ cup of the almonds and the 1 cup water in a microwave-safe bowl, cover with parchment paper, and cook on high until tender, 5 to 7 minutes.

2. Transfer to a blender and blend with the sherry vinegar until smooth and creamy. (This may need some more water, depending on evaporation during cooking.) Pour the mixture into a bowl. Whisk in the olive oil and almond extract. Season with salt and pepper. Let cool.

3. Place the lettuce in a large mixing bowl. Pour the dressing over the top and toss to coat evenly. Taste and season with additional salt and pepper, if needed. Arrange 3 halves of the lettuce on each of four salad plates. Top each salad with sliced radishes and the remaining tablespoon of toasted almonds, dividing them equally.

TIP

This salad pairs nicely with a lean grilled steak.

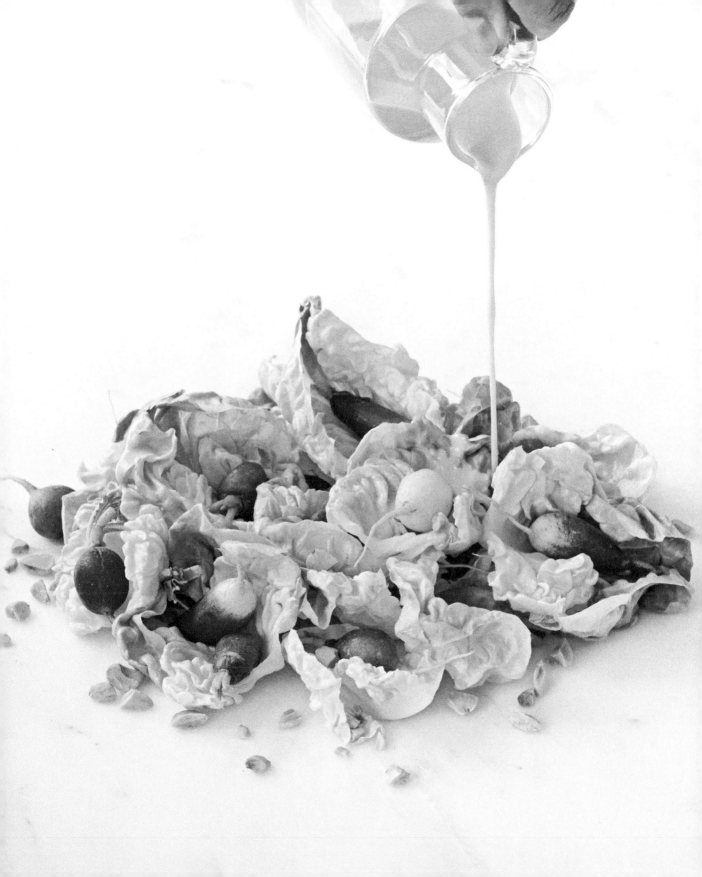

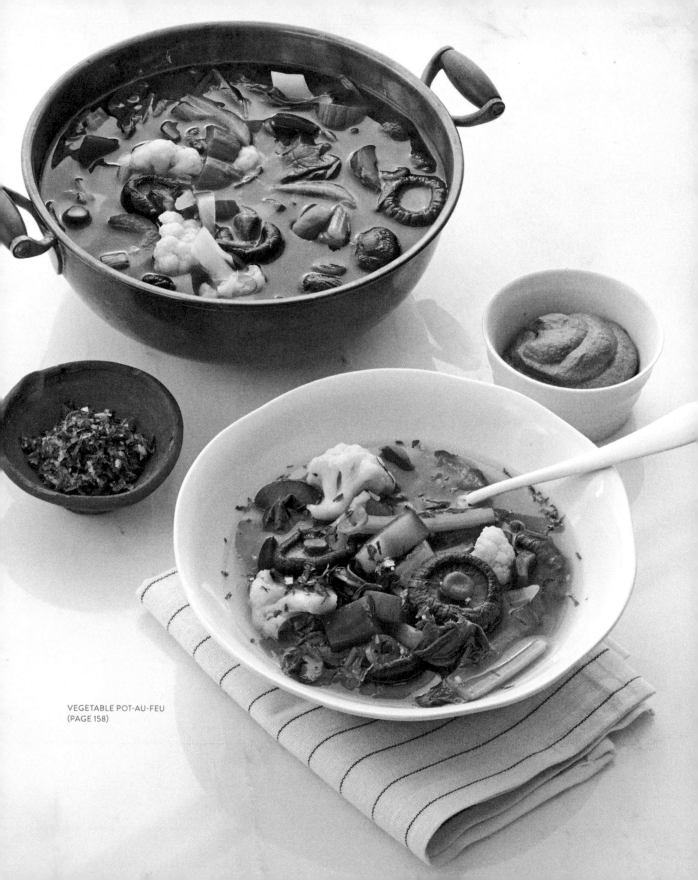

VEGETABLE POT-AU-FEU
(PAGE 158)

CHAPTER NINE

MAINS

Almond-Encrusted Flounder with Chopped Spinach and Clam Broth 152

Baked Chicken with Sweet-and-Sour Red Cabbage 156

Vegetable Pot-au-Feu 158

Beef-Stuffed Cabbage with Pepper and Tomato Goulash 160

Chicken with Mustard Greens, Quinoa, and Oranges 162

Eggplant Roll-Ups 164

Filet of Beef with Braised Kale and Black Olives 167

Flounder "a la Plancha" with Catalonian Eggplant Relish 170

Grilled Shrimp with Marinated Cucumbers, Kale, and Cauliflower 172

Meatballs with Mushroom and Spinach Gravy 174

"Pappardelle" of Chicken with Winter Pesto 177

Roasted Cauliflower with Green Peppers, Almond Curry, and Lime 180

Shiitake and Bok Choy Stir-Fry 182

Shrimp and Cabbage Hot Pot with Chile Peppers 184

Shrimp with Mustard Greens, Mushrooms, and Miso 186

Sliced Pepper Steak with Swiss Chard and Mushrooms 188

Spinach Pesto Pasta with Tomatoes 191

ALMOND-ENCRUSTED FLOUNDER WITH CHOPPED SPINACH AND CLAM BROTH

MAKES 4 SERVINGS
PREP TIME: 10 MINUTES
COOK TIME: 10 MINUTES

If you've ever wondered how to get a fried flavor on fish without deep-frying or using any carbs as coating—let me tell you about the magic of almonds. Crushed or blended into a meal, they make the perfect no-carb coating for fish, chicken, or any protein you choose. I've started using almonds more and more for this purpose, and the results are amazing. You get a satisfying crunch, plus negative calorie power. It's a win-win!

PER SERVING

164 calories
9.5g fat
36g protein
10.5g carbohydrates
5g fiber
250mg sodium

INGREDIENTS

12 ounces cleaned spinach

1 teaspoon extra-virgin olive oil

1½ tablespoons chopped garlic

24 littleneck clams, shucked, chopped, and juices reserved (yes, your fishmonger will do this for you, whew!)

Salt

1 teaspoon finely grated lemon zest

Crushed red pepper flakes

½ cup sliced almonds

Four 4-ounce flounder fillets

1 egg white, lightly beaten

Olive oil cooking spray

4 lemon wedges, for serving

METHOD

1. Preheat the oven to 350°F.

2. Place the spinach on a wire rack fitted over a rimmed baking sheet, and cook in the oven until wilted but not dried, about 3 minutes. Remove from the oven, and set aside to cool. When cool, squeeze out any excess water. Chop the spinach finely and set aside

3. Pour the olive oil into a medium nonstick skillet placed over medium-high heat. Add the garlic and cook until golden brown. Add the clams and their juices and bring to a simmer. Add the spinach and continue to simmer until it wilts, then turn off the heat and season with salt, lemon zest, and red pepper flakes. Set aside and keep warm.

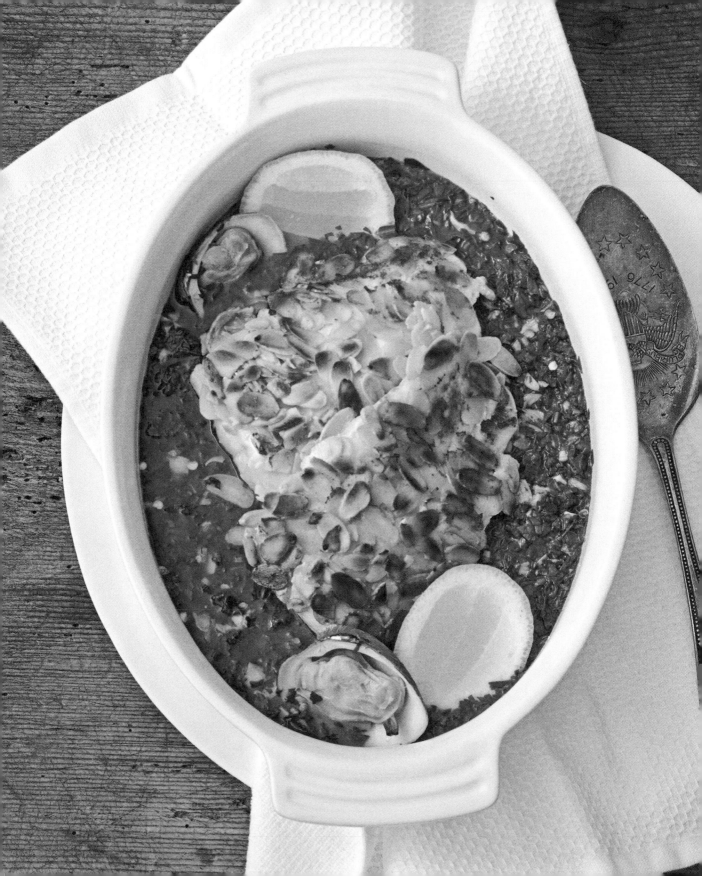

4. Place the sliced almonds on a plate. Season the flounder fillets with salt, brush the top with egg whites on one side, and flip directly onto the almonds, pressing to coat evenly. Repeat with the other fillets.

5. Lightly coat an oven-safe nonstick skillet with cooking spray and place it over medium heat until hot. Add the fillets, almond side down; transfer to the oven; and cook until the almonds have browned and the fish is cooked through. Spoon the spinach-clam mixture into four bowls, dividing it equally. Top with the fish, almond side up. Serve with lemon wedges.

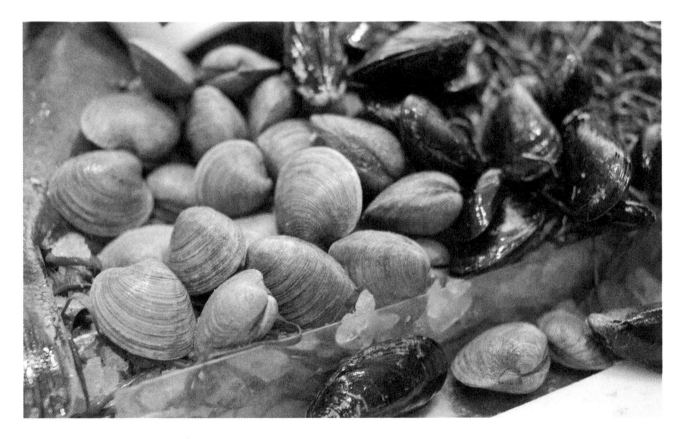

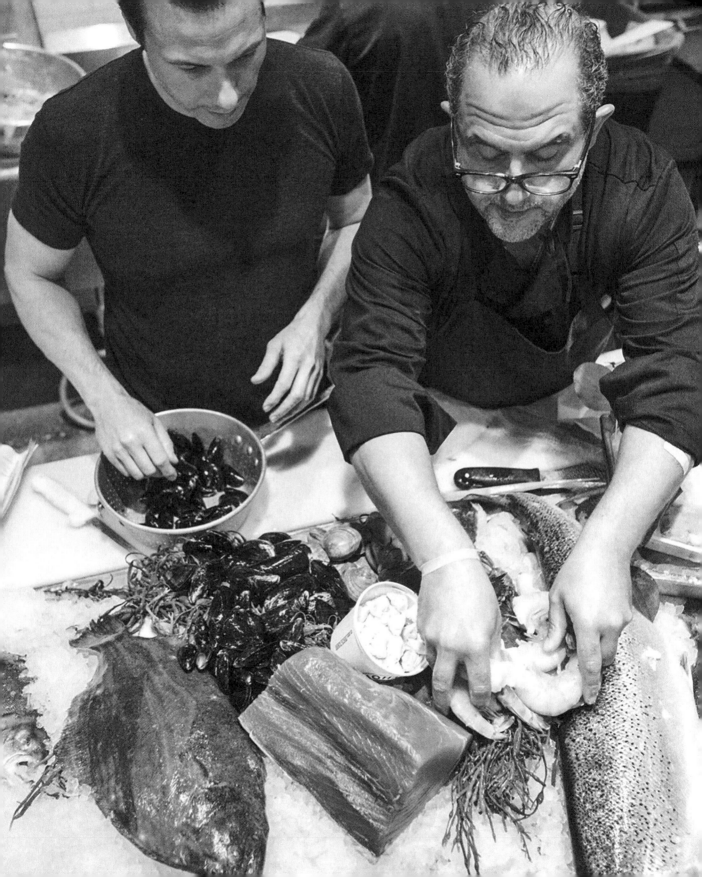

BAKED CHICKEN WITH SWEET-AND-SOUR RED CABBAGE

MAKES 4 SERVINGS
PREP TIME: 10 MINUTES
COOK TIME: 15 MINUTES

Cabbage is a true superfood—it is brimming with nearly forty healthy phytochemicals that may provide cancer protection, improve visual performance and brain function, and promote heart health. In this German-inspired dish, onion, apples, and a few caraway seeds transform otherwise humble ingredients into a tantalizing, simmered supper. Top with chives or serve with a side of horseradish for extra flavor.

PER SERVING

230 calories
7.5g fat
29g protein
26g carbohydrates
6g fiber
114mg sodium

INGREDIENTS

Olive oil cooking spray

Four 4-ounce skinless, boneless chicken cutlets

Salt

Freshly ground black pepper

1 cup thinly sliced onions

1 teaspoon chopped caraway seeds

2 large Red Delicious apples, grated on the large side of a box grater

8 cups shredded red cabbage

2 tablespoons apple cider vinegar

2 packets monk fruit extract (such as Monk Fruit In The Raw

METHOD

1. Preheat the oven to 350°F.

2. Lightly coat an oven-safe nonstick skillet with cooking spray and place over medium-high heat. Season the chicken and place in the hot skillet. Cook until browned on both sides, about 2 minutes per side. Transfer chicken to a plate.

3. Add the onions to the skillet and cook until softened, about 2 minutes. Add the caraway seeds, apples, and cabbage and cover the skillet. Transfer to the oven and bake until soft and tender, 6 to 8 minutes. Once the apples and cabbage are tender, stir in the vinegar and monk fruit extract. Season with salt and pepper. Place the chicken cutlets on top, cover, and continue to bake until the chicken is cooked through, about 2 minutes.

4. Spoon the cabbage onto four plates, and top with the chicken.

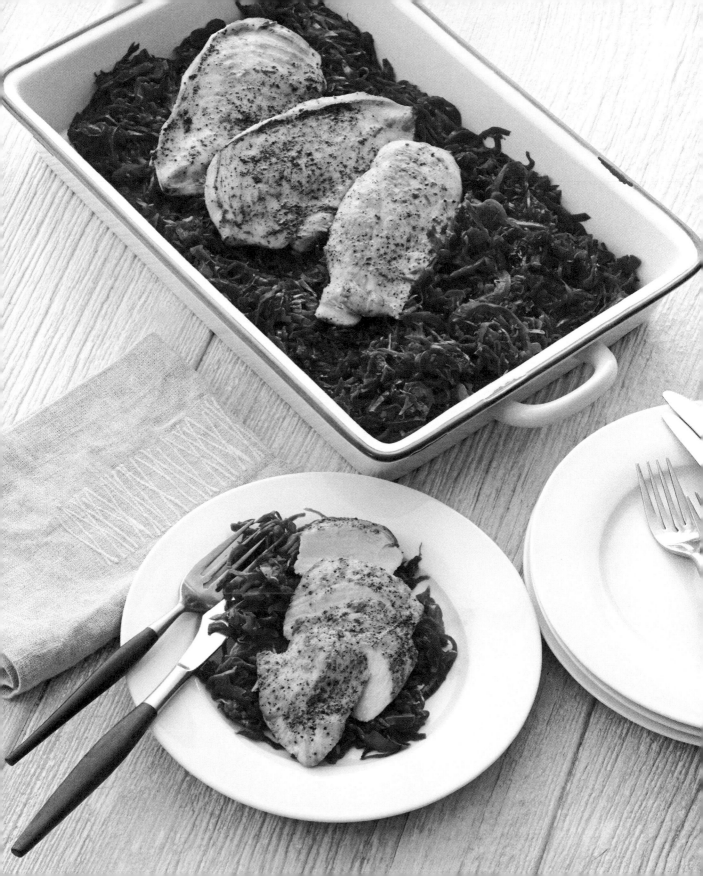

VEGETABLE POT-AU-FEU

MAKES 4 SERVINGS
PREP TIME: 10 MINUTES
COOK TIME: 30 MINUTES

Pot-au-feu is a French beef stew. The name translates to "pot on the fire"—in French households, the stew was traditionally left on the hearth to simmer all day long. My vegetarian version contains nine (count 'em) negative calorie foods—not only to heat up your metabolism but also to warm your heart and belly.

PER SERVING

169 calories
7g fat
9g protein
21.5g carbohydrates
7.5g fiber
187mg sodium

INGREDIENTS

4 cups unsalted vegetable stock
1 cup dried shiitake mushrooms, broken into bite-size pieces
½ cup toasted almonds
½ cup water
½ teaspoon smoked paprika
Salt
2 cups cauliflower florets
2 cups seeded diced cucumbers (1-inch dice)
1 cup thinly sliced onions
1 cup sliced bell peppers
½ cup sliced celery
4 cups cleaned spinach (or your favorite leafy green)
½ cup chopped fresh flat-leaf parsley
1 tablespoon finely grated lemon zest
2 tablespoons thinly sliced red jalapeños (Fresno chiles)

METHOD

1. Put the vegetable stock and dried mushrooms in an airtight container, seal, and transfer to the refrigerator. In a blender, pulse the almonds with the water and paprika until smooth. Season with salt and transfer the mixture to an airtight container. Refrigerate the mushrooms and the almond paste overnight.

2. The next day: Combine the cauliflower, cucumbers, onions, bell peppers, and celery in a large pot with the stock and mushrooms. Bring to a slow simmer and cook gently until the

vegetables are tender. Add the spinach and season with salt, then cover and turn off heat.

3. Mix together the parsley and lemon zest in a small bowl. Season with salt. Place the mixture on your dining table along with a small bowl of the almond mixture and the sliced jalapeños.

4. Ladle the vegetable stew into four warm bowls, dividing it equally, and serve with the condiments (which can be sprinkled over the stew).

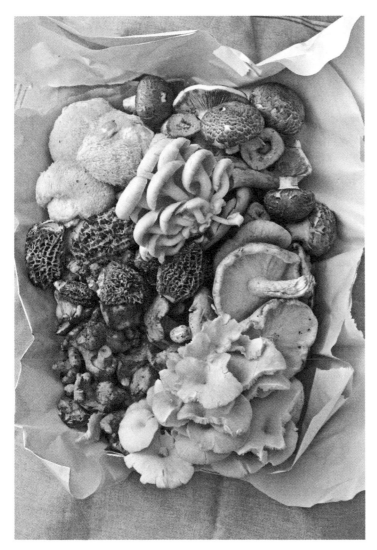

Coconut aminos are a liquid condiment I discovered for my clients who are allergic to soy and gluten. Available at organic, whole foods grocery stores, it is made from organic coconut sap, which is loaded with minerals, vitamin C, B vitamins, and amino acids. As such, coconut aminos have a higher amino acid content than soy-based sauces.

I use coconut aminos to replace soy sauce and Worcestershire sauce in recipes, and you can do the same. They deliver a delicious, deep, salty soy-sauce flavor, and make a terrific taste booster.

BEEF-STUFFED CABBAGE WITH PEPPER AND TOMATO GOULASH

MAKES 4 SERVINGS
PREP TIME: 10 MINUTES
COOK TIME: 10 MINUTES

There's a lot of fat-burning power going on in this dish with its thermogenic protein and black pepper, plus the red pepper and the high-fiber chickpeas. Savoy cabbage rounds out the team of negative calorie veggies: It's a lighter version of regular cabbage that is easy on the digestive system. This hearty dish is so tasty and simple to assemble, you'll want to make it again and again.

PER SERVING

262 calories
5g fat
31.5g protein
23g carbohydrates
7g fiber
210mg sodium

INGREDIENTS

1 head savoy cabbage, core removed

Olive oil cooking spray

16 ounces 96% lean ground beef (such as Laura's Lean)

Salt

Freshly ground black pepper

1 cup minced onions

1 cup chopped red bell peppers

½ cup no-salt-added chickpeas (garbanzo beans)

1 cup no-salt-added beef stock (such as Kitchen Basics)

1½ cups crushed tomatoes

1 tablespoon Hungarian paprika

METHOD

1. Preheat the oven to 350°F.

2. Place the cabbage on a microwave-safe plate and microwave on high until the leaves can be easily pulled off, about 2 minutes per layer. Reserve 8 whole leaves and chop the remaining cabbage.

3. Lightly coat a large nonstick skillet with cooking spray and place over medium-high heat. Season the beef with salt and pepper and add it to the hot pan; cook until browned, about 5 minutes. Transfer the beef to a plate. Add the onions, bell peppers, and chopped cabbage to the skillet and cook until softened, about 3 to 5 minutes. Add the reserved beef and the chickpeas and season again. Add the stock, tomatoes, and paprika and bring to a simmer. Cook until thickened and turn off the heat.

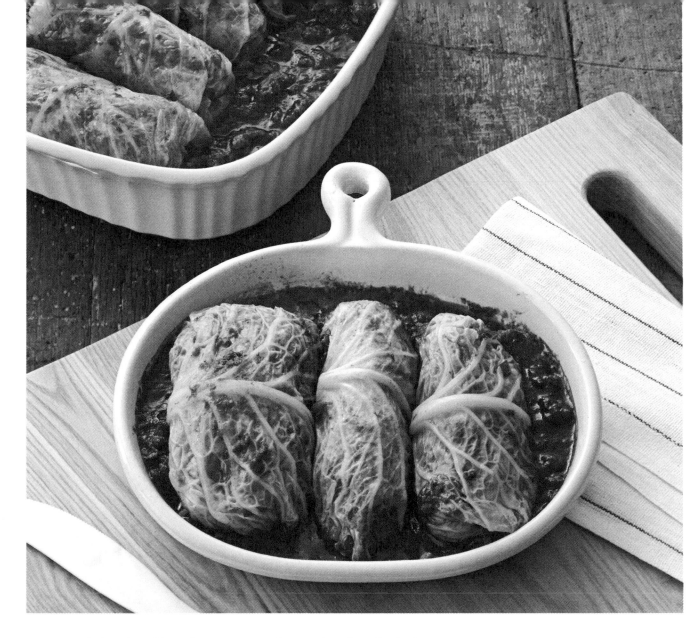

4. Lay the cabbage leaves out on a clean work surface. Strain the beef mixture through a colander, reserving the liquid. Transfer this sauce to a large baking dish. Working one at a time, evenly spoon the beef mixture onto each cabbage leaf, fold the sides over the filling, and roll into a pouch. Place each pouch seam side down in the baking dish. Transfer to the oven and bake until the cabbage is tender and the filling is hot, about 10 minutes. Place 2 pouches each on four plates and serve with sauce.

CHICKEN WITH MUSTARD GREENS, QUINOA, AND ORANGES

MAKES 4 SERVINGS
PREP TIME: 10 MINUTES
COOK TIME: 25 MINUTES

Mustard greens are full of some key fat-burners: calcium, fiber, and B vitamins that support metabolism. And the combination of mustard seeds, citrus, and soy sauce creates a delicious flavor profile. With protein-packed quinoa and chicken to keep you feeling full and satisfied, this is one weeknight dinner that will quickly become a part of your repertoire.

PER SERVING

241 calories
2g fat
18g protein
23g carbohydrates
6.5g fiber
337mg sodium

INGREDIENTS

1 tablespoon mustard seeds

2 cups orange segments, drained, with juices reserved

2 cups water

¼ cup quinoa, rinsed

Olive oil cooking spray

Four 4-ounce boneless, skinless chicken cutlets

Salt

Freshly ground black pepper

8 cups mustard greens, chopped

2 teaspoons Dijon mustard

1 tablespoon gluten-free, reduced-sodium soy sauce

METHOD

1. Place the mustard seeds and reserved orange juice in a small dish and set aside.

2. Bring the water to a boil in a saucepan. Add the quinoa and simmer until cooked, about 12 minutes. Set aside.

3. Lightly coat a large nonstick skillet with cooking spray and place over medium-high heat. Season the chicken and add to the skillet. Cook until browned, about 2 minutes per side. Transfer the chicken to a plate.

4. Add the mustard greens to the skillet and cook until wilted, 3 to 4 minutes. Add the orange segments and quinoa and cook until warmed through. Season with salt. Spoon the greens onto four plates. Add the orange–mustard seed mix, Dijon mustard, and soy sauce to the skillet and bring to a simmer. Add the chicken and warm through. Serve the glazed chicken over the greens.

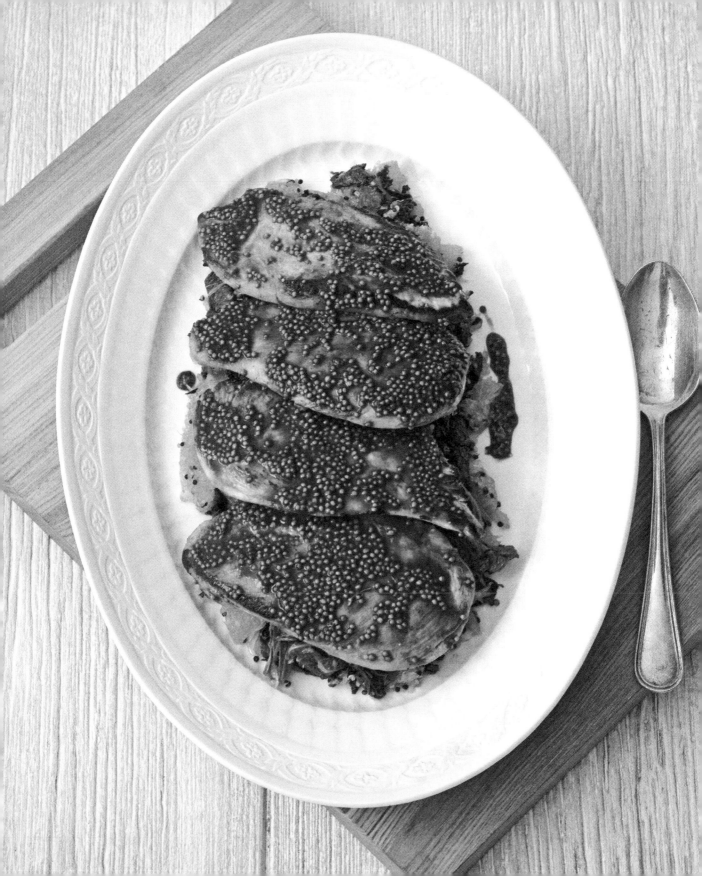

EGGPLANT ROLL-UPS

MAKES 4 SERVINGS
PREP TIME: 10 MINUTES
COOK TIME: 30 MINUTES

I'm Italian, and I love Italian food as much as (if not more than) the next umpteen million people. But I don't love the unhealthy effect of all the pasta that goes with it. Fortunately, an Italian dish doesn't need pasta in order to be delicious, and this recipe is a perfect example. These fun-to-make roll-ups let the negative calorie eggplant shine on its own.

PER SERVING

227 calories
12g fat
9.25g protein
24g carbohydrates
10.25g fiber
114mg sodium

INGREDIENTS

Olive oil cooking spray

½ cup chopped onion

1 cup diced red bell peppers

One 10-ounce bag washed spinach

1 tablespoon plus 2 teaspoons chopped garlic

Crushed red pepper flakes

1 cup fresh basil leaves, firmly packed

3 cups crushed tomatoes

1 large eggplant, cut lengthwise into ¼-inch-thick slices

Salt

½ cup toasted almonds, soaked overnight in enough water to cover

1 ounce Parmigiano-Reggiano cheese, finely grated on a Microplane grater

METHOD

1. Preheat the grill and the oven to 350°F.

2. Lightly coat a large nonstick skillet with the cooking spray, and place over medium-high heat. Add the onion and bell peppers to the hot skillet and cook until soft, 3 to 5 minutes.

3. Add the spinach and cook until wilted and the water has evaporated. Transfer the vegetables to a bowl and set aside. Spray the skillet again and place over medium-high heat. Add the garlic and cook until a deep golden brown. Add a pinch of red pepper flakes and half the basil leaves and sauté just long enough to wilt the basil. Add the tomatoes and cook until the mixture reaches a thick sauce consistency, 3 to 5 minutes.

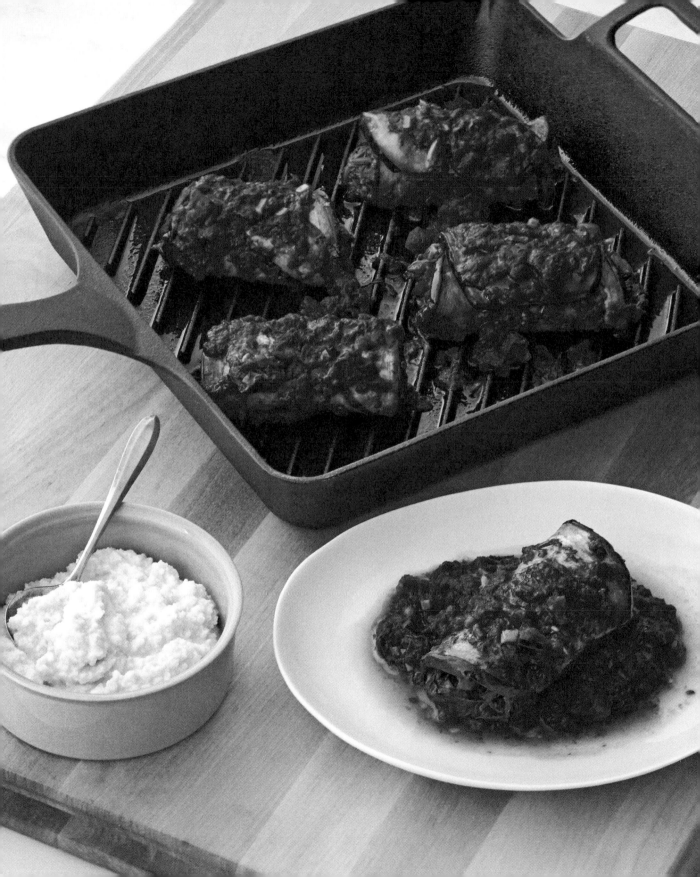

4. Spray the eggplant slices with cooking spray and season with salt. Grill the eggplant on each side until lightly charred, about 1 minute per side. Add ½ cup of sauce to the bowl with the vegetables, season with salt and red pepper flakes, and mix well.

5. Place the eggplant slices on a clean work surface, making 4 overlapping, 5-inch-wide x 10-inch-long rectangles. Place an even amount of the vegetables and some of the remaining fresh basil leaves on each rectangle and roll up. Place the rolls on top of the remaining sauce in the skillet and spoon some of the sauce over each roll. Transfer the skillet to the oven and bake until the eggplant is tender, about 10 minutes.

6. Place the almonds in a blender with just enough of the soaking water to blend them and process on high until it's a thick and smooth ricotta-like texture, about 1 minute. Remove from the blender and place in a small bowl, add the cheese, and season with salt. Pool a little sauce from the skillet on each of four plates, place 1 roll on top, and top each roll with the almond mixture.

TIPS

1. Add 1 teaspoon of freshly squeezed lemon juice to the almond mixture for more tang.

2. Remove the cheese from the recipe to create a vegan dish.

FILET OF BEEF WITH BRAISED KALE AND BLACK OLIVES

MAKES 4 SERVINGS
PREP TIME: 10 MINUTES
COOK TIME: 15 MINUTES

I've cut back on the amount of beef I eat, so when I do buy red meat, I'm picky about the quality and mindful of the fat content. These days I tend to go for filet of beef, which is very lean and super tender. This hearty beef recipe cooks up in only 20 minutes, and will leave you feeling satiated and energized.

PER SERVING

248 calories
12.5g fat
20g protein
14g carbohydrates
2.5g fiber
250mg sodium

INGREDIENTS

Olive oil cooking spray

Four 3-ounce filets lean beef tenderloin, trimmed of fat

Salt

Freshly ground black pepper

6 garlic cloves, thinly sliced

1 small onion, thinly sliced

Crushed red pepper flakes

5 cups curly kale (about 2 bunches), tough ribs removed and chopped into 2-inch pieces

1 cup water

¼ cup fat-free, salt-free crushed tomatoes (such as Pomi)

16 oil-cured olives, pitted

½ cup no-salt-added canned cannellini beans (such as Eden)

½ ounce pecorino Romano cheese, finely grated on a Microplane grater

METHOD

1. Lightly coat a large nonstick skillet with cooking spray and place over medium-high heat. Dry the beef with a paper towel and season each side with salt and black pepper. Add the filets to the skillet and cook until they are browned on one side, about 2 minutes. Flip them and brown on the opposite sides, about another 2 minutes. Transfer the filets to a wire rack set over a plate and set aside.

2. Reduce the heat to medium. Add the garlic to the skillet and cook until it is golden brown. Add the onions, red pepper

flakes, and kale and sauté, stirring constantly, until the kale has started to wilt, about 1 minute. Add the water and cover the skillet. Bring to a simmer and cook until almost all the water has evaporated, about 4 minutes.

3. Remove the lid from the skillet. Add the tomatoes, olives, and beans, and cook until the kale is tender and the sauce coats the leaves, about 1 minute.

4. Add the reserved filets to the skillet with all of the collected juice and let cook to the desired doneness (1 to 2 minutes for medium-rare).

5. Remove the beef and place 1 piece on each of four plates. Add the cheese to the kale, and season with salt, if needed. Spoon the kale next to each filet of beef on the plates.

TIP

Before you start to cook, remove the beef from the refrigerator and let it come to room temperature for at least 10 minutes. This technique lets the beef cook more evenly and faster.

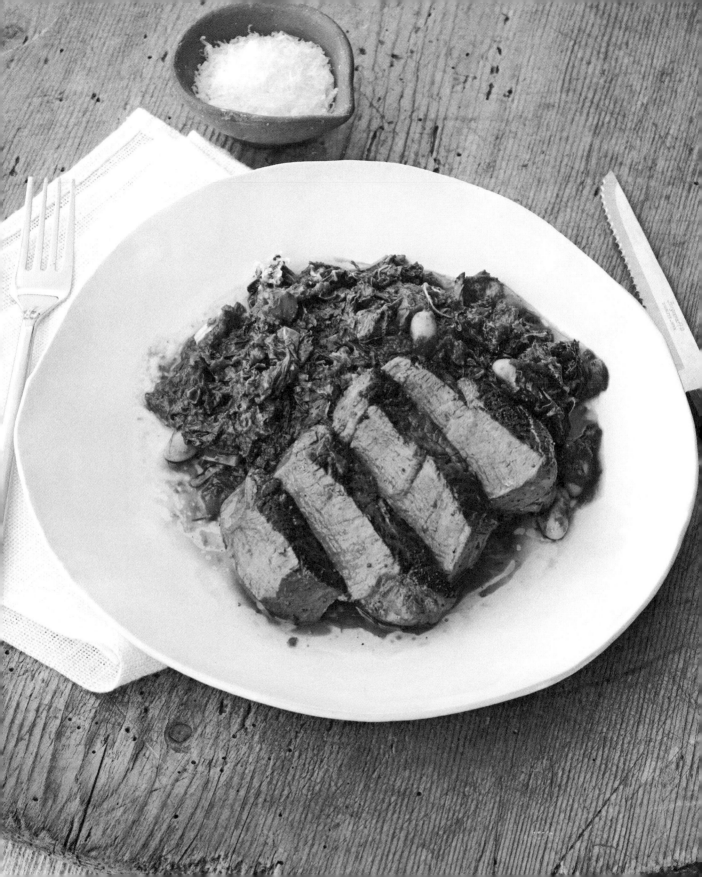

FLOUNDER "A LA PLANCHA" WITH CATALONIAN EGGPLANT RELISH

MAKES 4 SERVINGS
PREP TIME: 10 MINUTES
COOK TIME: 15 MINUTES

In Spain, seafood is often cooked *a la plancha*, which means that it is cooked simply and quickly, over high heat on a griddle. This Spanish-inspired dish incorporates aromatic Spanish spices with a Catalan-style eggplant relish. It is truly negative calorie food at its best and most flavorful!

For a truly authentic touch, try adding an anchovy fillet to the skillet once the garlic has browned.

PER SERVING

243 calories
7.25g fat
26.25g protein
19g carbohydrates
7.25g fiber
100mg sodium

INGREDIENTS

3 large Japanese eggplants, cut into ½-inch-thick rounds (4 cups total)

Olive oil cooking spray

Salt

1 teaspoon extra-virgin olive oil

1 tablespoon chopped garlic

¼ cup toasted almonds, chopped

Pinch of crushed red pepper flakes

1 cup small-diced green bell peppers

1 cup no-salt-added crushed tomatoes

¼ cup golden raisins

Dash of cinnamon

Dash of smoked paprika

Dash of ground coriander

Four 4-ounce flounder or fluke fillets

Lemon wedges, for serving

METHOD

1. Preheat the oven to 400°F.

2. Spread the eggplant out on a rimmed baking sheet, and spray the eggplant with cooking spray. Season it with salt and bake in the oven until browned and soft, 5 to 7 minutes. Remove from the oven and set aside.

3. Pour the olive oil into a large nonstick skillet and place it over medium-high heat. Add the garlic and cook until golden brown, about 2 minutes. Add the chopped almonds, red pepper flakes,

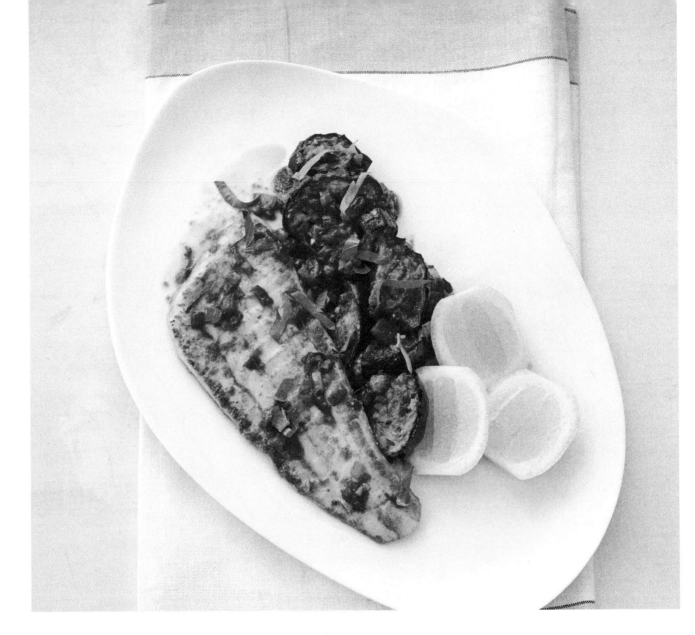

and bell peppers, and cook until soft, 2 to 3 minutes. Add the tomatoes, raisins, and eggplant and cook until everything is sticking to the eggplant as sauce would stick to pasta. Season with salt and the spices; set the relish aside and keep warm.

4. Place a cast-iron skillet over high heat. Spray the fish with cooking spray and season with salt. Place the fish in the hot skillet and cook until seared on both sides, about 1 minute per side. Place 1 fillet on each of four plates. Spoon eggplant relish onto the plate and serve with lemon wedges.

GRILLED SHRIMP WITH MARINATED CUCUMBERS, KALE, AND CAULIFLOWER

MAKES 4 SERVINGS
PREP TIME: 10 MINUTES
COOK TIME: 10 MINUTES

This recipe uses a Middle Eastern spice mixture called *baharat* that adds exotic flavor and depth to virtually any dish. One of the several spices in this blend is black pepper, known to promote a healthy metabolism. Add in three negative calorie veggies—kale, cauliflower, and cucumber—and you have a unique and delicious fat-burning meal.

PER SERVING

194 calories
6g fat
25.5g protein
9.45g carbohydrates
2.5g fiber
172mg sodium

INGREDIENTS

2 tablespoons freshly squeezed lemon juice

6 caper berries, lightly chopped

1 tablespoon extra-virgin olive oil

4 cups thinly sliced cucumbers

2 cups grated cauliflower (grated on large side of box grater)

1½ cups finely chopped kale, tough ribs removed

Salt

Baharat spice blend (available at ethnic stores and many grocery stores)

Olive oil cooking spray

16 ounces peeled, cleaned, and deveined shrimp

METHOD

1. Combine the lemon juice, caper berries, and olive oil in a large mixing bowl. Add the vegetables and toss to coat well. Season with salt and the *baharat* spice blend.

2. Preheat a grill or a grill pan to medium-high. Spray the shrimp with cooking spray, then season them with salt and the spice blend. Place on the grill and cook on each side until lightly charred and cooked through, about 2 minutes per side.

3. Add the shrimp to the bowl and toss quickly to combine. Spoon the mixture onto four plates, dividing it equally, and serve.

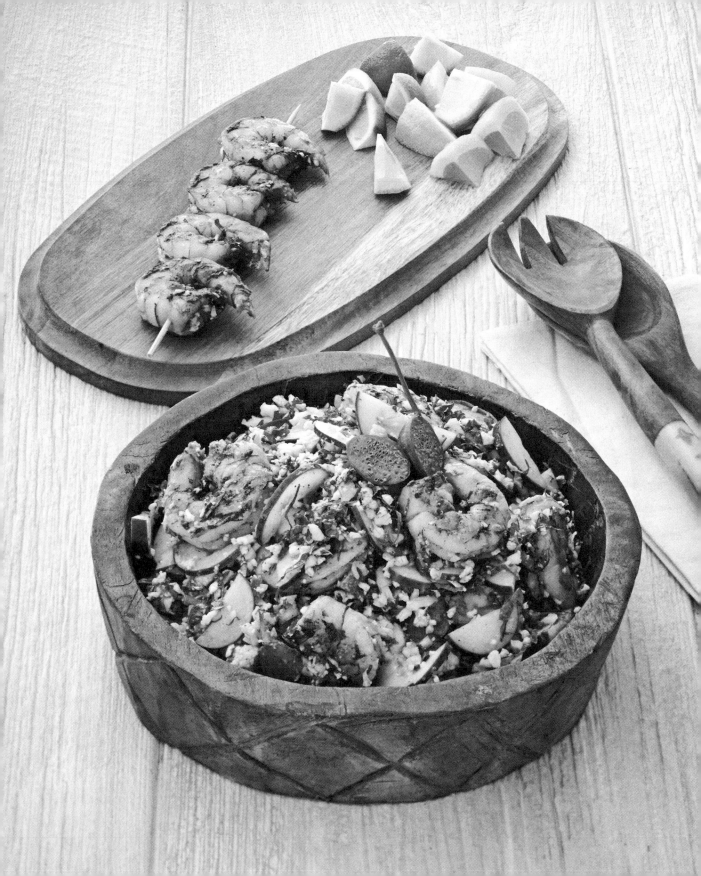

MEATBALLS WITH MUSHROOM AND SPINACH GRAVY

MAKES 4 SERVINGS
PREP TIME: 10 MINUTES
COOK TIME: 20 MINUTES

As an Italian, I was raised on meatballs, and quite honestly, I can't live without them. And that's good news for all of us. One of my passions has always been to make the food of my heritage into something that I could incorporate into a healthy lifestyle. This recipe proves that it is possible!

PER SERVING

226 calories
6g fat
29g protein
15.5g carbohydrates
2g fiber
290mg sodium

INGREDIENTS

12 ounces 96% lean ground beef (such as Laura's Lean)

1 cup finely chopped puffed brown rice (such as Arrowhead Mills)

4 cups unsalted beef stock (such as Kitchen Basics)

Salt

Freshly ground black pepper

Olive oil cooking spray

4 cups sliced cremini mushrooms

1 cup thinly sliced onion

8 cups washed spinach

2 tablespoons arrowroot, dissolved in 2 teaspoons of the stock

1 ounce Parmigiano-Reggiano cheese, finely grated on a Microplane grater

METHOD

1. Place the beef in a large mixing bowl, pushing it to one side. Add the rice and 1½ cups of the stock to the other side of the bowl. Season with salt and pepper and let the rice absorb the stock, about 1 minute. Using an electric hand mixer, mix the beef into the rice until homogeneous, about 1 minute. Adjust seasoning with salt and pepper. Form the mixture into 16 equal-size meatballs.

2. Coat a large nonstick skillet with olive oil cooking spray and place over medium-high heat. Once the skillet is hot, add the meatballs and brown on one side, about 1 minute. Turn the meatballs over and brown the opposite sides, about 30 seconds. Transfer the meatballs to a holding plate.

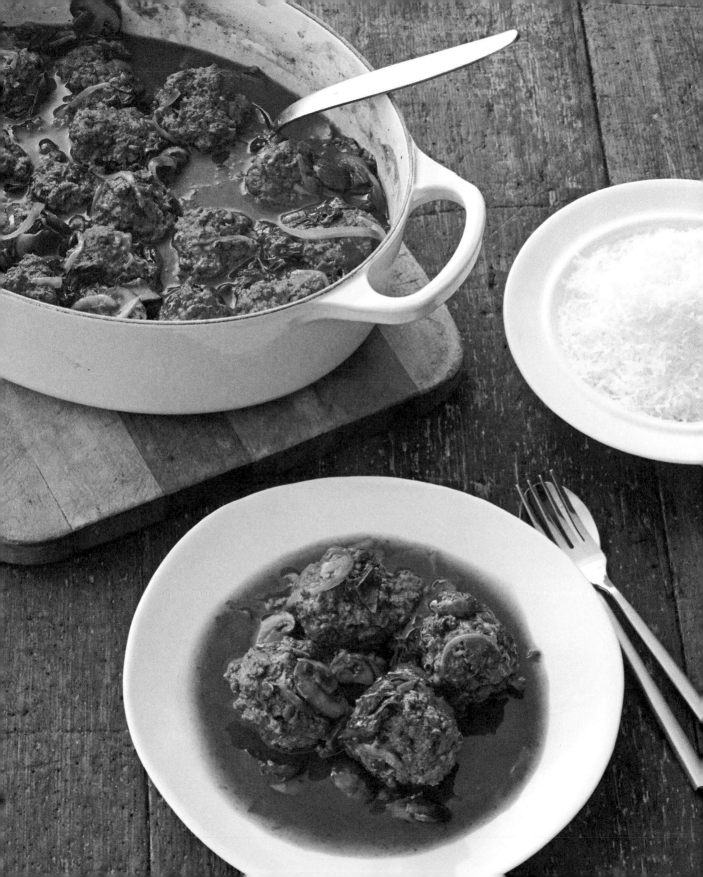

ARROWROOT

Arrowroot is a fine white powder you can use as a thickening agent to make gravies and sauces. I like it because it doesn't cause sauces to get cloudy or opaque. It also has a neutral flavor.

Be sure to dissolve arrowroot in a cold liquid before whisking into a hot liquid. This mixture is called a slurry.

Look for arrowroot in the spice section of the supermarket.

3. Spray the skillet again with cooking spray, and place back on the heat. Add the mushrooms and onion and cook until browned and softened, 3 to 4 minutes. Add the spinach and cook just to wilt, about 1 minute; then add the remaining stock and the arrowroot slurry and bring to a simmer while whisking until thickened. Add the meatballs and simmer until cooked through, 6 to 8 minutes. Spoon the meatballs and mushroom mixture into four bowls, distributing them equally; sprinkle with cheese; and serve.

TIP

Include some no-sugar-added dried cranberries if you want to liven things up a bit for an additional 20 calories per tablespoon.

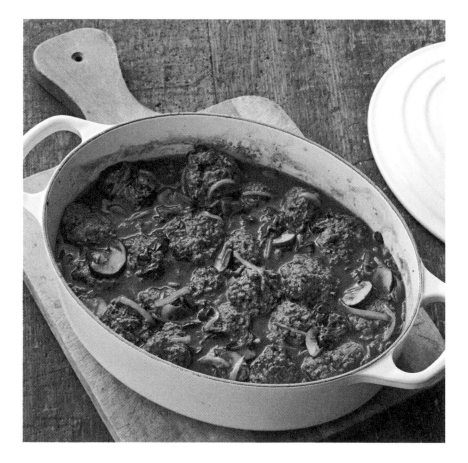

"PAPPARDELLE" OF CHICKEN WITH WINTER PESTO

MAKES 4 SERVINGS
PREP TIME: 15 MINUTES
COOK TIME: 15 MINUTES

The Italian word *pappardelle* derives from the Italian verb *pappare*, to gobble up—which is exactly what you'll do with this dish. As I was contemplating how to create it, it occurred to me: Why not make noodles out of the protein? Thinly sliced chicken cooked quickly makes a wonderful stand-in for the rustic pappardelle-style pasta. Dressed with nutritious escarole and a hint of winter spices, this recipe will not only bring you down from carb overload but energize you with a protein punch.

PER SERVING

176 calories
3g fat
28.5g protein
8.25g carbohydrates
2.5g fiber
267mg sodium

INGREDIENTS

2 quarts water

Olive oil cooking spray

6 garlic cloves, chopped

Dash of cinnamon

Dash of paprika

Crushed red pepper flakes

1 cup fresh basil leaves

1 small onion, thinly sliced

8 cups finely chopped escarole

4 cups unsalted chicken stock (such as Kitchen Basics)

Salt

12 ounces skinless, boneless chicken breast, sliced lengthwise into strips ⅛ inch thick

1 ounce Parmigiano-Reggiano cheese, finely grated on a Microplane grater

METHOD

1. Bring 2 quarts water to a simmer in a medium pot; you will be using this to poach the chicken strips.

2. Lightly coat a medium skillet with olive oil cooking spray and place over medium-high heat. Add the garlic and cook until golden brown. Add the cinnamon, paprika, red pepper flakes, basil leaves, and onion. Cook until the onion has softened, about 2 minutes. Add the escarole and cook until it has wilted and softened, another 2 minutes. Add the stock, bring to a simmer, cover, and cook until tender, about 5 minutes.

CELTIC SEA SALT

There are many different kinds of salt available these days, from plain old table salt to sea salt to kosher salt. A lot of people are starting to choose Celtic sea salt. It is the least processed of all salts, and retains as many as eighty-four minerals that were originally in the sea. You can buy Celtic sea salt in health food stores and natural foods stores. It tends to be pricey, but its fans love it for its purity.

3. Add a pinch of salt to the now-simmering water. Turn off the heat and add the chicken and stir so that all the strips are separated. Cook just until the strips have turned white; they will be half-cooked. Using a slotted spoon, transfer the strips to a plate to cool.

4. Check the escarole mixture; you want to cook it until most of the stock has evaporated and it looks like thick soup or sauce, then turn off the heat. Stir in half the cheese and season with salt to taste. Add the chicken strips, toss them to coat with the mixture, and continue to cook until the chicken strips have cooked through, about 90 seconds. Spoon the mixture onto four plates, dividing it equally; top with the remaining cheese; and serve.

TIPS

1. For a nutty, negative calorie protein, add 1 tablespoon of chopped walnuts to the skillet after the garlic has browned.

2. Place the chicken breast in the freezer for a half hour prior to slicing. It will be much easier to slice and you will get nice thin strips.

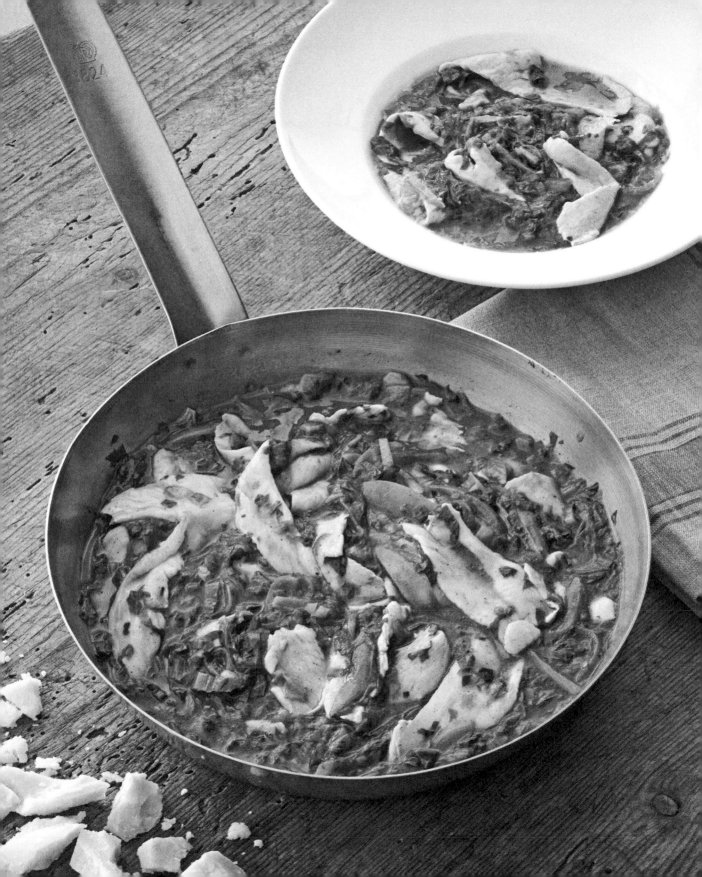

ROASTED CAULIFLOWER WITH GREEN PEPPERS, ALMOND CURRY, AND LIME

MAKES 4 SERVINGS
PREP TIME: 10 MINUTES
COOK TIME: 10 MINUTES

Gone are the days of boring old steamed cauliflower. Here's a rendition of roasted cauliflower that you'll love— the roasting brings out the delicate sweetness of the veggies. Cauliflower is packed with vitamin C, fiber, and antioxidants. The peppers add some heat, not only for flavor but also to turn up the burners on your metabolism.

You can personalize your curry any way you like. Add some ginger, fish sauce, or even some raw coconut nectar for sweetness.

PER SERVING

164 calories

7g fat

9.25g protein

22.5g carbohydrates

10g fiber

90mg sodium

INGREDIENTS

2 heads cauliflower, core removed, cut into large florets (about 2 inches across)

Olive oil cooking spray

Salt

2 green peppers (cubanelles for mild or poblanos for spicy), sliced crosswise into 1-inch-thick rounds

⅓ cup almonds, toasted and soaked overnight in water

1¼ cup unsweetened almond milk, or homemade almond milk (page 91)

2 packets monk fruit extract (such as Monk Fruit In The Raw)

1 tablespoon green curry paste (such as Thai Kitchen)

1 cup fresh cilantro leaves

1 tablespoon freshly squeezed lime juice

4 lime wedges, for serving

METHOD

1. Preheat the oven to 350°F.

2. Cut the cauliflower florets lengthwise and place in a mixing bowl. Spray them with cooking spray and season with salt. Spread the florets, flat side down, on a parchment-lined large rimmed baking sheet. Scatter the peppers near the edges and roast in the oven until the cauliflower is golden brown and tender, 10 to 15 minutes.

3. Put the almonds, almond milk, monk fruit extract, and curry paste in a blender and blend until smooth, about 1 minute. Strain through a fine-mesh sieve and then return the strained

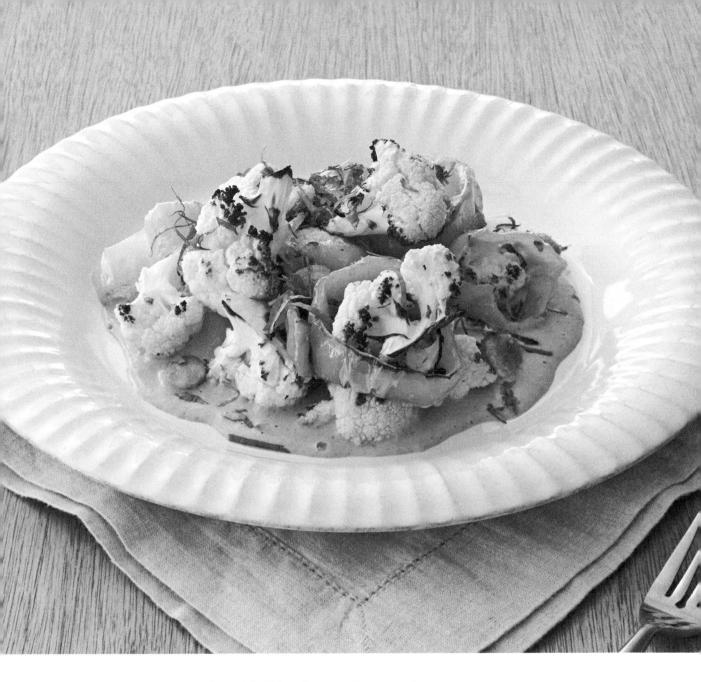

mixture to the blender with half the cilantro and puree until smooth. Season with salt and lime juice. Pour a pool of this sauce on each of four plates.

4. Distribute the cauliflower and peppers equally among the plates. Top with the cilantro and serve with lime wedges.

SHIITAKE AND BOK CHOY STIR-FRY

MAKES 4 SERVINGS
PREP TIME: 10 MINUTES
COOK TIME: 15 MINUTES

Here's a rice-free, killer stir-fry with a host of negative calorie foods. Now, I know what you're thinking: *Really? No rice?* Yes, you read that right. Bean sprouts stand in for the rice and do such a great job that you won't even miss it. The centerpiece, though, is beautiful green bok choy—a cruciferous vegetable loaded with nutrients and flavor.

PER SERVING

97 calories
1.5g fat
6.5g protein
17.5g carbohydrates
6.25g fiber
307mg sodium

INGREDIENTS

2 tablespoons plus 2 teaspoons coconut aminos

1 tablespoon chia seeds soaked in 2 tablespoons water

Olive oil cooking spray

2 cups bean sprouts, cut into rice-size pieces

6 cups bok choy, cut into bite-size pieces

1 cup thinly sliced red bell peppers

20 shiitake mushrooms, stems removed, caps thinly sliced

2 teaspoons chopped garlic

2 teaspoons chopped peeled fresh ginger

Salt

Crushed red pepper flakes

¼ cup chopped scallions

METHOD

1. In a large mixing bowl, combine the coconut aminos and the chia seeds. Set aside. Coat a large nonstick skillet with cooking spray and place over medium-high heat. Add the bean sprouts and cook, stirring, about 1 minute. Spoon the bean sprouts equally into four serving bowls.

2. Spray the skillet again with cooking spray and return it to the stovetop. Add the bok choy and bell peppers and cook until tender. Add the mushrooms and cook just until tender. Add the garlic and ginger and cook until aromatic, about 20 seconds. Toss everything together and add to the bowl with the chia seed sauce.

3. Toss the vegetables with the sauce to coat. Season with salt and red pepper flakes. Spoon the veggies on the top of the bean sprouts "rice," and top with the chopped scallions.

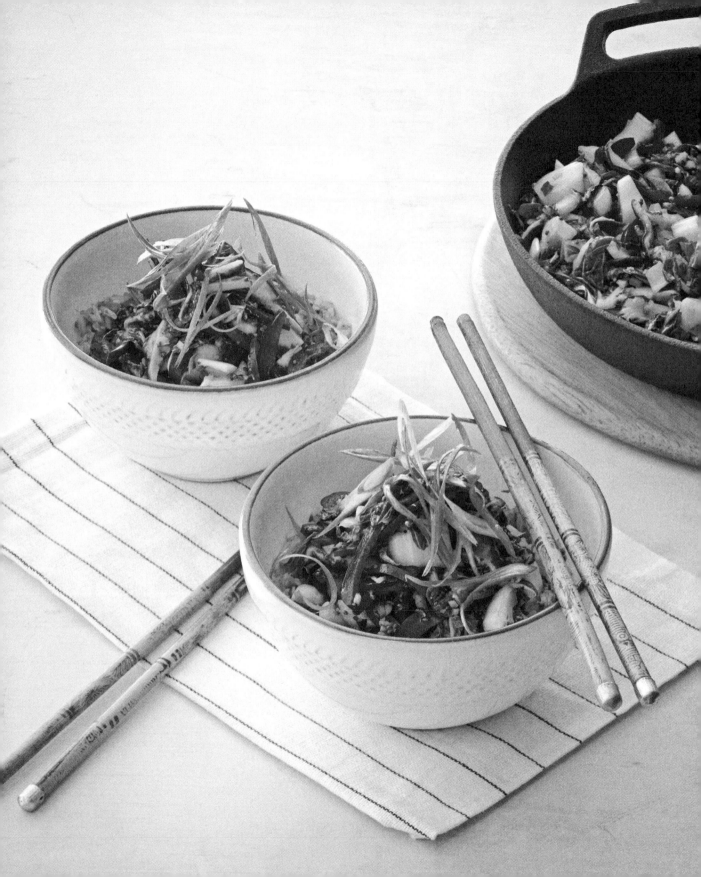

SHRIMP AND CABBAGE HOT POT WITH CHILE PEPPERS

MAKES 4 SERVINGS
PREP TIME: 10 MINUTES
COOK TIME: 20 MINUTES

Shrimp is a lean protein that is even more delicious when it's packing a little heat (at least for those of us who like our food spicy). This recipe adds some of that fiery flavor—a good thing for revving up the metabolism. The shrimp is paired with napa cabbage, which is a little sweeter than regular cabbage, and the sweet-spicy combination is in perfect balance.

PER SERVING

184 calories
2.5g fat
26g protein
15.3g carbohydrates
4g fiber
172mg sodium

INGREDIENTS

1 large tomato

½ cup orange segments

Olive oil cooking spray

1 tablespoon chopped garlic

1 tablespoon chopped peeled fresh ginger

½ cup chopped onion

2 cups chopped red bell peppers

8 cups chopped napa cabbage

1 cup water

16 ounces peeled, cleaned, and deveined shrimp

Salt

Crushed red pepper flakes

1 cup fresh cilantro, for serving

4 lime wedges, for serving

Chili garlic sauce, for serving

Reduced-sodium, gluten-free soy sauce, for serving

METHOD

1. Put the tomato and orange segments in a blender and puree until smooth.

2. Lightly coat a large pot with cooking spray. Place it over medium-high heat and add the garlic, ginger, and onion; cook until fragrant, about 1 minute. Add the bell peppers and cabbage and cook until softened, 3 to 5 minutes.

3. Transfer the puree to the pot. Add the water and bring to a simmer. Add the shrimp and simmer until they are cooked through. Season lightly with salt and red pepper flakes.

4. Ladle the stew into four soup bowls, dividing it equally. Serve with the cilantro, lime wedges, and condiments.

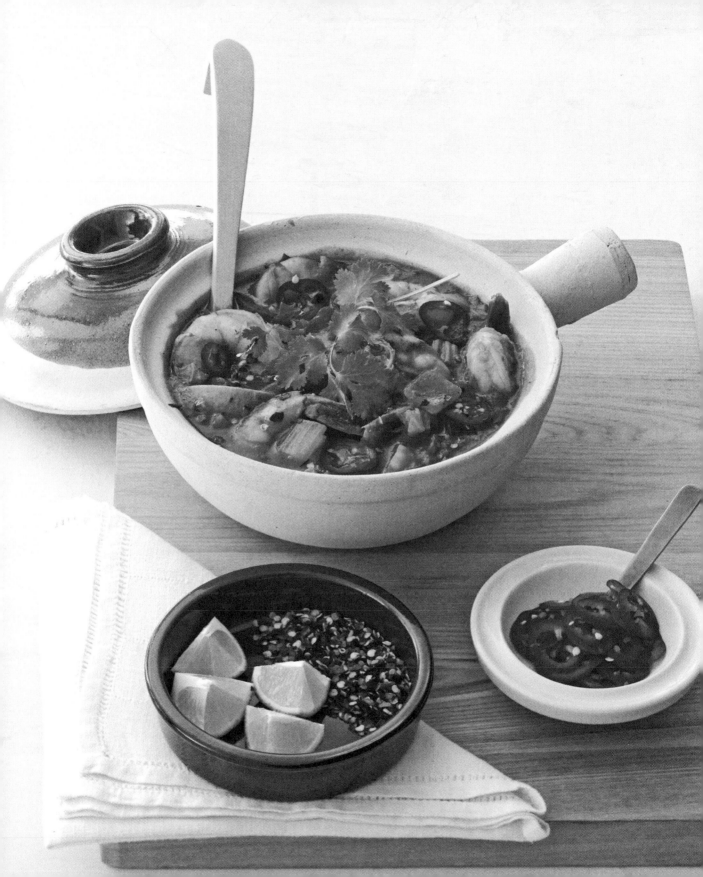

SHRIMP WITH MUSTARD GREENS, MUSHROOMS, AND MISO

MAKES 4 SERVINGS
PREP TIME: 10 MINUTES
COOK TIME: 10 MINUTES

I've loaded up this shrimp dish with two negative calorie foods: mushrooms and mustard greens. Mushrooms add a meaty texture, while the greens lend a robust taste. Mustard greens are classified as one of the "bitter" greens. For generations, Mediterranean cooks have "de-bittered" these vegetables by seasoning them lightly with salt and a bit of olive oil. In this dish, the garlic, miso paste, and other seasonings blunt any bitterness.

For extra bulk and a "noodlelike" effect, try adding 2 cups of bean sprouts to the pot.

PER SERVING

202 calories
3g fat
32g protein
14.45g carbohydrates
5g fiber
400mg sodium

INGREDIENTS

4 cups mushrooms

2 cups unsalted chicken stock (such as Kitchen Basics)

Olive oil cooking spray

1 tablespoon chopped garlic

8 cups chopped mustard greens, tough stems removed

2 tablespoons miso paste

1 pound cleaned, shelled, and deveined shrimp

Crab boil spice (such as reduced-sodium Old Bay)

Crushed red pepper flakes

¼ cup chopped scallions

4 lemon wedges, for serving

METHOD

1. Put half of the mushrooms and all of the stock in a blender and blend to a chunky puree.

2. Lightly coat a large pot with cooking spray. Place the pot over medium-high heat, add the garlic, and sauté until a deep golden brown, about 2 minutes. Add the mustard greens and cook until softened, about 5 minutes. Add the mushroom puree, the remaining mushrooms, and the miso to the pot and bring to a simmer. Continue to cook until the mixture is thick like a stew and the mustard greens are tender, about 5 minutes.

3. Add the shrimp to the mixture and cook through, about 2 minutes. Season with crab boil spice and red pepper flakes. Spoon the mixture into four soup plates, dividing it equally. Top with scallions and serve with the lemon wedges.

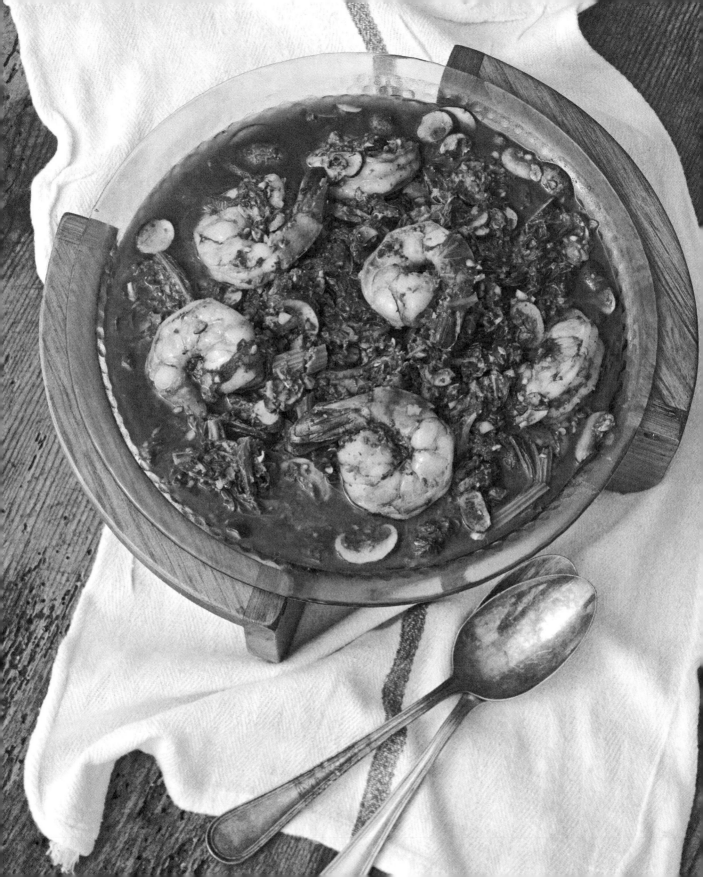

SLICED PEPPER STEAK WITH SWISS CHARD AND MUSHROOMS

MAKES 4 SERVINGS
PREP TIME: 10 MINUTES
COOK TIME: 20 MINUTES

I've eaten so much steak over the years that I know a good one when I taste it. One of my favorite ways to prepare it is as pepper steak, or as the French call it, *steak au poivre*. But ironically, I don't use the normal black pepper that is expected in this recipe—I use a pickled cherry pepper instead for a better zing than regular pepper gives. This recipe is low in everything, from fat to carbs, but super high in flavor.

PER SERVING

250 calories
8g fat
34.25g protein
23g carbohydrates
2g fiber
224mg sodium

INGREDIENTS

Olive oil cooking spray

One 16-ounce flank steak, trimmed of all visible fat

Salt

Chili powder

2 teaspoons chopped peeled fresh ginger

¾ cup minced onions

1 cup minced red bell peppers

¼ cup no-salt-added tomato puree

1 pickled cherry pepper, minced

2 cups sliced cremini mushrooms

4 cups chopped Swiss chard

METHOD

1. Preheat the oven to 350°F.

2. Lightly coat an oven-safe nonstick skillet with cooking spray. Place the skillet over medium-high heat. Season the flank steak with salt and chili powder and place it in the skillet. Cook until browned on one side. Flip the steak over and add the ginger, onions, and red bell peppers to the skillet. Transfer the skillet to the oven and cook the steak to the desired doneness, 5 to 7 minutes for medium-rare to medium. Remove the steak from the oven and let it rest on a wire rack placed over a baking sheet lined with aluminum foil. Add the tomato puree and minced cherry pepper to the pan and reserve.

3. Spray a separate skillet with cooking spray. Place the skillet over medium-high heat, add the mushrooms, and cook until

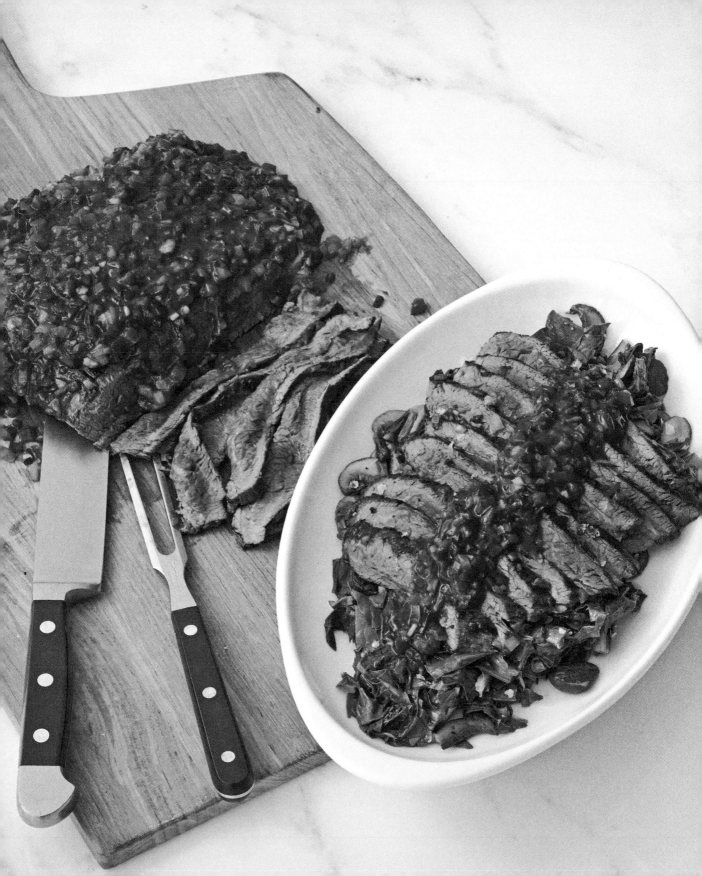

lightly browned, about 2 minutes. Add the Swiss chard and cook until tender, about 6 to 8 minutes more. Season with salt and place the vegetable mixture on four plates, dividing it equally.

4. Bring the cherry pepper mixture to a simmer and cook until it reaches the consistency of a thick sauce. Add the steak to the pan with any juices that accumulated on the foil and coat with the sauce. Transfer the coated steak to a cutting board and cut into thin slices. Place the slices on four plates, distributing them equally. Top with the remaining pepper relish.

TIPS

1. Allow the steak to come to room temperature before cooking.
2. This recipe can also be prepared with lean fish such as cod, flounder, or halibut.
3. Try adding a smashed anchovy fillet to the pepper relish for a burst of salinity.

SPINACH PESTO PASTA WITH TOMATOES

MAKES 4 SERVINGS
PREP TIME: 10 MINUTES
COOK TIME: 15 MINUTES

With this recipe, you're going to make your own pasta, and you won't even need a pasta maker. Heck, you won't even need any flour! The pasta you'll make has virtually no carbs and is gluten-free, but is packed with protein. Then it's all topped with tomatoes and pesto.

PER SERVING

135 calories
6g fat
12g protein
11.6g carbohydrates
4.75g fiber
238mg sodium

INGREDIENTS

Olive oil cooking spray

1 tablespoon plus 2 teaspoons chopped garlic

1 heaping cup fresh basil leaves

Crushed red pepper flakes

One 20-ounce bag washed spinach

¼ cup egg white powder (such as Deb El brand, available online or at many grocery stores)

1 tablespoon extra-virgin olive oil

3 cups cherry tomatoes, halved

1 ounce Parmigiano-Reggiano cheese, finely grated on a Microplane grater

Salt

METHOD

1. Preheat the oven to 350°F.

2. Lightly coat a large saucepan or skillet with cooking spray. Place the skillet over medium-high heat, and add 2 teaspoons of the garlic. Cook the garlic, stirring, until it is golden brown. Add half of the basil leaves, a pinch of the red pepper flakes, and the spinach. Cook until the spinach has wilted and all the excess water has evaporated.

3. Place the spinach mixture in a bowl over ice water to chill it down quickly. Once chilled, squeeze out any excess water and put the spinach and egg white powder in a blender and blend until smooth.

4. Place a piece of parchment paper or silpat liner in a baking sheet. Spread out the spinach mixture in a thin layer over the sheet and bake until cooked through, about 5 minutes. Let cool slightly. Remove the paper and spinach mixture from the baking sheet, then gently peel off the paper from the now solid spinach layer. Repeat with any remaining mixture. Carefully roll up the cooked mixture and cut into thin pasta-like strips (see pages 194–95).

5. Pour the oil into a nonstick skillet. Add the remaining garlic and cook until golden brown.

6. Add a pinch of red pepper flakes and the remaining basil leaves and cook until the basil has wilted. Add the tomatoes and cook until a loose sauce consistency forms. Add the spinach "pasta" and three-fourths of the cheese and toss to coat evenly. Taste and season with salt and additional red pepper flakes, if needed. Place an equal amount on each of four plates and top with the remaining cheese.

TIP

Try a splash of balsamic vinegar in the sauce for a "jammy" tomato flavor.

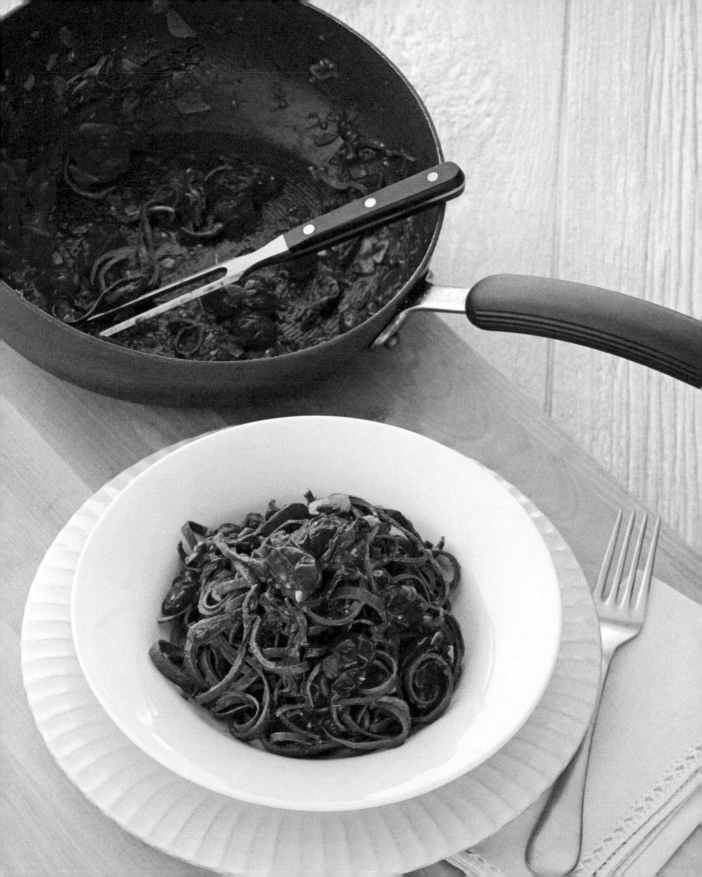

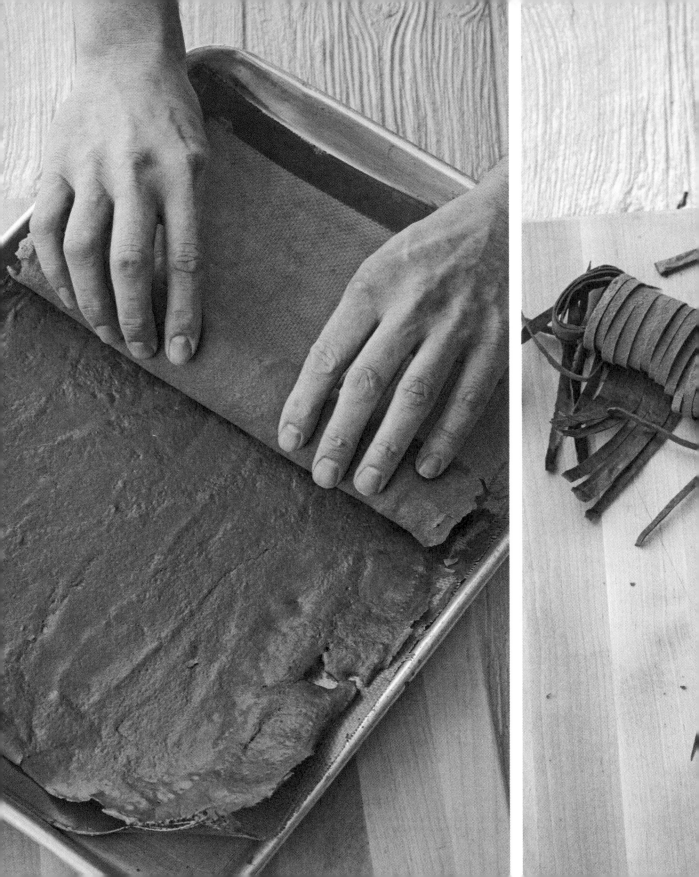

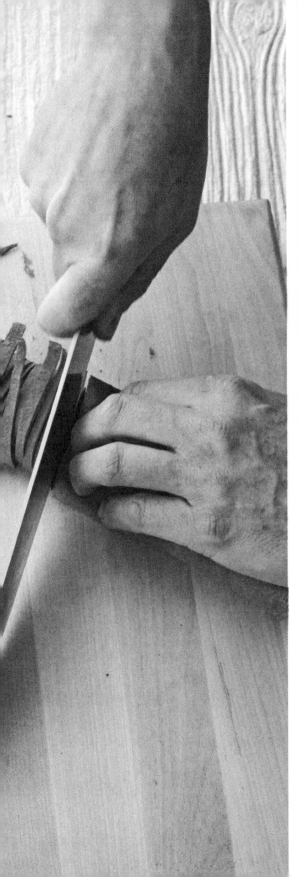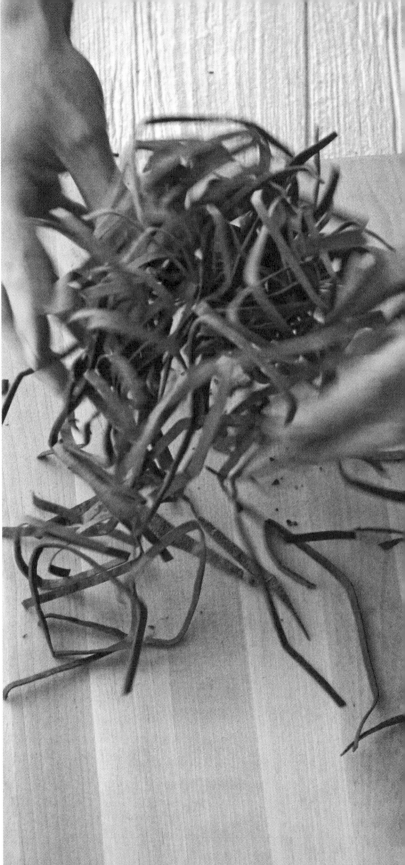

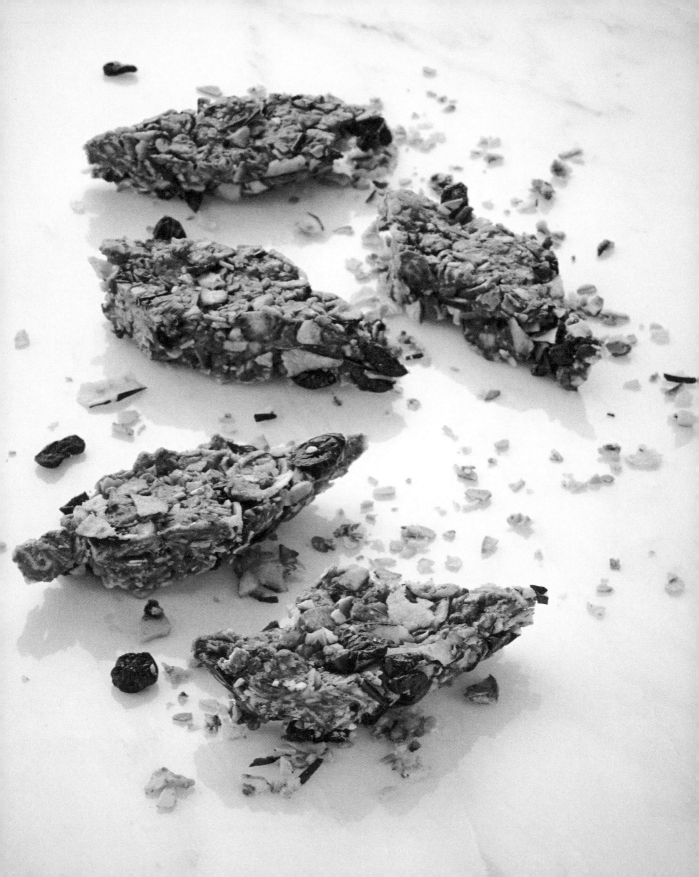

CHAPTER TEN

SNACKS

Cucumber and Almond Rice Sushi 198

No-Sugar-Added Organic Cranberry Sauce 200

Cauliflower and Apples with Thai Almond Butter Sauce 202

Eggplant and Almond Dip with Celery 204

Peanutty Apple Slices 206

Red Ants on a Log 208

Apple, Cranberry, and Almond Bars 210

Rocco's Raw Applesauce 212

CUCUMBER AND ALMOND RICE SUSHI

MAKES 4 SERVINGS
PREP TIME: 5 MINUTES
COOK/ASSEMBLY TIME: 15 MINUTES

Got a yen for sushi but don't feel like going out tonight? Try making your own. I know what you're thinking: *First he asked me to make pasta, now sushi . . . what does he think I am—a chef?* Don't worry. Making sushi is easy. In my version, slivered almonds stand in for the rice. And since this is veggie sushi, you don't have to worry about handling raw fish, either. The only raw ingredients here are cucumbers and avocado, and they're magnificent in this low-carb sushi.

PER SERVING

185 calories
12g fat
5.75g protein
11g carbohydrates
6g fiber
177mg sodium

INGREDIENTS

¾ cup slivered almonds, chopped to the size of cooked rice

1 cup water

Salt

2 packets monk fruit extract (such as Monk Fruit In The Raw)

1 tablespoon ground chia seeds

1 teaspoon rice wine vinegar

1 English cucumber, seeded and cut into matchstick-size pieces

¼ ripe avocado, pitted, peeled, and mashed

1 tablespoon plus 1 teaspoon wasabi powder, mixed with 1 tablespoon water

Nori (seaweed wraps)

1 tablespoon plus 2 teaspoons coconut aminos

METHOD

1. Place the almonds and water in a small saucepan over medium-high heat and bring to a simmer. Cook and stir until the water has almost evaporated and the almonds are soft, about 3 minutes. Pour the mixture into a bowl and season with salt and the monk fruit extract. Stir in the chia seeds and place in the refrigerator to thicken and cool. Once cooled, stir in the vinegar.

2. Mix the cucumber with the avocado and a little wasabi paste. Lay the nori on a clean work surface and spread the almond "rice" evenly on each sheet. Lay the cucumber down the middle in a neat line and then roll the sushi into tight rolls.

3. Cut each sushi roll into 6 pieces and serve with the remaining wasabi and coconut aminos for dipping.

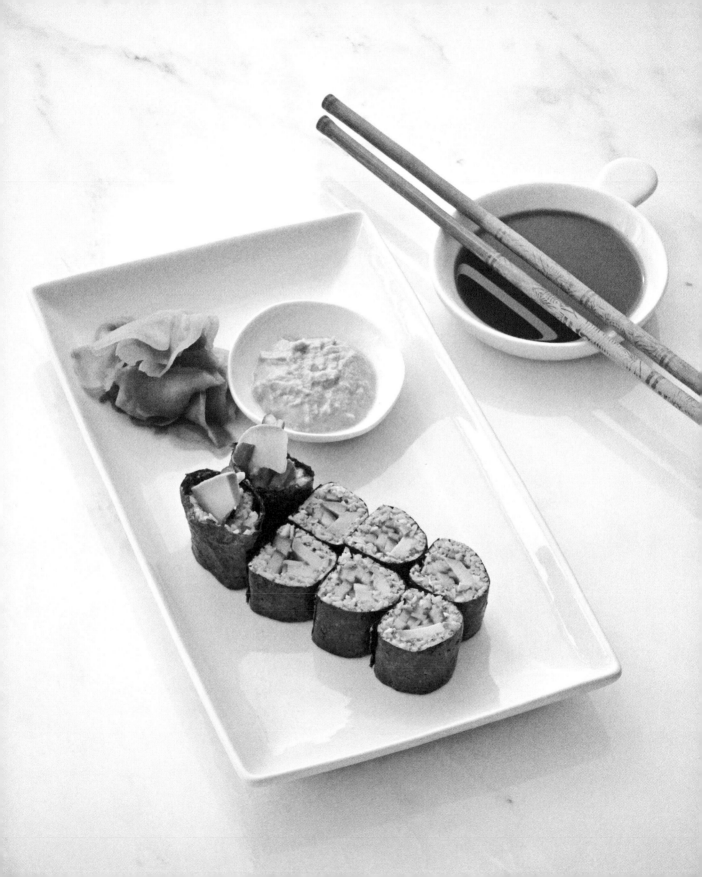

NO-SUGAR-ADDED ORGANIC CRANBERRY SAUCE

MAKES 4 SERVINGS
PREP TIME: 5 MINUTES
COOK/REST TIME: 10 MINUTES

Here's a great treat to have on hand year-round (not just in November!), and a terrific quick alternative to the sugar-laden cranberry sauce you'll find on most grocery store shelves. This sauce is designed for dipping—pair it with the rice thins, your favorite gluten-free crackers, or even celery.

Note that most pectin comes with a packet of calcium powder; this recipe does not use the calcium powder, so use just the pectin. If using Sure-Jell, double the amount of pectin.

PER SERVING

67 calories

0g fat

0.5g protein

16g carbohydrates

1.88g fiber

12mg sodium

INGREDIENTS

1 cup fresh cranberries

¾ cup water

1 tablespoon raw coconut nectar (see page 208)

¼ teaspoon finely grated orange zest

2 tablespoons freshly squeezed orange juice

5 packets monk fruit extract (such as Monk Fruit In The Raw)

½ teaspoon ground cinnamon

1 teaspoon citrus pectin (such as Pomona)

4 unsalted brown rice thins (such as Suzie's Thin Cakes)

METHOD

1. Place the cranberries in a large zip-top bag. Seal the bag and "pop" the berries by hitting them with a flat meat mallet or the bottom of a small pot. Transfer the berries to a microwave-safe bowl along with the water, coconut nectar, orange zest, orange juice, monk fruit extract, and cinnamon. Cook on high until the mixture is simmering, about 3½ minutes.

2. Remove the bowl from the microwave and carefully sprinkle in the pectin, while whisking immediately to dissolve and clear away any clumps. Microwave on high until simmering, about 1½ minutes.

3. Scrape the cranberry sauce into a stainless steel bowl. Place the bowl over another bowl that is filled with iced water to cool the cranberry mixture. Once cooled, the cranberry sauce will thicken.

4. Spread the sauce evenly over rice crisps and serve.

CAULIFLOWER AND APPLES WITH THAI ALMOND BUTTER SAUCE

MAKES 4 SERVINGS
PREP TIME: 5 MINUTES

Mark Twain once said, "Cauliflower is nothing but cabbage with a college education." Well, I'm giving it a PhD with this Asian-inspired recipe. You'll be dipping cauliflowers and apples—two fantastic negative calorie foods—into a tangy sauce that will satisfy your snack cravings in a heartbeat.

PER SERVING

153 calories
9g fat
6g protein
13.5g carbohydrates
4.5g fiber
278mg sodium

INGREDIENTS

⅛ teaspoon finely grated lime zest

1 tablespoon freshly squeezed lime juice

1 tablespoon Thai red curry paste (such as Thai Kitchen)

1 fluid ounce (2 tablespoons) coconut milk

2 tablespoons coconut aminos

2 packets monk fruit extract (such as Monk Fruit In The Raw)

¼ cup raw almond butter

2 cups cauliflower florets

1 cup apple slices

½ cup chopped fresh cilantro

4 lime wedges, for serving

METHOD

1. Put the lime zest, lime juice, and curry paste in a mixing bowl and whisk together. Add the coconut milk, coconut aminos, monk fruit extract, and almond butter. Whisk until smooth, adding water, if needed, to create a thick sauce-like texture.

2. Pour the sauce into four dipping dishes and place on four plates. Toss the cauliflower and apples with the chopped cilantro, and distribute equally among the four plates. Serve with the lime wedges. The sauce will keep in an airtight container in the refrigerator for up to 5 days.

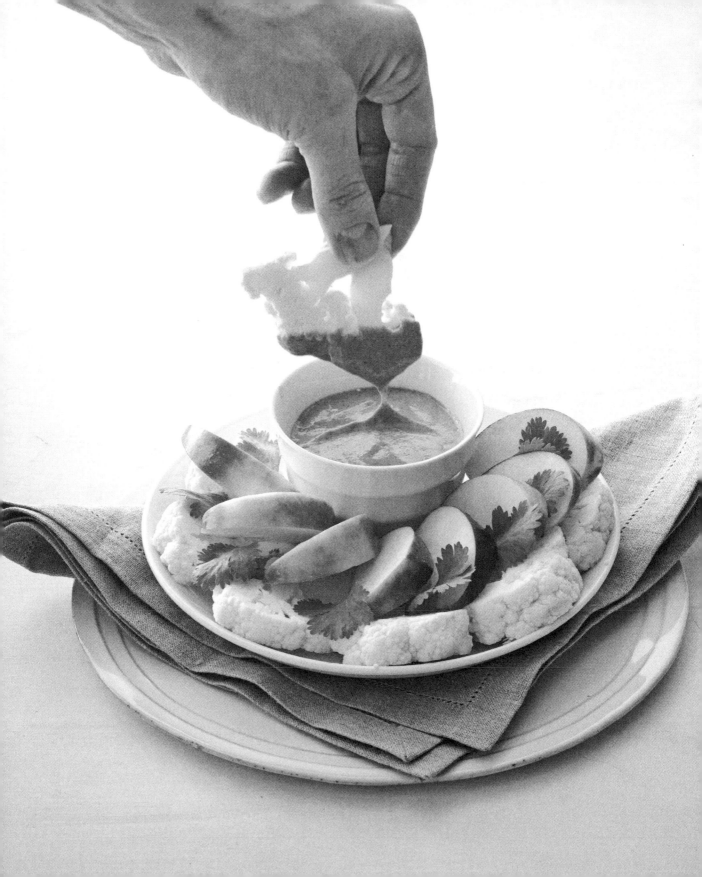

EGGPLANT AND ALMOND DIP WITH CELERY

MAKES 4 SERVINGS
PREP TIME: 5 MINUTES
COOK TIME: 15 MINUTES

Introducing the negative calorie version of *baba ganoush*, an eggplant dip with Middle Eastern roots that's a popular menu item in many Mediterranean restaurants. My version is ridiculously easy to whip together, and its smooth-spicy texture makes it the ideal dip for raw veggies like celery. Make it in large batches, if you want; it will last in the fridge for a week (unless your family or guests gobble it up before then!).

PER SERVING

89 calories
4.25g fat
3.5g protein
12g carbohydrates
6g fiber
150mg sodium

INGREDIENTS

1 medium Italian eggplant, cut in half lengthwise
Salt
2 tablespoons raw unsalted almond butter
2 tablespoons freshly squeezed lemon juice
½ teaspoon minced garlic (minced to a paste)
Chili powder
1 bunch celery cut into 5-inch-long sticks

METHOD

1. Preheat a grill, a grill pan, or a cast-iron skillet to high. Using the tip of a sharp knife, score a crosshatch pattern ½ inch deep on the cut side of the eggplant and season with salt. Place, cut side down, on the hot cooking surface and cook until slightly charred; flip and repeat. Transfer the eggplant, cut side down, to a microwave-safe plate and cook on high until tender, 4 to 5 minutes.

2. Scoop out the eggplant pulp and drain off any excess liquid. Process the pulp in a food processor until smooth. Transfer to a stainless steel bowl set over another bowl with iced water to cool.

3. Once chilled, add the almond butter, lemon juice, and garlic to the eggplant puree and stir to combine. Taste and adjust the seasoning with additional salt, if needed, and sprinkle with the chili powder. Serve as a dip with celery sticks.

TIP

Try adding different spices to your dip, such as za'atar, smoked paprika, or a spicy chili paste.

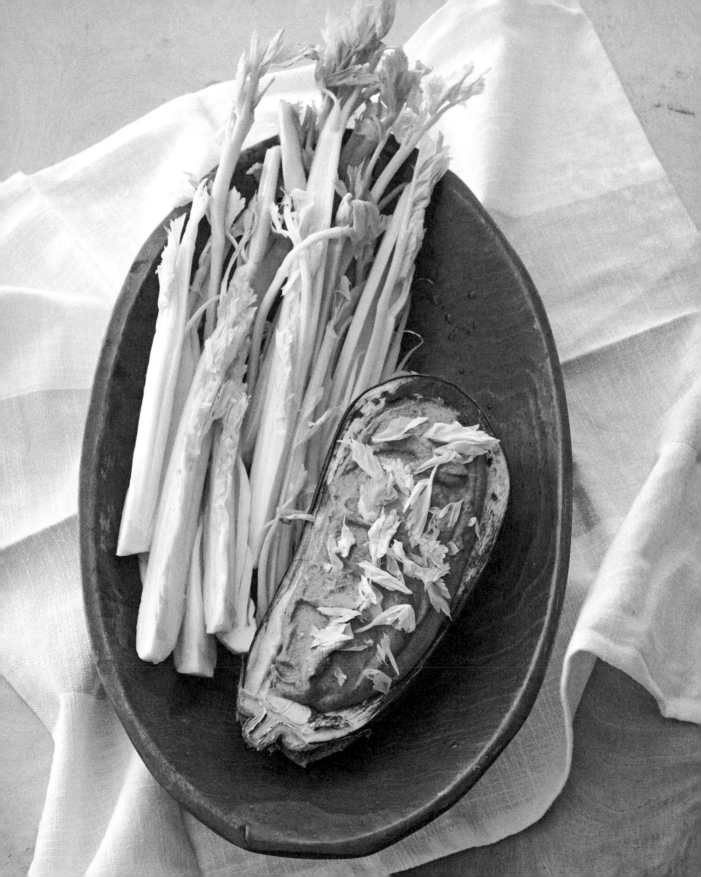

PEANUTTY APPLE SLICES

MAKES 4 SERVINGS
PREP TIME: 5 MINUTES

I have loved peanut butter ever since I was old enough to say, "A peanut butter and jelly sandwich, please." Peanut butter is delicious but super high in calories—and I don't know about you, but once it's in my house, I find portion control to be an issue! Peanut butter powder is a delicious alternative. It's a great ingredient for oatmeal, smoothies, and quick snacks like this one.

INGREDIENTS

4 medium apples (I like organic Honeycrisps), cut into slices

½ cup peanut butter powder (such as PB2)

METHOD

1. Place the apple slices on four small serving plates, dividing them equally.
2. Sprinkle the peanut butter powder over the top.

TIP

This dish can be packed up for an easy snack on the go.

PER SERVING

102 calories
0g fat
6.25g protein
18.5g carbohydrates
3g fiber
95mg sodium

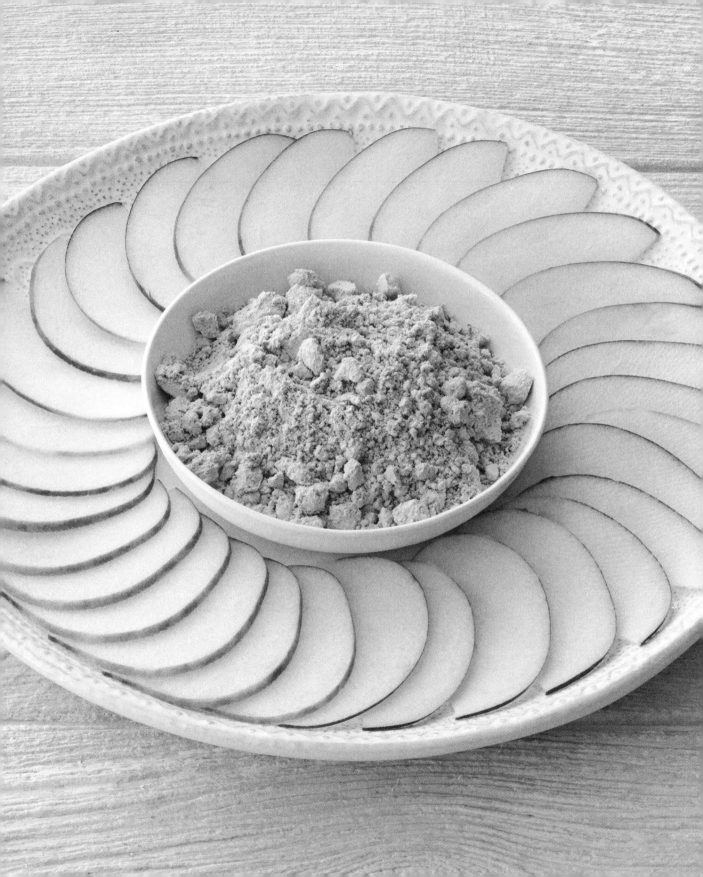

RED ANTS ON A LOG

MAKES 4 SERVINGS; 4 "LOGS" PER PERSON
PREP TIME: 5 MINUTES

Want to make healthy and negative calorie eating fun for the whole family? Try my version of "ants on a log," using almond butter to fill in the trenches of celery stalks that are then studded with dried cranberries (you could also substitute unsweetened dried cherries). Your kids will love this fun snack—it's perfect for class parties and playdates.

PER SERVING

72 calories
8g fat
4g protein
7.5g carbohydrates
3.25g fiber
50mg sodium

INGREDIENTS

¼ cup raw almond butter (such as Artisana)

1 tablespoon raw coconut nectar (such as Coconut Secret)

2 packets monk fruit extract (such as Monk Fruit In The Raw)

Salt

Twelve 5-inch-long celery stalks

2 tablespoons unsweetened dried cranberries

METHOD

1. Mix the almond butter, coconut nectar, and monk fruit extract in a small mixing bowl and season with salt.

2. Spread the almond butter in the cavity of the celery stalks, top with cranberries, and serve.

TIP

You can keep the almond butter mixture chilled in an airtight container in the refrigerator for up to 7 days.

INGREDIENT SPOTLIGHT
COCONUT NECTAR

Coconut nectar is another gift from the coconut. It's a syrup made from the sweet juice that drops off coconut flower buds. It contains nutrients not found in refined sugars: seventeen amino acids, as well as a bunch of minerals and vitamins B and C.

Coconut nectar has a mild, sweet flavor and is a great substitute for honey or maple syrup. Drizzle it on top of yogurt, stir it into tea, or even use it to sweeten your smoothies.

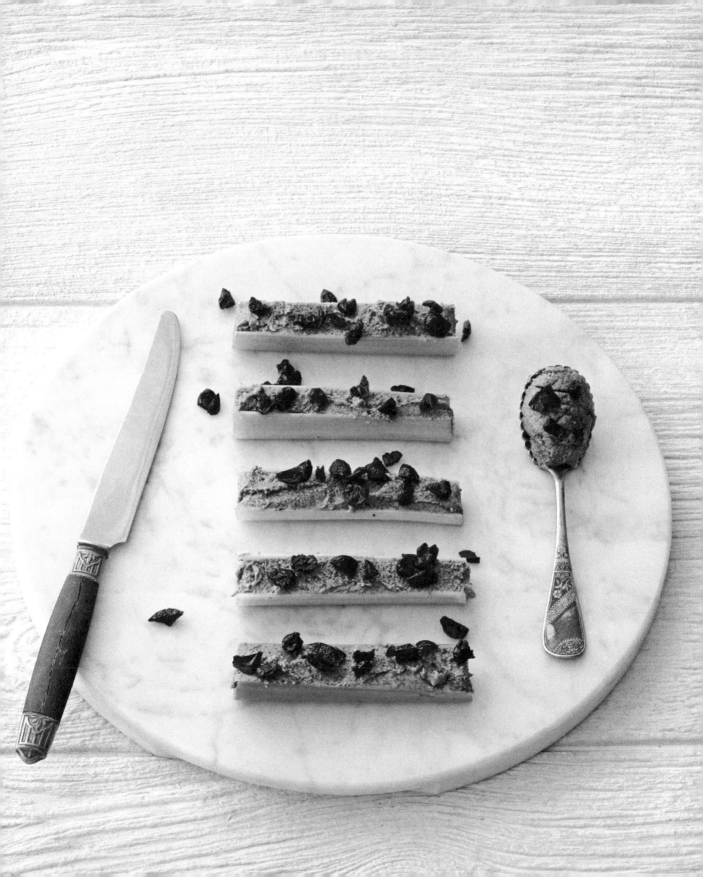

APPLE, CRANBERRY, AND ALMOND BARS

MAKES 4 BARS
PREP TIME: 5 MINUTES
PROCESSING TIME: 10 MINUTES

Store-bought granola bars are usually loaded with sugar and ingredients you can't pronounce—not to mention, they're usually superexpensive. With this easy recipe, you'll make your own protein bar in less time than it takes to run to the store to buy one. This is a raw, unadulterated protein bar with zero added sugar. You get the protein naturally from the almonds, and fiber from the oats and cranberries—a delicious combination of whole foods.

PER SERVING

211 calories
7.5g fat
3.5g protein
36g carbohydrates
7g fiber
11mg sodium

INGREDIENTS

2 cups freeze-dried apple chips (such as Bare Fruit Simply Cinnamon)
¼ cup toasted slivered almonds
¼ cup unsweetened dried cranberries
¼ cup toasted rolled oats
2 tablespoons raw almond butter
2 packets monk fruit extract (such as Monk Fruit In The Raw)
Salt
Cayenne pepper
1 tablespoon coconut nectar (such as Coconut Secret)

METHOD

1. Crush the apple chips, almonds, cranberries, and oats together in a mixing bowl. In another mixing bowl, combine the almond butter, monk fruit extract, and a pinch of salt and cayenne and mix until smooth. Add the coconut nectar to a small nonstick skillet and place over medium heat. Once it simmers, transfer the nectar to the almond butter bowl using a rubber spatula and mix well. Stir in the crushed ingredients and mix well to coat everything evenly.

2. Place a piece of plastic wrap at least 16 inches long on a clean work surface and lay the almond mixture down the middle of the wrap. Fold the wrap over the mixture and shape it into a long bar. Cut the bar into four pieces, and serve, or store in an airtight container in the refrigerator for up to 5 days.

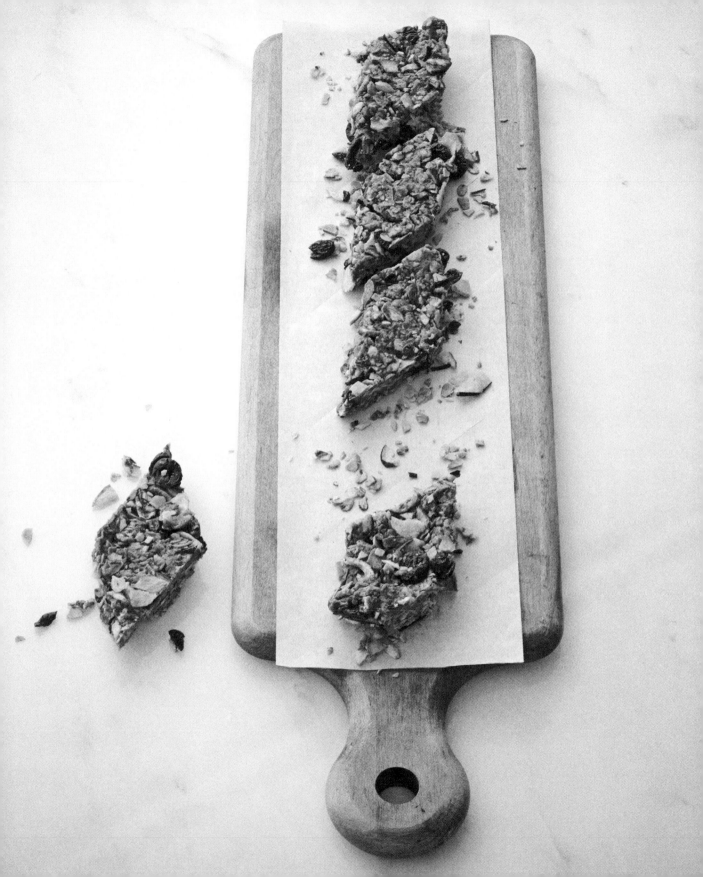

ROCCO'S RAW APPLESAUCE

MAKES 4 SERVINGS
PREP TIME: 15 MINUTES

You're probably wondering: *"Why make my own applesauce?"* Well, why not? You get to make it with your favorite apples. You get to make it without any additives. You get to save money by making it yourself. And you can do it in less time than it takes to wrestle the lid off a stubborn applesauce jar. Homemade applesauce always tastes better. Plus, my version is raw, so it keeps the glycemic impact lower than cooked versions. What's more, raw, homemade applesauce preserves precious nutrients and enzymes for a powerful health punch.

INGREDIENTS

4 medium apples (I prefer organic Honeycrisps)
2 packets monk fruit extract (such as Monk Fruit In The Raw)
½ teaspoon ground cinnamon

METHOD

1. Wash the apples well. Using a fine grater (such as a Microplane), grate the apples into a mixing bowl, stopping just short of grating the core or seeds.
2. Whisk in the monk fruit extract and cinnamon and serve.

TIPS

1. Experiment with different types of apples to suit your taste.
2. Try adding 1 tablespoon of chia seeds to this recipe for a healthy boost and a thicker sauce.

PER SERVING

93 calories
0g fat
0.5g protein
25g carbohydrates
4.5g fiber
1.75mg sodium

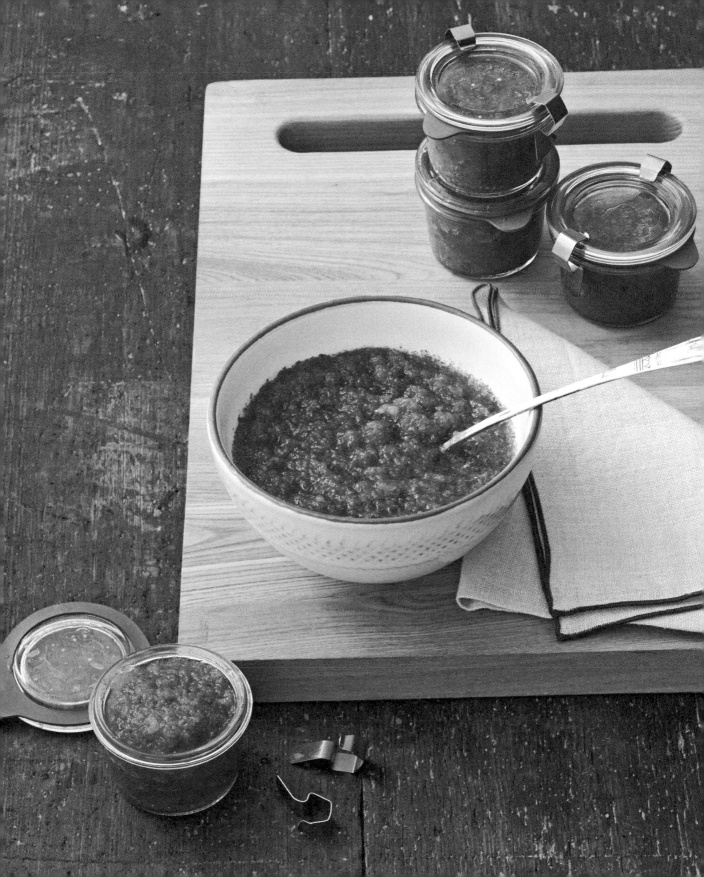

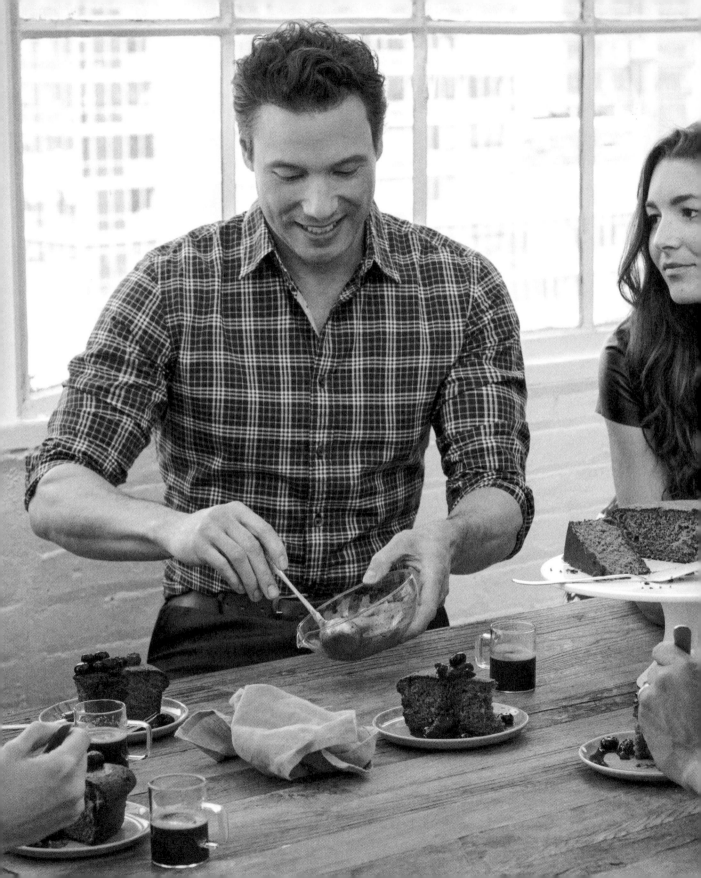

CHAPTER ELEVEN

DESSERTS

Chocolate and Almond Butter Truffles 216

Chocolate-Dipped Strawberries with Crushed Almonds 218

Cocoa-Dusted Almonds 220

Instant Almond Cake with Mixed Berries 222

Crepes Suzette with Oranges and Vanilla Cream 224

Citrus and Mixed Berry Bowl with Whipped Topping 226

CHOCOLATE AND ALMOND BUTTER TRUFFLES

MAKES 8 TRUFFLES; 4 SERVINGS; 2 TRUFFLES PER SERVING
PREP TIME: 2 MINUTES
PROCESSING TIME: 20 MINUTES

It is believed that the chocolate truffle was first cooked up—by accident—in the kitchen of the famed French chef Auguste Escoffier. One day his assistant was making pastry cream when he mistakenly poured the hot cream into a bowl of chocolate; he found that he could mold the chocolate-cream mixture into little balls. He then rolled the balls in cocoa powder, and they resembled the edible fungi called truffles. And so, he named them chocolate truffles. Here, I've substituted almond butter for the cream.

PER EACH TRUFFLE SERVING

123 calories
9.5 fat
3.5g protein
4g carbohydrates
7g fiber
50 mg sodium

INGREDIENTS

¼ cup plus 2 tablespoons raw almond butter

2 tablespoons raw coconut nectar (such as Coconut Secret)

3 packets monk fruit extract (such as Monk Fruit In The Raw)

Salt

1 no-sugar-added dark chocolate bar (such as Lily's)

METHOD

1. Mix the almond butter, coconut nectar, and monk fruit extract in a mixing bowl until smooth; season with a pinch of salt. Form the mixture into 8 equal-sized balls, stick a toothpick in each ball, and place on a piece of wax paper on a plate. Transfer to the freezer and chill until very firm, about 1 hour.

2. Place three-quarters of the chocolate in a microwave-safe bowl and cook on high until the chocolate has just melted, 30 seconds to 1 minute. Add the remaining chocolate and stir until smooth and still warm.

3. Remove the almond butter balls from the freezer and, using the toothpick as an aid, roll a truffle to coat with the chocolate until covered; then set on the wax paper–lined plate to cool. Repeat with the remaining truffles; place back in the freezer to set, about 5 minutes; and serve.

TIP

You can roll the truffles in ¼ cup of chopped almonds before they set for a prettier presentation and extra negative calorie power.

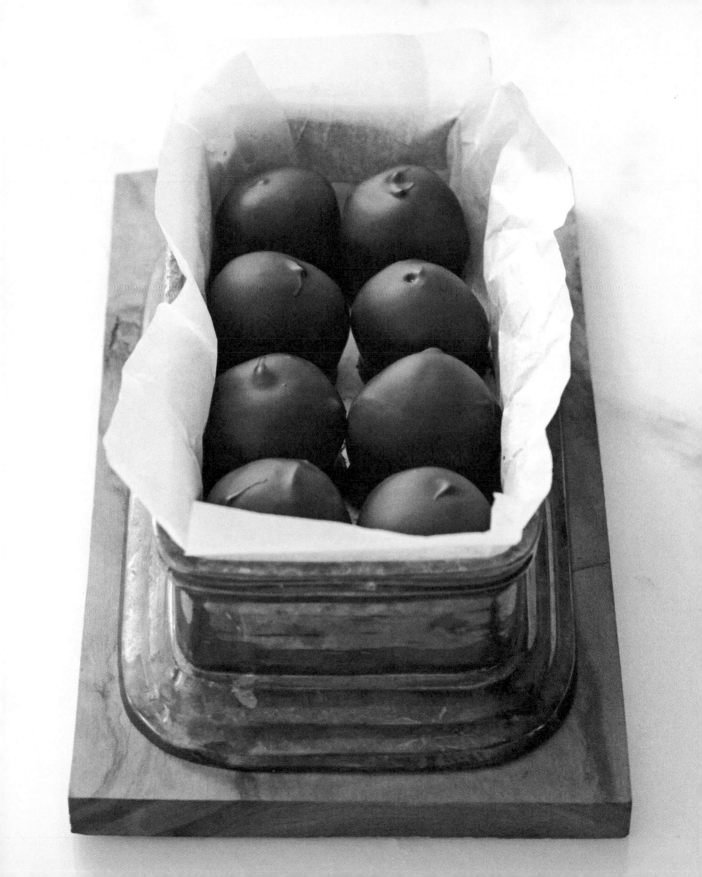

CHOCOLATE-DIPPED STRAWBERRIES WITH CRUSHED ALMONDS

MAKES 4 SERVINGS; 4 STRAWBERRIES PER PERSON
PREP TIME: 10 MINUTES
COOK TIME: 10 MINUTES

I'd like to reintroduce you to a classic dessert, the lovely Valentine's gift you've probably given or received many times in the past: chocolate-covered strawberries! This recipe coats luscious negative calorie strawberries with no-sugar-added dark chocolate and a sprinkle of protein-rich almonds. Indulge, please!

PER SERVING

131 calories
10.5g fat
3.5g protein
11g carbohydrates
5.5g fiber
2mg sodium

INGREDIENTS

1 bar no-sugar-added dark chocolate (such as Lily's)
¼ cup toasted and crushed almonds
16 medium strawberries

METHOD

1. Place three-quarters of the chocolate in a microwave-safe bowl and cook on high until the chocolate has just melted, 30 seconds to 1 minute. Stir in the remaining chocolate until smooth and still warm. Place the almonds on a plate.

2. Dip each strawberry in the chocolate to cover, roll in the almond mixture, and place on a piece of wax paper or parchment paper set over a plate. Move the finished berries to the refrigerator to cool and set. Serve chilled.

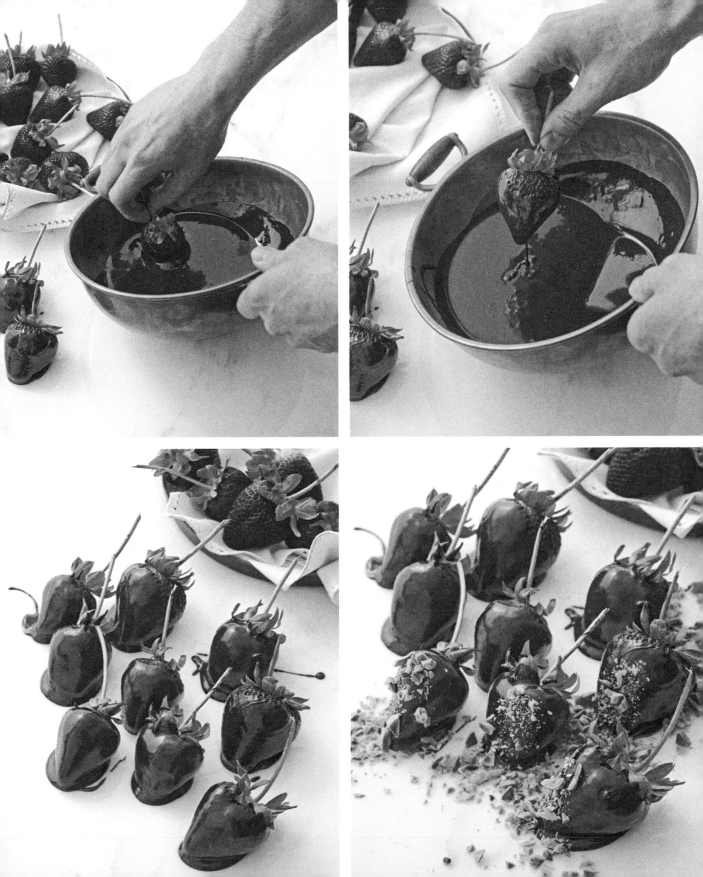

COCOA-DUSTED ALMONDS

MAKES 4 SERVINGS
PREP TIME: 10 MINUTES
COOK TIME: 10 MINUTES

This is just the thing to reach for when you're craving something sweet but you don't need a full-on "dessert." You can adjust the sweetness to your liking—less monk fruit for a bitter, dark chocolate flavor, and more for a sweeter chocolate taste. These almonds also keep well in the fridge.

PER SERVING

230 calories
18g fat
8g protein
12.5g carbohydrates
4.5g fiber
50mg sodium

INGREDIENTS

1½ tablespoons raw coconut nectar (such as Coconut Secret)

4 packets monk fruit extract (such as Monk Fruit In The Raw)

Salt

1 cup almonds (treat yourself to Marcona almonds if you can find them)

3 tablespoons unsweetened organic cocoa powder

METHOD

1. Preheat the oven to 350°F.

2. Combine the coconut nectar, half the monk fruit extract, and a pinch of salt in a large mixing bowl and set aside.

3. Place the almonds on a parchment paper–lined baking sheet and toast in the oven until golden brown. Transfer the almonds to the bowl and toss to coat well, and then place the almonds back on the lined baking sheet. Bake in the oven, stirring occasionally, until the coconut nectar is sticking all over the almonds, 5 to 8 minutes.

3. Transfer the almonds to a clean mixing bowl. Mix the cocoa powder and remaining monk fruit extract in a separate bowl. Add the cocoa powder mixture to the almonds and toss to coat well. Shake off the excess cocoa and place the almonds on a clean plate to cool. Serve at room temperature or chilled.

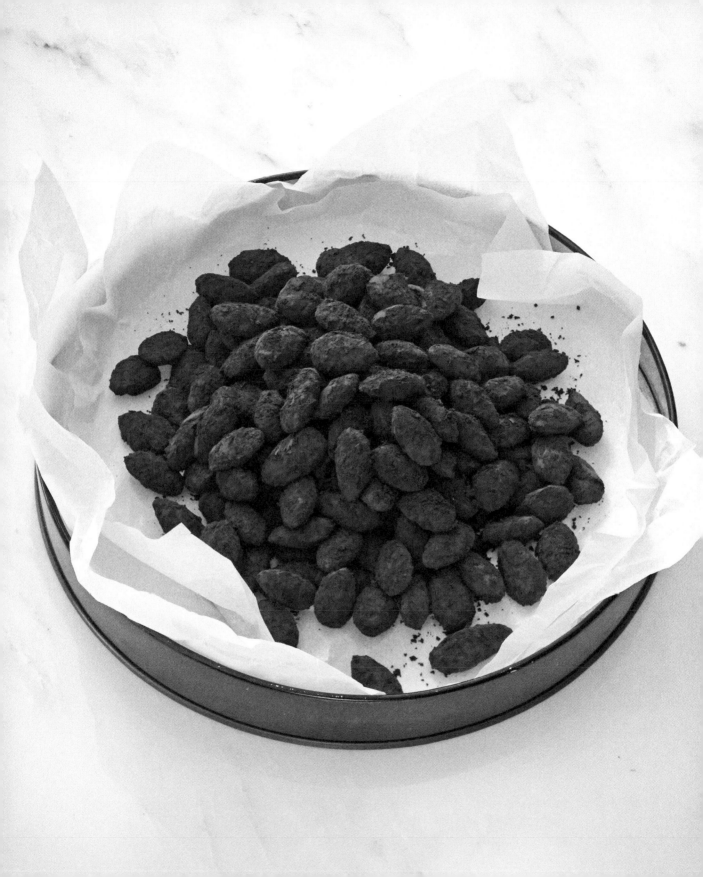

INSTANT ALMOND CAKE WITH MIXED BERRIES

MAKES 4 SERVINGS
PREP TIME: 5 MINUTES
COOK TIME: 7 MINUTES

This recipe will make 4 mini cakes in the microwave in just seconds. If you'd prefer to make a larger cake (like the one pictured here), just quadruple the ingredients and pour into a 10-inch nonstick cake pan (lightly coated with coconut oil cooking spray). Bake at 350°F until golden brown, about 10 minutes; then turn the oven down to 300°F and bake until fully cooked through, 15–20 minutes. Cool on a wire rack and serve, sliced, with the berries. The cake will serve 16.

PER SERVING

155 calories
7g fat
6.5g protein
17g carbohydrates
3g fiber
80mg sodium

INGREDIENTS

½ cup almond meal

2 eggs, separated; 1 yolk discarded

4 packets monk fruit extract (such as Monk Fruit In The Raw)

Four 6-ounce noncoated paper cups

Olive oil cooking spray

1 teaspoon vanilla extract

Salt

3 tablespoons raw coconut nectar (such as Coconut Secret)

1 cup mixed berries, mashed with a fork

METHOD

1. Preheat the oven to 375°F.

2. Place the almond meal on a baking sheet and bake in the oven until toasted and aromatic, 3 to 5 minutes. Remove from the oven and transfer the toasted meal to a cool baking sheet.

3. Put the egg whites and monk fruit extract in a mixing bowl and whisk until the egg whites form stiff peaks. Spray four 6-ounce noncoated paper cups with cooking spray. Poke holes in the bottom of the cups with a toothpick or fork.

4. Pour the cooled almond meal into a clean mixing bowl and add the egg yolk, vanilla, salt, and coconut nectar. Fold the egg whites into the almond mixture and spoon the batter into the prepared cups. Cook in the microwave about 30 seconds, then place the cups on their sides and cook until cooked through, about 45 seconds. Remove the cakes and place, upside down, on four serving plates; remove the cups and serve with the berries.

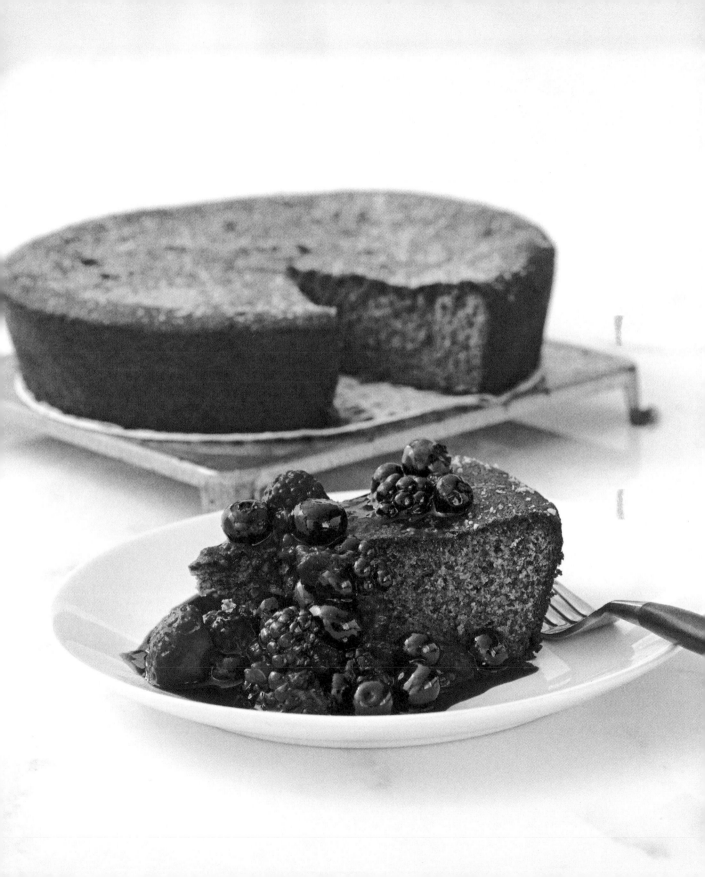

CREPES SUZETTE WITH ORANGES AND VANILLA CREAM

MAKES 4 SERVINGS
PREP TIME: 5 MINUTES
COOK TIME: 10 MINUTES

In 1895, the classic French dessert crêpes suzette was created serendipitously when a fourteen-year-old assistant waiter named Henri Charpentier was preparing dessert crepes for the Prince of Wales. Charpentier's dessert caught on fire, but the flames blended together several sweet flavors—and actually improved the taste. The prince loved it so much that he insisted the dessert be named after one of his dining companions, a beautiful Frenchwoman named Suzette.

PER SERVING

162 calories
3.5g fat
11g protein
23g carbohydrates
6g fiber
151mg sodium

INGREDIENTS

Olive oil cooking spray
¼ cup fat-free Greek yogurt
1 teaspoon vanilla extract
1½ cups cold water
2 tablespoons plus 2 teaspoons psyllium husk flakes (available in the natural section of most supermarkets in a variety of brands)
6 tablespoons plus 2 teaspoons egg white powder (such as Deb El)
1 teaspoon finely grated orange zest
1½ cups orange segments
3 packets monk fruit extract (such as Monk Fruit In The Raw)
3 tablespoons raw coconut nectar (such as Coconut Secret)
3 tablespoons toasted slivered almonds

METHOD

1. Preheat the oven to 350°F. Coat a 12-inch oven-safe nonstick skillet with cooking spray.

2. Mix the yogurt and vanilla and set aside. Pour the water into a large mixing bowl, add the psyllium husk flakes, and whisk until all the psyllium has dissolved and the water is slightly thickened, about 2 minutes. Add the egg white powder and whisk in slowly to dissolve the egg white but not to aerate it, about 1 minute.

3. Pour one-fourth of the mixture into the prepared skillet. Tilt the skillet so the mixture covers the bottom of the pan completely. Place over medium-high heat and cook until the bottom of the crepe is beginning to solidify, about 30 seconds. Transfer the skillet to the oven and bake until the top is cooked,

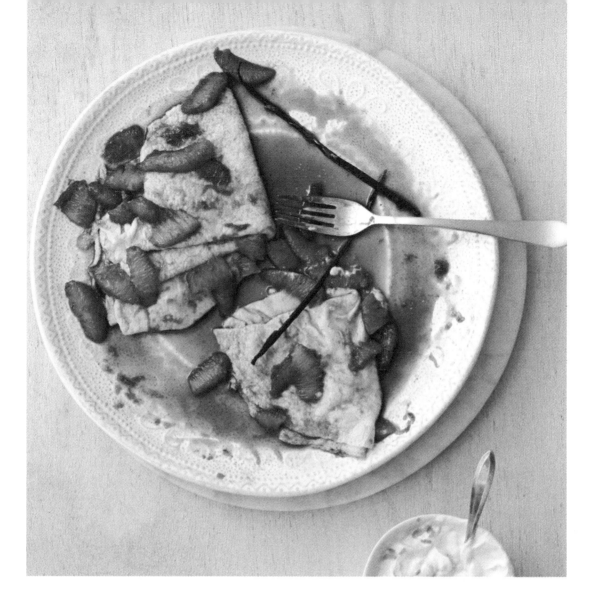

about 30 seconds. Place the skillet back on the heat on the stovetop, flip the crepe to lightly brown the other side, then slide off onto one of four serving plates and reserve. Repeat to make 3 more crepes and place each one on a serving plate.

4. Add the orange zest and orange segments to the skillet and cook until softened and warm. Turn off the heat. Add the monk fruit extract and coconut nectar. Using three-quarters of the filling, fill each crepe with the orange mixture. Fold the crepes in half, and then in half again. Top with the yogurt, the almonds, and the remaining orange mixture.

CITRUS AND MIXED BERRY BOWL WITH WHIPPED TOPPING

MAKES 4 SERVINGS
PREP TIME: 10 MINUTES
COOK TIME: 15 MINUTES

When I was growing up, my mom would whip up clouds of luscious whipped cream. Of course, back then it was loaded with sugar. These days, we know how to make whipped cream much healthier but keep that dreamy, delicious quality intact. Here's one way to do it.

PER SERVING

128 calories
1.5g fat
5.6g protein
4.7g carbohydrates
7g fiber
64mg sodium

INGREDIENTS

1 cup unsweetened vanilla almond milk, or homemade almond milk (page 91)

1¾ teaspoons gelatin powder

4 packets monk fruit extract (such as Monk Fruit In The Raw)

1 tablespoon coconut nectar

1 vanilla bean, split lengthwise

½ cup fat-free Greek yogurt

4 cups mixed berries

½ cup orange segments cut into bite-size pieces

METHOD

1. Pour 1 tablespoon of the almond milk into a small bowl. Pour the gelatin over the milk and set aside.

2. Pour the remaining milk, monk fruit extract, and coconut nectar into a small saucepan. Using the tip of a small knife, scrape the seeds from the vanilla bean into the pot and bring the mixture to a simmer. Scrape the gelatin mixture into the hot milk and whisk to dissolve. Pour the mixture into a stainless steel bowl and stir in the yogurt. Fill a larger bowl halfway with ice water and place it underneath the bowl of the almond milk mixture, using it as an ice bath.

3. Using a handheld mixer, start whipping the mixture on low, then increase to high speed. As the mixture cools, it will gain volume and become a thick whipped topping. Continue to whip until aerated and stiff, about 3 to 5 minutes. Distribute the mixed berries and orange segments equally among four bowls and top each with the topping. Serve immediately.

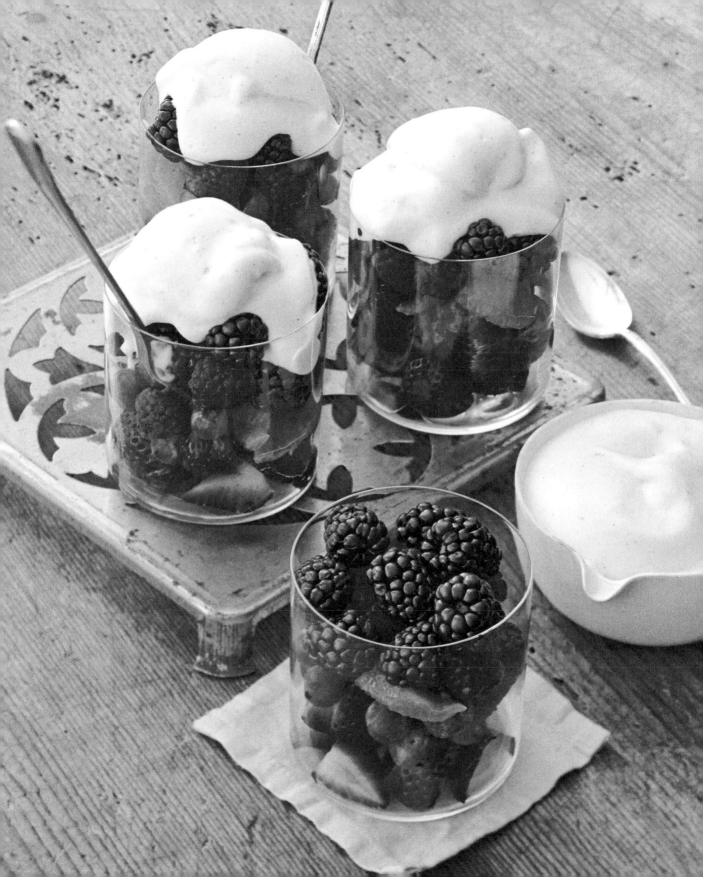

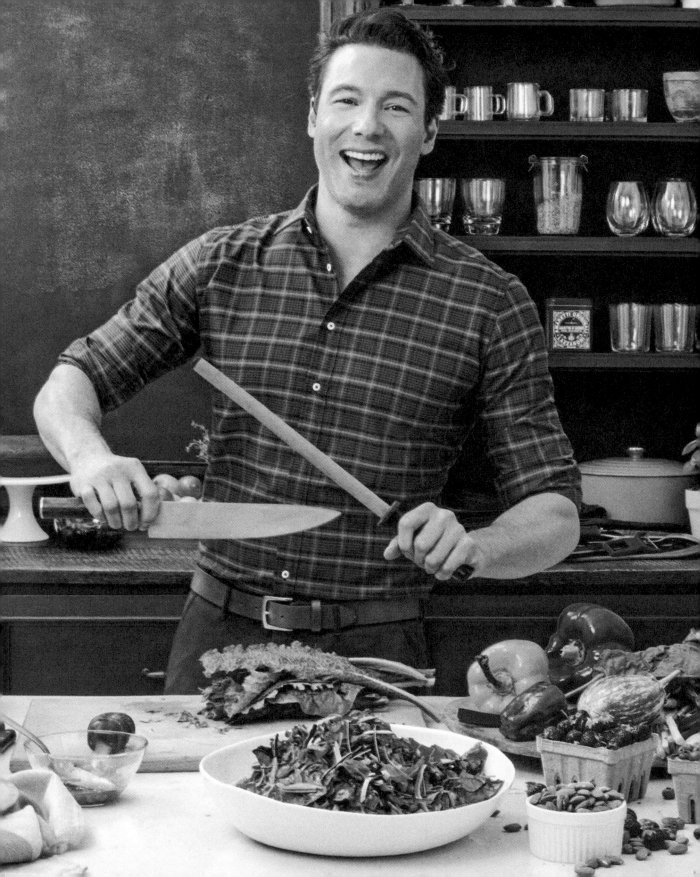

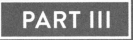

PART III

THE NEGATIVE CALORIE LIFESTYLE

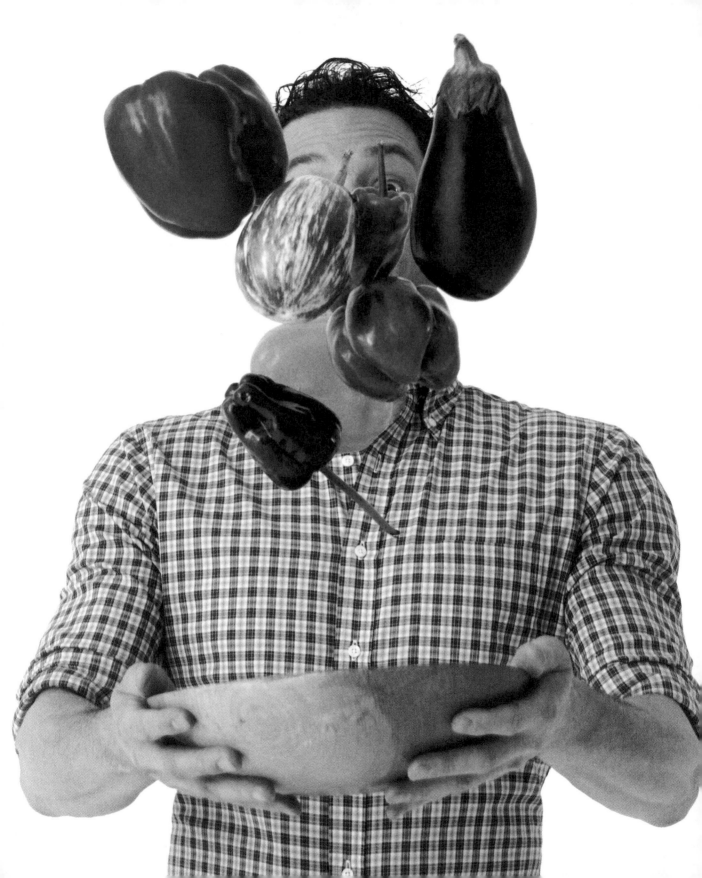

CHAPTER TWELVE

GOING MEATLESS

IN the past, vegans and vegetarians may have been regarded with skepticism, but these days, with our increased understanding of the health benefits conferred by a plant-based diet, going meat-free is practically chic. When people ask me if the vegetarian entrées on this plan taste as good as the meat dishes, I say, "Yes! And most of the time, you can't even tell the difference." When I whip up a vegetarian meal at home, even my carnivore guests can't believe how satisfying and delicious a meatless meal can be.

One reason plant-based diets have become so popular is that they are incredibly nutritious and can be a wonderful choice for weight loss. Plant-based diets are rich in fiber, water, and phyto-nutrients; they exclude animal fats and animal protein and instead include clean, plant-based protein sources such as beans, legumes, whole grains, nuts, and other proteins that we all should be eating.

Vegetarians often weigh significantly less than meat eaters. In fact, a 2013 study at the University of South Carolina found that participants who followed vegetarian and vegan diets lost more weight than dieters who ate meat. (Vegans eat no animal products of any kind, while vegetarians may eat cheese and other dairy products.)

In this study, 63 men and women were randomly assigned to one of five eating styles: vegan, vegetarian, pesco-vegetarian (plant-based plus fish), semi-vegetarian (plant-based with some animal foods), and regular "omnivorous" eating. All five diets emphasized low-fat, low-carb unprocessed foods. No one had to count calories.

At the two-month point, the dieters who went on the vegan and vegetarian diets dropped an average of 8 to 10 pounds. In contrast, those eating some meat or fish lost 5 pounds on average.

At the six-month point, the vegans had dropped about 7 percent of their weight, the semi-vegetarian group had shed about 4 percent, and the pesco-vegetarian group and the meat eaters had both lost about 3 percent.

Plant-based diets include a lot of negative calorie foods, so it's easy to see why these diets can be so effective when it comes to weight loss.

THE 10 BEST FAT-BURNING VEGETARIAN PROTEINS

If you're in the veggie camp, you're in luck, because all 10 negative calorie foods are vegetables and fruits. When you eat two or more of these foods at your main meals, you'll keep your body in a fat-burning mode.

But what about protein?

A common myth about plant-based diets is that it's tough to get enough protein. But there are many wonderful plant-based proteins that have weight-control benefits. Here are the 10 best I've found.

1. CHICKPEAS

Like other beans, chickpeas (also called garbanzo beans) are full of fiber and protein, which promote fullness. Chickpeas are also high in "resistant starch," a type of fiber that is impossible for the body to digest, and instead winds its way through the digestive system intact. Along the way, it helps produce fatty acids that stimulate fat-melting enzymes (particularly in the belly), and it helps promote fat-burning in your liver.

One of my favorite chickpea-based snacks is hummus—it is always in my refrigerator! What I love about the stuff is that it is a nutritional slam dunk. It's easy to buy at the store, of course, but it's just as easy to prepare at home and, in my opin-ion, it tastes much better when homemade. Just put a can of chickpeas, a little tahini (a sesame-seed butter), garlic, freshly squeezed lemon juice, and a bit of olive oil in a blender or food processer, and give it a whirl. You can season and flavor the hummus to your taste. Like it spicy? Add in some minced jalapeño or red pepper flakes. Like it milder? Cut back on the garlic and add more lemon juice, or an herb like basil or oregano. It takes about five minutes to make yourself a batch that you'll have all week long.

USE IT TO LOSE IT There are lots of ways to eat chickpeas besides in hummus. Try them in soups and salads, or just by their lonesome on the plate. Spice them, garlic them, or herbify them . . . just keep them coming.

2. HEMP SEEDS

This plant food probably doesn't immediately spring to mind when you think of veggie proteins, but hemp seeds are an excellent source of plant-based protein because they are a *complete protein*. That means they provide all of the amino acids your body needs to support metabolic function. (Your body can't make certain amino acids on its own, so you need to provide them with your food choices!)

Hemp seeds are particularly rich in the amino acids methionine and cysteine. Both are involved in the repair and growth of lean body tissue, particularly in response to exercise. The branched chain amino acids leucine, isoleucine, and valine—nicknamed by their acronym BCAAs—are also plentiful in hemp. BCAAs are known for their fat-burning and muscle-building power.

Another quality of hemp I like: It's never genetically modified, so you don't have to worry about GMOs here. And to address the elephant in the room: no, hemp seeds will not make you high. Hemp food products, from seeds to protein powders, contain undetectable levels of THC (the mind-altering chemical found in marijuana), so you're not going to get a buzz from your protein smoothie!

USE IT TO LOSE IT It's easy to incorporate hemp seeds in your diet: Sprinkle them on cereal and salads. Add them to smoothies. You can also make your own hemp milk in seconds by blending or food-processing ½ cup seeds, 1½ cups water, 2 teaspoons coconut nectar, and 1 teaspoon vanilla extract. It will keep in a jar in the refrigerator for up to a week. Simply shake it well just prior to serving it. Use the milk in smoothies or pour it over cereal.

3. KIDNEY BEANS

I'm definitely a bean boy. I'm not sure what it is I like best about kidney beans—whether it's their flavor (so rich, so delicious) or their versatility—the fact that they can be made into anything from soups to chili to salads to brownies (yes, they make a delightful flourless base for these beloved treats).

Studies show a strong association between eating the common bean (*Phaseolus vulgaris*—which includes kidney beans, black beans, pintos, and others) and losing body fat and improving body composition.

Beans also rank low on the glycemic index. By definition, this indicates that they produce a relatively low rise in blood glucose after a meal compared with high-glycemic index foods such as white rice, which sharply elevate glucose. Other studies have found that beans improve satiety.

Eating lots of beans may not be the best practice for your next date or social event (along with beans do come, for most people, some digestive issues). It's better to load up on kidney beans in the privacy of your own home!

USE IT TO LOSE IT Some of the best ways to prepare kidney beans are in chili, stews, and soups. They taste so meaty that no one will know you've served a meatless dish. If you buy uncooked beans, it's a good idea to soak them overnight. This helps prevent the gassy, bloated feeling some of us get after eating beans. As for canned beans, rinsing them well under cold running water in a colander, and then draining them, also reduces the chance of digestive distress.

4. LENTILS

Thinking about lentils might make you yawn, but hear me out—these legumes are underrated. Lentils have so much flavor, and are loaded with fat-burning fiber and protein. What I love the most about lentils is how quick and easy it is to cook them. In 30 to 40 minutes lentils are ready to serve; no overnight soaking is necessary. I'm not advocating a lentil-heavy diet. But I strongly suggest that you make lentils a pantry staple if you haven't done so already, and cook with them often.

Studies have found that consuming lentils increases satiety. The reason lentils fill you up is threefold: (1) they contain slowly digestible starch; (2) they are rich in protein; and (3) they are high in fiber, which helps make you feel full.

USE IT TO LOSE IT Lentils are great in stews, in soups, and as the base for veggie burgers. They require very little prep work. However, I advise checking for, and discarding, any of the tiny stones or stems that are often found in lentil packaging. After inspecting the lentils, place them in a strainer and rinse; they're ready to cook. You don't have to soak them like dried beans. Season lentils with spices such as cumin, garlic powder, or allspice.

5. PEAS

I love peas. They're among my favorite legumes by a Manhattan mile, and my freezer is full of them. Peas are rich in vitamins and contain a variety of disease-fighting phytochemicals.

Scientists have recently begun to study, and isolate, protein in peas, and that is why you now find pea protein powder at many health food stores. Pea protein is one of the few vegetable protein sources that does not trigger food allergies; nor does it contain gluten. And peas are not genetically modified, either. Pea protein powder also supplies BCAAs, the fat-burning, muscle-building amino acids also contained in hemp seeds.

As for satiety, pea protein shines here, too. In one study, 39 healthy subjects supplemented with either pea protein, whey protein, or a control of milk protein. The participants who were given the pea protein reported feeling less hungry than participants who consumed other types of protein. Peas rule!

USE IT TO LOSE IT Like most legumes, peas are delicious in soups and stews, or as a side dish. You can even puree them with garlic, freshly squeezed lemon juice, and a little olive oil to create a lovely green hummus for dipping with negative calorie veggies such as celery, raw cauliflower, or raw broccoli. Try adding pea protein powder to your smoothies, too.

6. PISTACHIOS

Pistachios have earned the nickname "the skinny nut," and rightly so. One of the most interesting studies on pistachios proved once again that a calorie is not a calorie. Researchers from UCLA decided to find out if near-equivalent numbers of calories from either pistachios or pretzels would produce any significant body composition changes when eaten as part of a calorie-modified, 12-week fat-loss diet. The volunteers—a group of obese men and women—were instructed to go on a reduced-calorie diet. Along with it, they were randomly assigned to a protocol that included a mid-afternoon snack of either 2 ounces of unsalted pretzels (220 calories), or 3 ounces of in-shell pistachios (240 calories; about 75 nuts).

At the end of the study, the researchers measured everyone's body mass index (BMI). Both groups had lost weight. But the results showed that the pistachio group had better success at reducing body mass index (BMI), compared with the pretzel group. The volunteers on the pistachio protocol went from a 30 BMI to a 28.8 BMI, which meant that they were no longer considered obese, versus the pretzel eaters, who moved from only a 30.9 to a 30.3 BMI, still considered obese.

Note that the pistachio snack contained more calories than the pretzels, and the dieters eating pistachios were the weight-loss winners. A calorie is not a calorie! The pistachio is definitely among the negative calorie nuts. In fact, the fat calories in these nuts may not be completely absorbed by the body, making them effectively lower in calories than previously thought.

Pistachios are also a treasure trove of nutrients: protein, good fats, fiber, potassium, magnesium, vitamin E, and a number of phytochemicals. Clearly, pistachios should be a part of any healthy weight-loss plan.

USE IT TO LOSE IT A handful of these little green nuts makes a great-tasting snack. Or crush them and sprinkle over oatmeal, yogurt, or salads.

7. QUINOA

Though often praised as a healthy grain, quinoa is not technically a grain at all, but rather a seed. It originated in South America and dates all the way back to the Incan Empire.

Like hemp seeds, quinoa delivers a complete protein package, offering all of the amino acids your body requires. Quinoa has a low glycemic index (very similar to vegetables), so it won't spike your blood sugar. Quinoa is also brimming with fiber, making it a great choice for weight loss, and for anyone with diabetes.

I love to cook with quinoa—it has a unique flavor often described as a cross between brown rice and oatmeal, with a subtle, nutty nuance. And

because it is gluten-free, it makes a great substitute in all kinds of grain-based dishes.

USE IT TO LOSE IT Not only is quinoa a superfood, it's also quick and easy to prepare and so versatile that it can be eaten at any meal. Try cooking it for breakfast in some almond milk as a substitute for oatmeal, or swap it into any dish that calls for rice or pasta.

8. CHIA SEEDS

I used to feel sorry for chia seeds. That was back in the days when this nutritional treasure trove was consigned to late-night TV commercials selling clay "pets" with the seeds that sprouted to look like fur.

But in the last decade, chia seeds have burst onto the health scene not as hair plugs for a kooky pet but as a functional food that is loaded with protein, fiber (just 2 tablespoons contain nearly 30 percent of your daily requirement!), healthy fats, and fat-burning minerals like calcium. Who knew?

Well, now the world knows, and chia seeds are one of the best entries into the world of healthy nutrition. I cook with them a lot because they pack such a powerful nutritional wallop.

The main reason I love chia seeds is that they fill me up and keep me from getting hungry. In that regard, I classify them in the negative calorie food category. They are satiating. After you digest them, they start absorbing a lot of liquid in your stomach to form a gel that keeps you satiated (in fact, the gelatinous coating is what bonded the seeds to that clay pet). Research published in 2010 in the *European Journal of Clinical*

Nutrition showed that chia seeds curb your appetite for two hours after you eat them—plus, they help reduce the blood sugar spikes that typically occur after a meal.

Chia seeds may be among the newest nutritional kids on the block, but they've been around since ancient days. They were a food source for the Mayas and cultivated by the Aztecs as a cash crop more than five hundred years ago. Both cultures considered chia a medicine, as well as a food. You're going to see chia seeds in a lot more products soon. Stay tuned.

USE IT TO LOSE IT Chia seeds are amazingly versatile. Sprinkle them on oatmeal, salads, Greek yogurt, quinoa, or rice. You can also blend them into smoothies.

9. TOFU

I've always supported the idea of tofu as being healthy, but until recently, I didn't really cook with it. My typical MO was, "This tofu stir-fry recipe sure looks delicious." Then I'd proceed to toss in strips of beef, chicken, or fish instead.

But now I really like tofu, and I enjoy cooking with it because tofu probably is one of the most versatile ingredients in a plant-based diet. Like tempeh, tofu is made from soybeans, the only beans that contain more protein than carbohydrates. As such, soy protein ranks right up there with animal protein in terms of thermogenic effect. Soy protein also improves insulin resistance, the hallmark of obesity.

Soy coaxes your body into releasing the hormone glucagon, which unlocks fat and carb stores to keep your body lean and supplied with energy, thereby controlling hunger. A 2006 study published in the journal *Appetite* revealed that tofu, in particular, is as satiating as chicken and keeps you feeling full for several hours after a meal.

The many varieties of tofu you'll find at the grocery store differ mostly in how much water they contain. Silken tofu, which I prefer, has the highest quantity of water. That's why it's so soft and creamy.

USE IT TO LOSE IT Tofu absorbs the flavors of anything it is cooked with, yet retains a distinctive, almost meaty texture. Use tofu in salads, stir-fries, and smoothies for extra protein. It also makes a great substitute for cheese in traditional Italian dishes such as lasagna.

10. WALNUTS

One ounce of walnuts contains 4 grams of protein, so these tasty nuts are a great protein alternative. Walnuts are also rich in healthy fats, including alpha-linolenic acid (ALA). This omega-3 fat is a key player in maintaining healthy brain biochemistry and stabilizing mood. (Some say there's a reason why walnuts seem to resemble the shape of the human brain!) A 2011 study in the *American Journal of Clinical Nutrition* found that for every half-gram increase of ALA eaten per day, a person's risk of depression fell by as much as 43 percent.

Another thing going for walnuts: They trigger a reaction in the body that slows the rate at which your stomach empties. That means—you guessed it—they perform well as a natural appetite suppressant. And speaking of tummies, research with walnuts has shown that they can also help reduce your waistline.

USE IT TO LOSE IT Try snacking on a handful of walnuts a half hour prior to mealtime; they can help control your appetite. Sprinkle walnuts on yogurt or oatmeal, or toss them into salads and stir-fries for a quick source of veg-friendly protein.

VEGGING OUT

As you can see, the Negative Calorie Diet is totally adaptable to a vegetarian or vegan lifestyle. Just start with a base of negative calorie fruit and vegetables, and follow this simple 3-step process to create all of your meals.

STEP 1: CHOOSE YOUR APPROACH

Select the most practical form of plant-based eating that's right for you. Technically, a vegetarian is a person who doesn't eat meat but may eat other animal products such as cheese, milk, or eggs. A vegan, on the other hand, doesn't go near or use any products originating from animals, including eggs, milk, chocolate, yogurt, or cheese. Also egg-free are lacto-vegetarians, a group that can be a little more flexible than their vegan counterparts when it comes to eating animal by-products. Ovo-vegetarians allow eggs while at the same time avoiding all dairy products, so eggs are as animal as they get.

Then there are flexitarians: people who subsist primarily on plant-based foods, but aren't strictly veg. No hard-and-fast rules determine the amount of meat a person must eat to be considered a flexitarian.

STEP 2: PERSONALIZE YOUR PLAN

No matter what level of vegetarianism you choose, the basic principles of nutrition remain the same. Protein is a must. A weight-loss diet must include sources of healthy protein. The 10 protein-rich foods listed in this chapter are a great place to start if you're opting for a meat-free lifestyle.

If you don't care to cut meat completely out of your diet, I still recommend scaling back on your meat consumption when you're looking to lose weight. Try substituting tofu for chicken, or beans for ground beef, in your favorite recipes.

I've had a number of clients who are vegans and vegetarians, and I find it fun to think of creative meal ideas for them. You can do the same by trying different low-starch, high-fiber, protein-packed recipes. I don't like to use fake "vegetarian meats" in my recipes; I'd rather stick to natural plant-based proteins and a variety of fresh, organic, and seasonal ingredients.

STEP 3: PLAN NEGATIVE CALORIE MEALS

For a plant-based weight-loss plan, combine negative calorie foods with proteins and healthy fats. Use this basic configuration to plan your meals: 2 or more negative calorie foods + 1 lean protein + a small amount of optional fat such as extra-virgin olive oil.

At breakfast, for example, you might have one of my negative calorie smoothies blended with pea or hemp protein powder; or a bowl of oatmeal or quinoa made with almond milk and topped with berries.

For lunch, make yourself a generous salad of leafy greens, chopped tomatoes, chopped celery, sliced cucumbers, or other negative calorie vegetables, topped with tofu, walnuts, or beans. Drizzle it with olive oil, plus some vinegar and maybe a fat-burning spice or two, and you've just made yourself the perfect vegetarian negative calorie salad. Or you can turn to page 151 and try some of my meatless lunch recipes.

At dinnertime, match up a vegetarian protein like quinoa or lentils with some cooked or raw negative calorie vegetables, and you've got a meal that will keep you full until the next day. It's fine to include a variety of vegetables outside those in the negative calorie category, too—you can find a list of those on page 48. Strive to have at least two negative calorie foods at main meals. Top dinner off with one of my negative calorie desserts.

Snacks are also a cinch; try negative calorie fruits such as apples, citrus fruits, or berries, or any negative calorie veggie. Pair these with some almonds, walnuts, pistachios, or hummus.

SAMPLE ONE-WEEK MEATLESS MENU

Here's a look at how to plan a Negative Calorie meatless menu:

MONDAY

BREAKFAST

Apple and Cinnamon Breakfast "Risotto" with Oat Bran and Almonds (add a tablespoon of hemp seeds for extra protein) or any Negative Calorie Smoothie made with pea or hemp protein powder

LUNCH

Charred Thai Style Broccoli Salad with Almonds and Lime

DINNER

Eggplant Roll-Ups

SNACK

Cucumber and Almond Rice Sushi

TUESDAY

BREAKFAST

Blueberry and Quinoa Porridge with Mint or any Negative Calorie Smoothie made with pea or hemp protein powder

LUNCH

Shaved Brussels Sprouts with Warm Toasted Garlic, Almond, and Lemon Dressing (omit the cheese)

DINNER

Vegetable Pot-au-Feu

SNACK

Apple, Cranberry, and Almond Bars

WEDNESDAY

BREAKFAST

Breakfast Citrus Salad with Cucumbers and Basil or any Negative Calorie Smoothie made with pea or hemp protein powder

LUNCH

Mushroom Bouillon with Leeks, Tofu, and Wasabi

DINNER

½ cup cooked kidney beans + Shaved Brussels Sprouts with Warm Toasted Garlic, Almond, and Lemon Dressing

SNACK

Handful of pistachios + 1 medium apple

THURSDAY

BREAKFAST

Breakfast Pizza with Mushrooms and Broccoli or any Negative Calorie Smoothie made with pea or hemp protein powder

LUNCH

The Grate Salad Bowl with Chia Seed Dressing

DINNER

Soup and salad dinner:

1 cup organic lentil soup + Strawberry and Spinach Salad with Almonds and Basil

SNACK

Red Ants on a Log

FRIDAY

BREAKFAST

Breakfast Bowl with Quinoa and Berries or any negative calorie smoothie made with pea or hemp protein powder

LUNCH

Leafy Green Salad with Creamy Almond Dressing and Radishes

DINNER

Shiitake and Bok Choy Stir-Fry

SNACK

Handful of walnuts + 1 medium orange

SATURDAY

BREAKFAST

Apple and Cinnamon Breakfast "Risotto" with Oat Bran and Almonds (add 1 tablespoon of hemp seeds for extra protein) or any Negative Calorie Smoothie made with pea or hemp protein powder

LUNCH

Mixed Leafy Green Soup "Caldo Verde" with Chickpeas

DINNER

Roasted Cauliflower with Green Peppers, Almond Curry, and Lime

SNACK

Eggplant and Almond Dip with Celery

SUNDAY

BREAKFAST

Blueberry and Quinoa Porridge with Mint or any Negative Calorie Smoothie made with pea or hemp protein powder

LUNCH

Vegetable Pot-au-Feu

DINNER

Eggplant Roll-Ups (omit the cheese or use a nondairy cheese)

SNACK

Peanutty Apple Slices

There you have it: a simple and satisfying menu of meatless choices, supercharged with negative calorie foods. Each week, purchase a variety of negative calorie foods and my recommended plant-based proteins. The key is to keep your pantry and fridge stocked for success and follow the plan as long as you need to meet your goal.

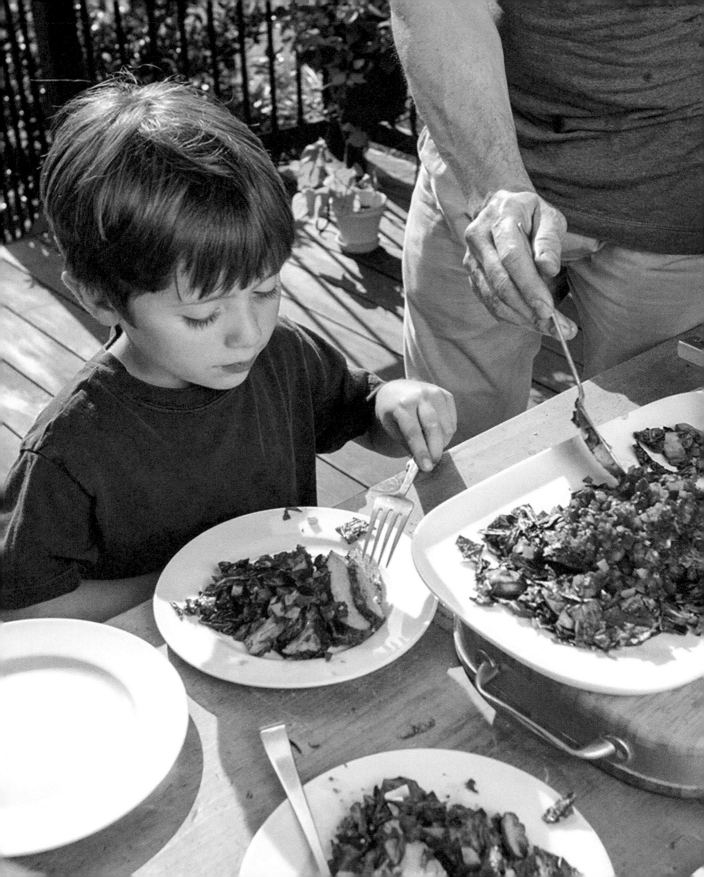

CHAPTER THIRTEEN

THE FAMILY PLAN

DIETING is an infamously solo endeavor. The problem is, eating is a social activity. We sit down to dinner with our families at the end of a long day; we share a special meal with our spouses; we go over to our aunt's or sister's or grandmother's house for her legendary cooking on the weekends. We eat with our families. But we "diet" without them.

Quite often, going it alone can be precarious. Without the support of others following the same plan, it's all too easy to revert back to old, unhealthy habits. How many times have you blown your diet because other people have led you astray? A diet would be really easy to follow if you lived alone on a desert island, but here in the real (populated) world, the family and friends who are not dieting with you can pose real challenges to your focus and resolve.

Let's take a look at some strategies for Negative Calorie Diet success, no matter how large or small your household is.

IF YOU'RE THE ONLY ONE ON THE DIET

It may be that your spouse and kids don't need to lose weight, or simply have no interest in dieting. That's fine, because you can do the Negative Calorie Diet all on your own, and the good news is that everyone in your family will benefit from this healthier way of eating. Here's what I suggest to make things easier if you're going solo:

- Serve your family what they want, but in the healthiest way possible: Grill, bake, or roast rather than panfry, for example. Include plenty of negative calorie vegetables prepared simply.

- Don't cook your family something completely different from what you're having. Otherwise, you may be tempted to nibble on what you're preparing for them.

- Have on hand low-sugar, reduced-sodium, high-fiber versions of the foods your family loves. Buy reduced- or lower-sodium sauces, stocks, soups. Choose organic, whole-grain varieties of breads and breakfast cereals.

- Keep snacks such as nuts and fruits readily available at home, but don't push. Let your family taste the healthier snacks on their own. Chances are they will enjoy how satiating these are, and begin choosing healthier snacks on a regular basis.

- If your kids resist these changes, take it one step at a time. Begin with the rule that nourishing food comes before junk food. Allow kids the choice to eat healthy food or not. Ignore angry reactions. Never get into food fights. Be patient and persistent. Your efforts will pay off.

- Accept the fact that you may have to go it alone—at least for now. Just don't try to change everything all at once. If you do, it might feel too overwhelming for family members, and they will rebel.

- Ask for support. If you feel that your family might be knowingly or unknowingly sabotaging your diet, send them an e-mail or text enlisting their help. Tell them about behaviors that drive you to cheat, like constantly asking you how many pounds you've lost, or keeping junk food in plain sight. For example, "You might think your questions about my weight are helpful, but I take them as pressure and feel frustrated when I can't report weight loss every time you ask." Or sit down with your family and have a rational discussion about why it's important for you to lose weight and emphasize health reasons. Explain that they don't have to modify their way of eating, but they should at least support what you're doing.

- Assemble a support team outside the family. Enlist friends and coworkers to diet with you.

- Set a good example for your children. They learn from you. If they see you enjoying fruit and veggies, they will often try to emulate that—and they'll see that the diet is a positive change.

Your lifestyle can inspire your family and friends to make the leap—and ultimately feel so much healthier and energetic. You can't ask for much more than that!

A REASON TO DIET TOGETHER AND GET WELL

Since the early 1970s, the percentage of American kids and teens defined as overweight or obese has more than tripled, to about 17 percent, according to the Centers for Disease Control and Prevention (CDC). Three out of every four overweight adolescents stay heavy into adulthood.

It isn't just a cosmetic issue, either. Childhood obesity leads to immediate and long-term health problems. If you're a parent, be aware that if your children or teens are obese, the Centers for Disease Control says they are more likely to:

- Be at a higher risk for cardiovascular disease, such as high cholesterol or high blood pressure.

- Develop prediabetes, a condition in which elevated blood sugar levels indicate a greater risk for full-blown diabetes.

- Become more prone to bone and joint problems, sleep disorders, and poor self-esteem.

Stemming the tide of childhood and teen obesity is one soapbox I believe in jumping on. If you love your kids—and I know you do—I hope you'll do everything in your power to give them a long, healthy life. I do believe that the Negative Calorie Diet, with its emphasis on organic fruits and vegetables, lean proteins, and healthy fats, can offer a path to health for many families.

THE NEGATIVE CALORIE DIET, FAMILY-STYLE

If your family could stand to lose a little weight and get a little healthier, why not diet as a family unit? It's a lot easier to shop and cook when you're all on the same plan—and it's a lot more fun when everyone is working toward a shared goal.

Another benefit of dieting as a family is that it increases your odds of success. Researchers at the University of Pittsburgh School of Medicine divided a study of dieters into two groups: One group was assigned to dieting alone; the other

CLEANSE WITH A BUDDY FOR 10 DAYS

The 10-Day Negative Calorie Cleanse can also be a lot more fun—and effective—if you have a partner. Whether it's a friend, neighbor, colleague, or coworker, it's great to have someone in the trenches with you who can relate to your experience. Here are some tips:

- Don't be afraid to ask for a buddy or two to do the cleanse with you. I'm sure you can find plenty of people in your life who would love to do it—and need to.

- Share feedback on which smoothies, salads, and soups you like best.

- Get together several times during the 10 days to eat together or sip your smoothies.

- If one of your cleanse buddies is a guy and you're a woman, don't be too competitive. Men lose weight faster than women.

- Have your buddy meet you for light workouts, such as walking or doing yoga or Pilates.

- Make a pact to call each other for a pep talk, especially if either of you feels like diving into a pint of ice cream.

- Keep a running list of all the positive effects of the cleanse, such as glowing skin, weight loss, better sleep, more energy, and so forth—share your experiences with each other.

group was assigned to diet with family or friends. After 16 weeks, the dieters who had support dropped more weight than did those who had dieted alone. After nearly 10 months, 66 percent of the group with support had maintained their weight loss; only 24 percent of the lone dieters kept their weight off.

I recommend, too, that you try to dine together as much as you can. Even if you don't have time for a long meal during your workweek, almost every recipe in this book is simple enough to make at the end of a long day. But make it a priority to sit down for dinner at least once a week. Traditionally, for my family, this is what Sundays were all about.

There were always twenty to thirty family members over for dinner. Most of the time was spent cooking and eating. We played cards or boccie while the pasta simmered, the meat roasted, and the desserts baked—all recipes that had been handed down over generations and were deeply woven into our way of life. Everyone made sure that these gatherings were a time when we all felt good, revived, nurtured, and loved.

Family meals don't have be fancy, high-maintenance extravaganzas. In fact, they shouldn't be, especially if you're the cook. You should be able to relax and enjoy your family.

Unfortunately, family mealtimes like those I experienced as a kid have gone the way of manual egg beaters—and it is hurting children and teens. A group of pediatricians and psychotherapists, writing in *Canadian Family Physician* in 2015, studied this issue and concluded that infrequent family meals are associated with eating disorders, alcohol and drug abuse, depression, or thoughts of suicide in teens, and added, "There is a positive relationship between frequent family meals and increased self-esteem and school success."

Studies like this are certainly food for thought. To me, coming together as a family for meals is an easy, natural, and instinctive way of expressing love and family values, which kids today need more than ever.

If your family members express an interest in going on this program together, it's a good idea to sit down and talk about your plan before you begin. Make sure the focus, especially for kids, is on getting healthy, having fun, and feeling better—not just weight loss.

Here are some suggestions to make the Negative Calorie Diet a positive family affair:

- Let your children get involved in choosing what goes into their lunch boxes. Sometimes you might find that you just have to pack them the peanut butter and jelly they're begging for—and that's OK. Choose natural peanut better, a no-sugar-added jam, and whole-grain bread. Construct the best versions of their "kid foods" that you can.

  That said, fitting in with their peers at the lunch table can be overrated. My mom used to send me to school with a few pieces of her delicious homemade bread, a hunk of provolone, and an apple or a banana for dessert. While everyone else was eating PB&J and Twinkies, I was biting down on my little Italian lunch, and they gawked at me as if I were an alien. But you know what? They got over it. And eating this way taught me to love food, to see the value in whole foods and ingredients.

• Gradually introduce some of the negative calorie soups, salads, entrées, and desserts into your meal schedule. These are foods everyone should be eating more of anyway. Realistically, though, few children are going to eat every kind of fruit and vegetable under the sun. Even if your kids start off eating just a couple of fruits or vegetables every day, that's still better than nothing. Their tastes will develop as they get used to the foods.

• See if your kids want to try some of the negative calorie smoothies, such as the Strawberry Shortcake Smoothie (page 88) or Spiced Apple Pie Smoothie (page 92). If your children like milk shakes, they'll probably like smoothies. Also, you and the kids can experiment with smoothies, blending one or two servings of vegetables (think kale, arugula, or spinach) with sweet fruits like negative calorie berries or apples.

• Get the whole family on board by doing some fun projects like growing your own vegetables. Helping you sow, tend, and harvest the plants will make them excited to eat the foods they've worked so hard to raise.

• Take your kids along on visits to the grocery store or farmers' markets. Allow them to select new fruits or vegetables they find appealing. Invite them into the kitchen with you and let them help you prepare meals. I loved helping my mother in the kitchen as a kid, and there was plenty of trial and error. Unbeknownst to me, I was training and developing my palate. When I was in my early teens, my mother worked until five or six o'clock at night, so my brother and I would have to fend for ourselves in the kitchen. Those times with her and on our own were an incredibly valuable education in food and nutrition.

• Remind each other of your motivation. Losing weight is part of a plan to stay healthy and enjoy a long life together as a family.

It's always great to diet and take charge of your health, whether as an individual or as a family. Getting healthy as a family offers a host of rewards. Once you make a lifestyle change together, you'll find that other healthy habits soon trickle down as well—things like more cooking at home, more exercise, more time spent outside, and new family traditions and activities. And you'll definitely be a happier, more bonded family, which should be enough to keep you motivated forever.

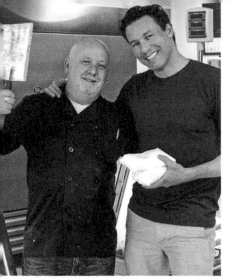
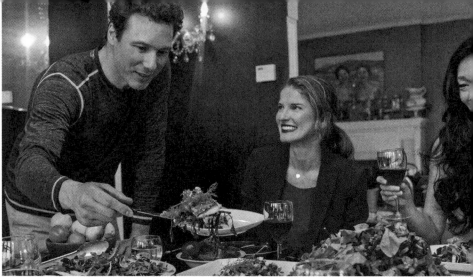
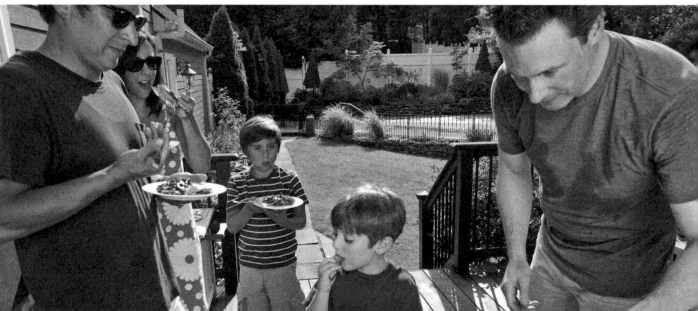
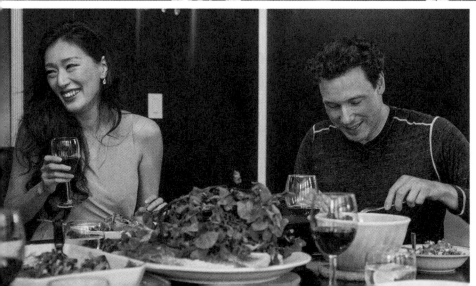
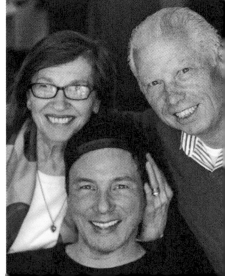

CHAPTER FOURTEEN

EATING OUT AND ON THE GO

I'T'S not where you eat, it's what you eat. With the Negative Calorie Diet, you can eat at any restaurant while dining out, traveling, sitting around in airports, or vacationing because just about every single eating establishment on the planet cooks with, and serves, negative calorie foods. It doesn't take the discipline of a navy SEAL—only creativity and confidence. Don't be timid or quiet when it comes to tailoring your order in the name of your weight!

When building your meals at restaurants, avoid fattening fare and keep the following configurations in mind.

Breakfast: 1 lean protein (such as egg white) + negative calorie veggies like spinach, tomatoes, and mushrooms OR 1 grain + a negative calorie fruit OR 1 lean protein + a negative calorie fruit.

Lunch: 1 lean protein + 2 or more negative calorie vegetables (including a green leafy salad) + 1 negative calorie fruit, if desired.

Dinner: 1 lean protein + 2 or more negative calorie vegetables (including a green leafy salad) + 1 negative calorie fruit, if desired.

On-the-Go Snacks: Carry with you small baggies of nuts, cut-up raw negative calorie veggies, and some fresh negative calorie fruits such as apples or berries.

For more specific guidance on what to eat when you're dining out, I've put together the following guidelines, which cover a full range of restaurants. For each, I've compiled a list of 10 sample negative calorie meals you can build at these establishments, and also called out what you want to avoid. Use this information to plan ahead and identify negative calorie food choices so you don't become overwhelmed by huge menus and won't give in to impulse ordering.

AMERICAN-STYLE CHAIN RESTAURANTS

(Such as Applebee's, Chili's, Ruby Tuesday, or TGI Fridays)

I used to think these chains were absolutely off-limits, but now that some of them have modified their menus, I've modified my stance—they are okay as a last resort if you order responsibly. That means sticking to whole foods that are organic whenever possible, and made fresh. Look for offerings on the menu listed as "light" or "guiltless." Here are some common examples of choices that fit the Negative Calorie bill:

1. Grilled sirloin and portobello mushrooms
2. Grilled chicken salad with oil and vinegar dressing on the side
3. Seafood salad (such as fresh greens topped with grilled shrimp) with oil and vinegar dressing on the side
4. Grilled salmon with broccoli, or any fresh fish dinner, and seasonal vegetables and a garden salad with oil and vinegar dressing on the side
5. Grilled sirloin with roasted tomatoes and mixed greens with oil and vinegar dressing on the side
6. Grilled chicken, steamed vegetables, and a salad with oil and vinegar dressing on the side
7. White bean chicken chili
8. Apple, cranberry, and spinach salad with oil and vinegar dressing on the side
9. Grilled turkey burger with steamed broccoli
10. Veggie trio: Choose three negative calorie sides to create your own meatless meal: steamed broccoli, roasted tomatoes, and a side salad, for example.

WHAT TO AVOID Fried entrées, fatty beef burgers, sandwiches, and anything laden with sauces

ASIAN RESTAURANTS

When I was a kid growing up in the Jamaica neighborhood of Queens, we sometimes went to a Chinese take-out place near our house. We always ordered the exact same things: wonton soup, shrimp with lobster sauce, and roast pork fried rice—complete with a side of egg rolls, of course. The meal was always fantastic, and the food was an inspiration to me—a gateway to Asian flavors, which became a huge part of my repertoire as a chef. So Asian food is near and dear to my heart. I love it even more these days because so much of it is healthy and easy to include on a weight-loss plan. The main thing to be aware of when you're ordering Asian food is that it tends to be sauce-heavy. Try to avoid anything coated in sauce, and limit your intake of soy sauce, which is high in sodium (even the low-sodium version is very salty). Here are some suggestions for what to order while you're following the Negative Calorie Diet:

1. Carb-free vegetarian lettuce wraps, or summer rolls, made with items such as wok-seared tofu, red onions, nuts, and water chestnuts, or other vegetables
2. Soup (healthy choices include broth-based soups such as egg drop, miso, or hot and sour soup), and seaweed salad
3. Steamed dishes, such as chow mein, lo mein, or chop suey, with steamed brown rice on the side

4. Sushi made with raw fish, vegetables, and preferably brown rice. Avoid sushi made with mayonnaise or suspect "spicy" sauces.

5. Sashimi and seaweed salad, a cucumber salad, or a simple house salad with carrot-ginger dressing on the side

6. Szechuan-style bean curd with steamed vegetables

7. Steamed edamame (soybeans in pods) and seaweed salad, a cucumber salad, or a simple house salad with carrot-ginger dressing on the side

8. Teriyaki chicken or beef with steamed vegetables

9. Vegetable-based entrées if steamed or stir-fried using a minimal amount of oil

10. Moo shi (steamed vegetables, chicken, and shrimp)

WHAT TO AVOID Spareribs, duck, General Tso's chicken, egg rolls, fried wontons, orange chicken, sesame chicken, sweet-and-sour entrées, fried entrées, and anything coated with sticky, heavy sauce

BARBECUE RESTAURANTS

When you think of barbecue joints, you probably think juicy, meaty ribs. It doesn't get much better than that, right? But if you eat too many BBQ ribs, you'll be barely able to see or touch your own. Even so, don't be afraid to venture into a barbecue restaurant. With so many grilled proteins on the menu, there are plenty of healthy options available. Here are a few ideas:

1. Roasted chicken with a side of green beans
2. Char-grilled chicken breasts with a side of green beans or vinegar-based coleslaw

3. Beef brisket with a simple house salad with oil and vinegar dressing on the side, or vinegar-based coleslaw

4. Grilled shrimp and a simple house salad with oil and vinegar dressing on the side

5. Blackened catfish and a simple house salad with oil and vinegar dressing on the side

6. Baby back ribs with green beans

7. Smoked barbecue turkey with vinegar-based coleslaw, sliced onion, and dill pickle

8. Pulled pork with vinegar-based coleslaw, sliced onion, and dill pickle

9. BBQ chicken over a bed of greens, with oil and vinegar dressing on the side

10. Grilled salmon with a side order of green beans or a simple house salad with oil and vinegar dressing on the side

WHAT TO AVOID Spareribs, wings, fried entrées, sandwiches, and anything laden with barbecue sauce

BREAKFAST RESTAURANTS

I love eating breakfast out. Have someone serve me piping hot espresso and scrambled eggs or a perfect omelet, and I'm in food heaven. Apparently I'm not the only fan of dining out in the morning. According to a consumer analyst firm called NPD Group, nearly 14 percent of us have breakfast away from home each day. If you rank among this group and regularly eat breakfast out, aim for meals that contain fiber and lean protein. Here are your 10 best negative calorie bets for breakfast:

1. Vegetable omelet with spinach, tomatoes, and mushrooms

2. Scrambled egg whites with vegetables (such as spinach, tomatoes, and mushrooms)
3. Turkey bacon and seasonal fresh fruit
4. Oatmeal and seasonal fresh fruit
5. Grits and seasonal fresh fruit
6. Turkey sausage and seasonal fresh fruit
7. Greek yogurt with a sprinkling of nuts and seasonal fresh fruit
8. Scrambled eggs and sliced tomato
9. Lox and seasonal fresh fruit
10. Smoothie made with plenty of negative calorie fruits and even some greens, if possible

WHAT TO AVOID Fried eggs, hash browns, pancakes, waffles, country ham, muffins and pastries, sausage, bacon, quiche, and crepes.

DELI RESTAURANTS

I love delis. As a New Yorker I grew up with some of the best delis in the world at my doorstep, and the simple, inexpensive food served in these places never goes out of style. And there's plenty of it on most delis' extensive menus—including numerous choices that fit right into the Negative Calorie lifestyle.

1. Broth-based soups such as chicken, vegetable, and barley soup
2. All-vegetable salad, in which you choose a leafy-green base and pile your favorite fresh negative calorie veggies as high as you would like.
3. Grilled chicken over fresh greens with oil and vinegar dressing on the side
4. Smoked salmon (lox) with a green salad with oil and vinegar dressing on the side

5. A Greek salad (go easy on the feta) with oil and vinegar dressing on the side
6. Fresh fruit and low-fat Greek yogurt parfait (hold the granola)
7. Chicken breast or rotisserie chicken
8. Veggie or turkey burger with lettuce, tomato, pickles, and no bun
9. A bowl of chicken or turkey chili
10. A lettuce wrap made of lean deli meat such as fresh turkey or chicken with mustard and pickles

WHAT TO AVOID Sandwiches, pasta, mayo-based salads, fatty meats such as pastrami and corned beef, Reuben sandwiches, and french fries

FAST FOOD

I'll probably go to chef hell for even mentioning fast food restaurants, but there are some choices that will allow you to eat fast food and still stay true to the Negative Calorie Diet. Keep in mind, too, that many fast food meals pile on enough food for an army, even though they pretend to be a "single serving." Stay away from those heavily advertised supersized and value-sized meals, and go for the smallest portion—even a child's portion, if you have to. Better choices include:

1. Southwest salad (no tortilla bowls or strips)
2. Chicken Caesar garden salad
3. Grilled chicken breast, green beans, and coleslaw (at a fried chicken establishment)
4. Grilled chicken with a side salad
5. Rotisserie chicken with steamed vegetables

6. Any broiled hamburger (toss out the bun) with a side salad
7. Salad bar entrée salad, choosing mostly negative calorie vegetables and lean protein
8. Roast beef (skip the bun) with a side salad
9. Charbroiled turkey burger (skip the bun) with a side salad
10. Baked fish with steamed vegetables

WHAT TO AVOID Everything except what I've listed!

FRENCH RESTAURANTS

If I were on death row and had to order my last meal, it would be a French dish, swimming in cheese sauce. But before my mouth starts watering too much, let me say that you shouldn't be intimidated by French food, nor do you have to succumb to cheese or cream sauces. A lot of French food is really not that rich or fattening at all, and can be worked into the Negative Calorie Diet any day of the week. Take a look:

1. Bouillabaisse: a broth-based fish stew
2. Salmon tartare with a salad and a light vinegar-based dressing
3. Navarin: a lamb and vegetable stew
4. Any roasted meat or poultry and a vegetable salad with a light vinegar-based dressing
5. Any braised meat or poultry and a vegetable salad with a light vinegar-based dressing
6. Grilled fish and a vegetable salad with a light vinegar-based dressing
7. Steak au poivre and a vegetable salad with a light vinegar-based dressing
8. Salade niçoise—skip the potatoes

9. Grilled frog legs and a vegetable salad with a light vinegar-based dressing
10. Beef bourguignon with sautéed vegetables

WHAT TO AVOID Any entrée that is fried or served in a heavy sauce; and, of course, it's better to skip the cheese plate and desserts!

GREEK RESTAURANTS

I love Greek food, and the world can't have enough Greek restaurants, in my opinion. Whenever I see a Greek menu and I'm trying to eat healthy, I fall more in love with this vegetable- and lean protein–rich cuisine. You can rarely go astray at a Greek restaurant. Here are a few of my top picks:

1. Vegetable kebabs
2. Souvlaki (kebabs made of chicken, lamb, or pork)
3. Charbroiled portobellos, zucchini, peppers, onions, and tomato, served with a small Greek salad, with oil and vinegar dressing on the side
4. Dinner-size Greek salad
5. Quinoa salad
6. Serving of hummus with cucumbers or other veggies for dipping—nix the pita bread
7. Stuffed grape leaves (dolmades), served with a small Greek salad, with oil and vinegar dressing on the side
8. Vegetarian plate with hummus, *baba ganoush*, and raw vegetables for dipping, served with a small Greek salad with oil and vinegar dressing on the side
9. Kakavia soup: a traditional Greek fisherman's soup, typically made with the catch of the day,

or whatever is seasonal, like snapper, mullet, or whitefish

10. Any seafood meal that is grilled, pan-seared, or broiled, and not fried, and offers a side of fresh vegetables or a salad

WHAT TO AVOID Gyros, moussaka, spinach pie, and baklava

INDIAN RESTAURANTS

When I'm not in my own kitchen and I have a rare evening off, I like to drop in at an Indian restaurant. Like most ethnic foods, Indian food has a good side and a bad side. The good side is that this cuisine includes lots of grains, is high in fiber, and has less fatty animal protein. Legumes and vegetables are also commonly used—another plus, especially if you're a vegan or vegetarian. The bad side is that much of the food is fried or sautéed. However, there are plenty of healthy selections you can make:

1. Chicken or shrimp cooked tandoori style
2. Dal: a lentil dish low in fat that is made with two negative calorie vegetables, tomatoes and cauliflower. When ordering dal, skip the rice.
3. Curried chickpeas
4. Curried fish, as long as it isn't fried
5. Lentil soup
6. Chicken or beef tikka (this is a roasted, mildly spiced dish)
7. Gobhi matar tamatar (this is a great vegetarian dish made with cauliflower, peas, and tomatoes—all helpful in fat-burning)
8. Curried vegetables
9. Chicken vindaloo

10. Lassi—here's a dessert that is basically a smoothie, made by blending together fruit, ice, and yogurt

WHAT TO AVOID Items made with coconut milk or cream; fried or fat-laden bread (papadums, chapati, naan, kulcha, or roti); heavily fried entrées

ITALIAN RESTAURANTS

It's Friday night and your friends want to meet at an Italian restaurant. The worried monologue in your head begins: *"How am I going to manage eating well with all that pasta?"* Here's how, with these choices:

1. Tuscan grilled steak and a side salad with oil and vinegar dressing on the side
2. Chicken cacciatore without pasta (Always check to see if you can substitute spaghetti squash for pasta.)
3. Minestrone and a side salad with oil and vinegar dressing on the side
4. Caesar salad with grilled chicken or shrimp with dressing on the side
5. Cold vegetable salads can be a delicious choice; drizzle with a little olive oil
6. Grilled chicken and a side salad, with oil and vinegar dressing on the side, or a tomato-cucumber salad
7. Grilled fish and side salad with oil and vinegar dressing on the side, or a tomato-cucumber salad
8. Grilled veal and a side salad with oil and vinegar dressing on the side, or a tomato-cucumber salad

MY 10 TRIED-AND-TRUE TIPS FOR EATING OUT, NEGATIVE CALORIE STYLE

1. When ordering a salad, ask for the dressing on the side. Select a simple vinaigrette, or ask for oil and vinegar.

2. Request healthier substitutions such as side salads, fresh fruit, or steamed vegetables for fried options such as fries, onion rings, or hash browns.

3. Eat baked or grilled chicken instead of fried chicken. The same goes for broiled or baked or grilled fish instead of fried fish.

4. Know the label lingo. Entrées described as fried, batter-fried, breaded, creamy, crispy, scalloped, or au gratin are going to be heavy on the calories. The same goes for dishes that come in butter or cream sauce.

5. Be assertive and request special orders. Restaurants want to make you happy and earn repeat customers—you're spending the bucks—so generally they will accommodate you by tweaking a dish to make it healthier or by offering substitutions. All you have to do is speak up and ask. For instance, you can ask to skip the sauce, or have the dressing on the side. Ask the server to not even bring the bread basket or dessert menu.

6. Learn to share. Portions in restaurants are as big as Jupiter. Split your entrée with a friend, or have half of it boxed up for tomorrow's lunch or dinner.

7. Pump the fluids. Remember, water is the ultimate negative calorie nutrient. When your server asks you, "What would you like to drink?" ask for water with some fat-burning lemon wedges.

8. Plan ahead. A little research goes a long way. Put together a list of your favorite restaurants that serve great negative calorie choices, even in the towns or cities you visit while traveling.

9. Travel light. Dieting while traveling amounts to a dietary no-man's-land. Here's what I suggest: When going on the road, make up a snack kit, filled with nuts, trail mix, and some fruit. Always have your kit with you to avoid eating garbage while traveling and to dodge food traps at airports. At restaurants, use the techniques I've suggested here to assemble a proper negative calorie meal.

10. Let people know. Informing hosts, relatives, and business associates ahead of time that you're watching your weight can help you avoid uncomfortable situations.

9. Chicken or veal marsala and side salad with oil and vinegar dressing on the side, or a tomato-cucumber salad

10. Lightly sautéed squid (no breading), with a side of Italian vegetables such as grilled zucchini or eggplant

WHAT TO AVOID Antipasto salads, entrées made with cream- and cheese-based sauces, chicken parmigiana, garlic bread, ravioli, eggplant parmigiana, meat lasagna, spaghetti with meatballs, fettuccine Alfredo, and gnocchi

MEXICAN RESTAURANTS

Mexican restaurants get an undeserved doubtful reputation, but only because of the ever-present and bottomless tortilla chips, cheese, and high-calorie margaritas. But the fact is, Mexican food *can* be enjoyed while you're on the Negative Calorie Diet. Order one of these the next time you go out for Mexican:

1. Ask for your fish to be steamed and/or covered with fresh tomatillo sauce

2. Grilled fish with a side salad with oil and vinegar dressing on the side

3. Mexican-seasoned grilled chicken with a side of vinegar-based (not creamy) coleslaw and pico de gallo

4. Black beans with a side salad with oil and vinegar dressing on the side

5. Fajita chicken, beef, or shrimp—hold the tortillas

6. Vegetable fajitas—hold the tortillas

7. Taco salad—skip the sour cream and the deep-fried, bowl-shaped tortilla

8. Carnitas (marinated grilled beef strips) with a side salad with oil and vinegar dressing on the side, or a vinegar-based (not creamy) coleslaw

9. Grilled chicken or vegetable tacos with soft corn (not fried) tortillas

10. Chicken mole—hold the rice and refried beans

WHAT TO AVOID Entrées labeled *grande*, *supreme*, or *combo*; fried stuff like tortilla chips, chimichangas, sour cream, and burritos

STEAK HOUSES

It's always a good idea to read the nutrition information published by restaurants, if you can. I did this one time with a steak house and was shocked to learn that a char-grilled rib eye had nearly 800 calories. (We're not counting calories, but that amount at one meal will mess with your diet.) So you have to be careful at steak houses. Watch your portion sizes, too. You don't have to eat the whole animal! Each serving of protein should be no bigger than the palm of your hand or a deck of cards. For protein, veer toward filet mignon, sirloin, chicken, or fish, paired up with veggies. For example:

1. Filet mignon or petite sirloin, a vegetable medley, and a tossed side salad with oil and vinegar dressing on the side

2. Grilled chicken breast, a vegetable medley, and a tossed side salad with oil and vinegar dressing on the side

3. Grilled salmon or tilapia, a vegetable medley, and a tossed side salad with oil and vinegar dressing on the side

4. Lobster tails or snow crab legs, a vegetable medley, and a tossed side salad with oil and vinegar dressing on the side

5. Grilled shrimp, a vegetable medley, and a tossed side salad with oil and vinegar dressing on the side

6. Large ahi tuna appetizer and a tossed side salad with oil and vinegar dressing on the side

7. Any entrée salad, or salad bar salad, but skip the croutons, cheese, and bacon, and choose a vinegar-based dressing

8. Grilled kebabs made with beef, chicken, or shrimp, and negative calorie vegetables such as bell peppers, tomatoes, and mushrooms

9. Plate of various types of steamed veggies, including negative calorie vegetables

10. Shrimp cocktail and a side salad with oil and vinegar dressing on the side

WHAT TO AVOID Huge portions of fatty meats such as rib eyes or prime rib; fried foods; any food laden with sauces; sides such as mashed potatoes, creamed spinach, or steak fries

Once you practice these negative calorie choices a few times, you'll create healthy habits that will become automatic when you are eating out. Remember, if you eat out infrequently, and especially if you are on maintenance—enjoy yourself. Allow yourself to have a special, memorable meal. If you eat out a lot and you're still trying to lose weight, then try to stick to the guidelines in this chapter to make sure you don't derail your progress.

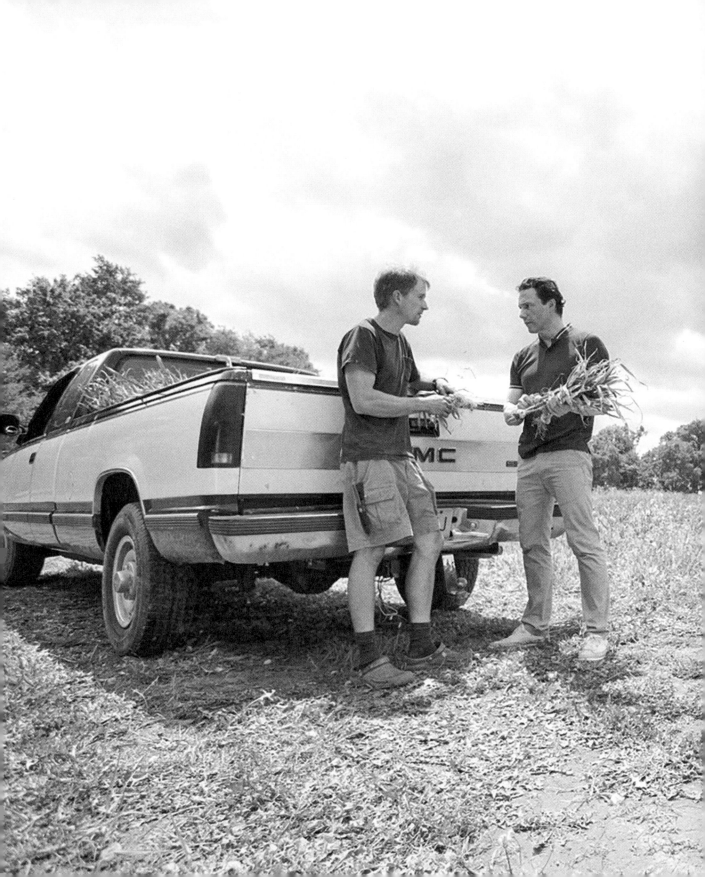

CHAPTER FIFTEEN

MAINTAIN—THE NEGATIVE CALORIE WAY

LOSING the weight is one thing; keeping that weight off is another endeavor altogether. I believe that weight maintenance, compared with pure dieting, is the new battleground in the war on obesity, which takes approximately 300,000 lives annually in the United States and racks up $100 billion in health costs each year. A diet can help us win the battle, but maintenance wins the war.

A lot of experts say that the hardest part of losing weight is keeping the pounds off over the long haul, and it's true that many people do struggle to maintain weight loss after a traditional "diet" ends.

One of the nice things about the Negative Calorie Diet is that it is sustainable as a lifestyle. This is because you're not eschewing any major food groups or drastically cutting back on your food intake; you're just switching over to healthier—but still delicious—foods. After spending 20 days following this plan, my clients are con-

verted; they feel great, they have more energy, their sugar cravings are gone, and their taste buds have changed. They don't want to go back to their old, unhealthy ways!

Weight maintenance, like weight loss, is dependent upon eating a diet rich in nutritious, thermogenic, and satiating foods—that means an emphasis on fruits, vegetables, and lean proteins. Don't fall into the trap of counting calories now that you're not following an official "plan"—you didn't need numbers before, and you don't need them now. It's just too darn easy to obsess over calories and lose focus on the bigger picture of nutrition. It can also be seductive to bargain with your food, *"Hmmm . . . I can have a piece of cheesecake for 350 calories, or six ounces of chicken breast for 320 calories."* Remember: a calorie is not a calorie. You want to eat for quality, not quantity.

THE NEGATIVE CALORIE MAINTENANCE PLAN

Now that you've reached your target, how do you avoid putting the pounds back on? The Negative Calorie Maintenance Plan simply builds on your new healthy habits. There is no mega change involved, no shaking up your lifestyle. Let common sense guide you, too, and choose mostly whole foods.

On maintenance, you get to add more variety back to your diet by reintroducing a wider range of quality starchy vegetables including potatoes, sweet potatoes, beets, turnips, winter squash, and additional beans and legumes. Be sure to keep portion sizes in mind—one portion is an average baking potato, sweet potato, beet, or turnip; ½ cup of beans or legumes; and 1 cup of winter squash. Have one portion a day if you wish.

BEANS, LEGUMES, AND STARCHY VEGETABLES

◊ Azuki beans
◊ Black beans
◊ Black-eyed peas
◊ Broad beans
◊ Chickpeas (garbanzo beans)
◊ Cranberry beans
◊ Fava beans
◊ Great northern beans
◊ Lentils
◊ Lima beans
◊ Navy beans
◊ Pink beans
◊ Pinto beans
◊ Red kidney beans
◊ Split peas, yellow or green
◊ White kidney beans
◊ Artichokes
◊ Beets
◊ Carrots
◊ Corn
◊ Parsnips
◊ Potatoes
◊ Peas
◊ Pumpkin
◊ Rutabaga
◊ Turnips
◊ Sweet potato
◊ Winter squash

You may also start to reincorporate more whole-grain foods such as pasta, brown rice, bread, and cereal. A portion is ½ cup of pasta, rice, or cooked cereal; 1 to 2 slices of bread, 1 bun, or 1 roll; 4 to 6 whole-grain crackers. Have one portion a day if you wish.

WHOLE-GRAIN FOODS

◊ Barley
◊ Brown rice
◊ Bulgur
◊ Couscous
◊ Miracle noodles and rice
◊ Oatmeal
◊ Oat bran
◊ Quinoa
◊ Pastas (try to stick with whole-grain, gluten-free, quinoa, or vegetable-based pastas, rather than refined white pastas)
◊ Wild rice

◇ Whole-grain, gluten-free, and sprouted-grain breads, buns, or rolls

For a healthy fat, you can eat more avocados on the maintenance plan: ¼ to ½ of a fruit daily, if you wish. You may also incorporate additional cheeses, if desired, such as goat cheese, feta, mozzarella, cheddar, or other hard cheeses—aim for no more than 2 ounces daily; and for cottage cheese or ricotta, no more than ½ cup daily.

Once you're down to your target weight, you can also add in some treats if you feel that you can enjoy them in moderation without overindulging. I like to suggest that people focus on eating clean during the week and save their treats for the weekends.

Naturally, you'll have to be careful with treats. If you continue with the negative calorie principles, you shouldn't experience cravings, but it can still be tricky to add in high-sugar or high-carb foods because they tend to lead us to overeat. Here are a few suggestions for how to handle treats:

• **Alcohol.** If you want a glass of wine, beer, or a cocktail with your evening meal, go ahead. Skip sugary concoctions and opt for a simple vodka, tequila, rum, gin, or whiskey on the rocks or mixed with club soda. As for wine, resist the urge to order a whole bottle. Just have a glass, sip it slowly, and alternate your sips with sips of water. If you want to be social but choose not to drink in situations where alcohol is flowing, do what I do: I have a tumbler of sparkling water or club soda, garnished with a wedge of lemon or lime, or blushed to a pale pink with a splash of cranberry juice.

• **Chocolate.** Choose dark chocolate that contains at least 60 percent cocoa, though 70 percent or greater is ideal, and preferably organic. This type of chocolate contains antioxidants, magnesium, and iron. Enjoy a couple of small squares a day, if you wish.

• **Desserts.** Allow yourself an occasional dessert. I'd be cautious here, though, because it's easy to reactivate a sweet tooth. Have no more than 2 (small) desserts a week, if any. If possible, choose desserts made with healthy ingredients such as organic eggs, whole meal or legume flour, healthier sweeteners like maple syrup or agave nectar, and so on. That way you'll be getting iron, fiber, B vitamins, magnesium, and other nutrients. If you eat healthy 90 percent of the time, you can afford the occasional treat.

SAMPLE MEAL CONFIGURATIONS ON THE NEGATIVE CALORIE MAINTENANCE PLAN

The food you'll eat on the maintenance plan won't be all that different from what you have been eating for the past 20 days. Take maintenance breakfasts, for example. The major difference now is that they can include cereal or a high-fiber muffin. Maintenance lunches are about the same as diet lunches. And maintenance dinners are similar to the ones on the diet plan, with the exception that meat portions are a bit larger and there is almost always a starch or carb, and an occasional dessert, if desired.

Let's take this meal by meal, and you'll see how Negative Calorie Maintenance works in real life.

MAINTENANCE BREAKFASTS

These can include any one of the following:

- **A NEGATIVE CALORIE SMOOTHIE** This makes the ultimate light on-the-go breakfast, and I encourage you to enjoy smoothies on maintenance. They start your day with a negative calorie punch of fruit, vegetables, and protein, as well as vitamins, minerals, antioxidants, and fiber, in one press of the blender button.

- **A HIGH-PROTEIN BREAKFAST** This may include several scrambled egg whites, or a couple of scrambled eggs, maybe some turkey bacon or sausage, plus a slice of whole-grain toast. Always include a serving of fresh fruit, preferably a negative calorie fruit. For variety, I like to have a different fresh negative calorie fruit each morning. But maintenance will work just as well if you have your favorite fruit every morning.

- **CEREAL AND FRUIT** This might include a bowl of oatmeal, quinoa, or some whole-grain cereal with berries or sliced banana. Add some unsweetened nondairy milk, such as almond milk, coconut milk, hemp milk, flax milk, or cashew milk for, an extra pump of flavor and protein.

- **NEGATIVE CALORIE DIET BREAKFAST RECIPES** Continue to include your favorites at breakfast. Don't ditch the recipes just because the "diet" part is over. These recipes will help you maintain your weight loss, and you're already a pro at making them!

For any breakfast, have your choice of tea (green is best) or coffee. Add a splash of nondairy milk if you like.

MAINTENANCE LUNCHES

You have a variety of choices here:

- **SALADS** You can't go wrong with leafy greens. When building a salad, choose as many negative calorie veggies as possible and top it off with a lean protein (either animal or plant-based). Add in some healthy fats like avocado slices and a simple dressing of olive oil and freshly squeezed lemon juice, and you've got a salad that will keep you full all day long.

- **SOUP** Here's another hearty, fat-burning bet. Stick with broth-based soups like vegetable soups, as well as protein-rich soups like lentil or pea soup. Avoid creamy soups such as "cream of" anything, bisques, or heavy chowders. Pair a bowl of soup with a small salad for a full meal.

- **SANDWICHES** Enjoy sandwiches now that you're on maintenance. Between two slices of whole-grain or sprouted-grain bread, place veggies, tuna, leftover chicken, mashed avocado, hummus, or whatever you like.

- LIQUID LUNCH Some days when I'm slammed for time, it's more convenient to drink my lunch, and that means a negative calorie smoothie, made at home and packed in a thermos. My negative calorie smoothies make terrific meal replacements.

- NEGATIVE CALORIE DIET LUNCH RECIPES Keep these in your lunch repertoire as go-to meals you already know and love!

MAINTENANCE DINNERS

I recommend eating a lean protein at dinner, such as grilled, roasted, or baked fish, shellfish, chicken, turkey, lean beef, or a vegetarian protein source. Pair your protein of choice with a heap of negative calorie vegetables and a green salad. You can also include a moderate serving of starch: ½ cup of brown rice perhaps, ½ cup of whole wheat or quinoa pasta, a baked potato or sweet potato, ½ cup of beans or legumes, or a cup of a starchy vegetables such as mashed winter squash, turnips, or parsnips. A dessert is permissible, too, up to twice a week. Or enjoy one of my negative calorie desserts, which are unlimited.

MAINTENANCE SNACKS

You'll rarely be hungry on maintenance if you continue to follow negative calorie principles, but when hunger does strike, you have lots of options:

- A negative calorie smoothie
- Fresh fruit and nuts
- A cup of broth-based soup, including any of my negative calorie soups

- Sliced cucumbers or other raw veggies to dip in hummus
- 2 ounces of cheese and 4 to 6 whole-grain crackers
- Fresh fruit with ½ cup of cottage cheese
- 2 cups of air-popped popcorn
- 2 ounces of dark chocolate (about 2 small squares)
- Any one of my negative calorie snacks

DON'T FORGET YOUR FLUIDS

On maintenance, it's key to drink plenty of water throughout the day—I recommend 8 to 10 glasses. Water helps keep your metabolism running in high gear, improves digestion, hydrates your body, and tames hunger and cravings by keeping your stomach partially filled.

USE THE NEGATIVE CALORIE CLEANSE ON MAINTENANCE

Successful maintainers don't take any chances and don't let pounds creep up on them. If you gain a few pounds, or if your clothes start to feel tight, do something about it right away. It's as simple as resuming the Negative Calorie Cleanse for three to five days. When you infuse your body with whole, nutritious foods it will begin to purge toxins naturally—and burn fat, where toxins are often stored. You can drop 3 to 5 pounds, maybe more, by doing the cleanse on a short-term basis. Use the cleanse as often as you wish to lose pounds you've regained, and keep using it as a weight-control tool.

THE EXERCISE FACTOR

Another vital tool in weight control is exercise, an important factor that helps put you in a negative calorie balance.

Exercise builds lean muscle mass. The more muscle you have, the faster your metabolism is and the more efficiently your body burns stored energy. As well as burning fat and accelerating your metabolism, exercise can help boost energy and immunity and reduce stress—all of which can only help with weight control and maintenance.

I'm no trainer, but I think the key to staying in shape is to incorporate both cardio and resistance training into your workout regimen. Cardio is a real fat-burner, so choose an activity you enjoy, or alternate among several. For fat loss, you probably want to exercise about four times a week. Research has found that many successful maintainers keep their weight off by walking four miles a day, seven days a week, on average. Others do more vigorous activity such as jogging, running, or aerobic dancing to keep their weight in check. For even greater fat loss and more lean muscle mass, add resistance training to your workouts, using weights, resistance bands, or even your own body weight.

Another good way to increase your metabolic rate is to stay as active during the day as possible. Park an extra block from work and walk up the stairs instead of taking the elevator or escalator. If you sit in an office all day, try to break up your day and stand for part of it. If you can expend energy every day through simple activities, you'll tip your energy balance into the fat-burning column.

One final suggestion regarding exercise: Time a negative calorie smoothie with your exercise session. If you drink one of my smoothies within 30 to 60 minutes after exercising (especially after resistance training), you'll help maximize muscle growth and replace spent energy stores.

Here's how: The smoothie contains proteins and carbs, all with their own distinct jobs. Protein supplies amino acids, essentially the building blocks used to manufacture muscle. While exercise breaks down muscle fibers, muscle growth doesn't start until after your workout. That's when protein comes in. If you supply your body with protein shortly after exercising, amino acids are pulled into the muscle, priming it to repair and build after a hard bout at the gym.

As for carbs, they replenish muscle glycogen (stored carbohydrates that supply energy). The addition of protein assists this process, so you see, both nutrients work together to generate muscle recovery and development.

LIVING A DELICIOUSLY HEALTHY LIFE

For me, living as long as I can means living as well as I can—maintaining a vibrant mind and sound body well into my golden years. I know I can increase my odds of achieving that goal by eating a nutritious diet, staying at a healthy weight, and working out consistently. Almost weekly, researchers report on the long-term advantages of maintaining a healthy lifestyle. Here are just a few reasons why it pays to clean up your diet:

LOWER CANCER RISK

The American Cancer Society (ACS) recently published a paper titled "Body Weight and Cancer Risk," enumerating the types of cancers related to being overweight or obese. These include the following kinds of cancers:

- Breast (in postmenopausal women)
- Cervix
- Colon and rectum
- Endometrium (lining of the uterus)
- Esophagus
- Gallbladder
- Kidney
- Liver
- Multiple myeloma
- Non-Hodgkin's lymphoma
- Ovary
- Pancreas
- Prostate (aggressive forms of prostate cancer)

The ACS explains that excess body weight increases cancer risk in several ways, namely by weakening the immune system, increasing inflammation in the body, affecting the balance of certain hormones (such as insulin and estrogen), misregulating cell division, and interfering with proteins that influence how the body uses certain hormones.

Scientists are still learning how shedding weight can help lower your risks, but there is growing evidence that weight loss can cut your risk of many cancers. Losing weight by eating nutritious foods can be preventive medicine. Who wouldn't want to decrease the risk of cancer just by eating a healthy, whole foods diet? It's a no-brainer.

BETTER HEART HEALTH

I know firsthand about the impact of weight loss on heart health. About ten years ago, my doctor took a look at my blood pressure and cholesterol numbers and asked if I had plans to buy a burial plot anytime soon. I was shocked. At the time, I was working as a restaurant chef, eating and tasting great but fattening food all day long, and the weight had crept on, especially around my stomach. So I had this big belly. That was scary because I knew that weight carried around the middle is the most dangerous to health. Needless to say, I changed my diet and started exercising. I even competed in a bunch of marathons. The weight came down, and so did the blood pressure and cholesterol numbers.

Losing weight—even just 5 to 10 percent of your weight—confers several benefits on the heart. First, weight loss reduces the workload of the heart so that there's less pressure on blood vessels. When you drop pounds, your blood pressure drops back into a healthy range, too.

Then there's the issue of blood fats: triglycerides, LDL cholesterol (the "lousy" kind), and HDL cholesterol (the "happy" type). Losing weight can reduce your triglycerides, lower your LDL, and increase your HDL. When all three events occur, you've got more good cholesterol and less bad cholesterol and fat roaming around in your bloodstream. This means your body is less likely to form plaque that can clog your coronary arteries.

Weight loss can also prevent the formation of abnormal blood clots, which can form when blood flow throughout the body slows down. Blood clots are deadly because they can travel to your heart, lungs, or brain and cause a heart attack or stroke. Maintaining a healthy weight and normal blood pressure means a reduced risk of blood clots.

When I started to shape up all those years ago, the first positive thing I noticed was that I was losing belly fat. A 2013 study reported in *Internal Medicine News* explained that it's not obesity per se that raises cardiovascular risk; it's where the excess body fat is stored. And the worst kind of storage fat is "visceral abdominal fat," which is located deep within the stomach area—and was the kind I had. The study found that people with a lot of this visceral fat who were younger than 40 years old (that was me!) had a greater risk for cardiovascular disease than did those over 40. This tells me that visceral abdominal tissue is riskier for the young. Great lesson: The earlier you lose that beer belly or muffin top, the better!

STAY SHARP

If you're bulking up around your waist, that spells trouble for your brain, too. Being overweight or obese can harm cognitive abilities, especially as a person ages. The good news is that there is evidence that losing weight might help reverse some of these adverse effects.

In a study published in the *Journal of the American College of Nutrition* in 2012, researchers assessed 50 obese men and women before and after they followed a diet at the weight-loss clinic. The scientists administered tests of cognitive function and found that after the dieters lost 8 to 12 percent of their body weight, their scores on the cognitive tests significantly improved. The

scientists concluded that "weight loss can significantly affect public health strategies for the prevention of dementia."

Why does obesity hurt the brain? One reason, researchers believe, is that obesity causes inflammation, which may be linked to the deterioration of blood vessels in the brain.

Certain negative calorie foods not only help you shed weight but also may protect your brain. These foods include cruciferous and green leafy vegetables as well as fruits like berries and oranges. All of these foods are high in antioxidants, which have been shown to decrease inflammation in the body. Other brain-protecting foods include fish, which contain omega-3 fatty acids, and nuts, which are a great source of vitamin E (another antioxidant).

BOOST YOUR MOOD

Researchers aren't clear about whether obesity causes depression or depression causes obesity. But a study published in *Diabetes Care* in 2014 suggests that losing weight could help improve mood.

Scientists investigated whether losing weight could ease depression in the short term and long run. They assessed levels of depression in individual who were both obese and diabetic, prior to the study, annually at years 1 through 8, and again at year 8. Initially, the participants were put on a diet of 1,200 to 1,800 calories a day, designed to help them lose 7 percent or more of their body weight over a year.

By the end of the first year, the study found that the diet and the weight loss it produced significantly reduced mild and more severe depression. Over 8 years of follow-up, the weight loss also helped prevent depression and reduced the risk of more severe depression in people who had mild symptoms.

According to many nutritionists and doctors, what you eat while losing weight can also affect your mood. There are foods, for example, that boost serotonin—the natural "feel-good" chemical in the brain. Kiwi fruits, bananas, plums, pineapple, cherries, tomatoes, and walnuts all help to increase serotonin production.

Adding tryptophan to your diet has also been shown to improve your mood, as it increases serotonin production in the brain. Foods high in tryptophan include poultry, fish, cottage cheese, nuts, eggs, and legumes.

Finally, you want to eat plenty of foods rich in vitamin B_6. This vitamin is essential for the creation of brain chemicals such as dopamine and serotonin. Foods rich in this vitamin include brown rice, chicken, eggs, green leafy vegetables, legumes, nuts, and peas.

Clearly, being overweight may make you vulnerable to life-shortening diseases, cognitive decline, mood problems, and other conditions. But I don't want to dwell too much on the risks. I'd rather think about how maintaining a healthy weight and eating whole foods can help your heart, brain, and other organs stay healthy and carry you through a long, happy life.

As for me, working in the healthy food and lifestyle business has truly changed my life; I'm healthier than ever before, and every day I learn something new about nutrition and how we can harness the power of whole foods to live better. It's also incredibly rewarding for me to witness the positive changes in my clients who ditch processed foods and switch over to a diet of fresh, organic whole foods. They are walking, talking proof that if you put the effort into taking care of your body, you can change your life.

A healthy, delicious lifestyle is about what you do most of the time—making smart food choices, buying the best-quality food you can find and afford, and getting in plenty of physical activity whenever you can. When you live like this, you feel inspired to stay the course, and you have the energy and vitality you need to do everything you love and dream about.

I hope that the Negative Calorie Diet will become a positive lifestyle change for you and your family. My highest wish is for you to use the information in this book to become the healthiest and happiest possible version of you—and to love your healthy, delicious life more than you ever thought possible.

My best to you,
Rocco DiSpirito

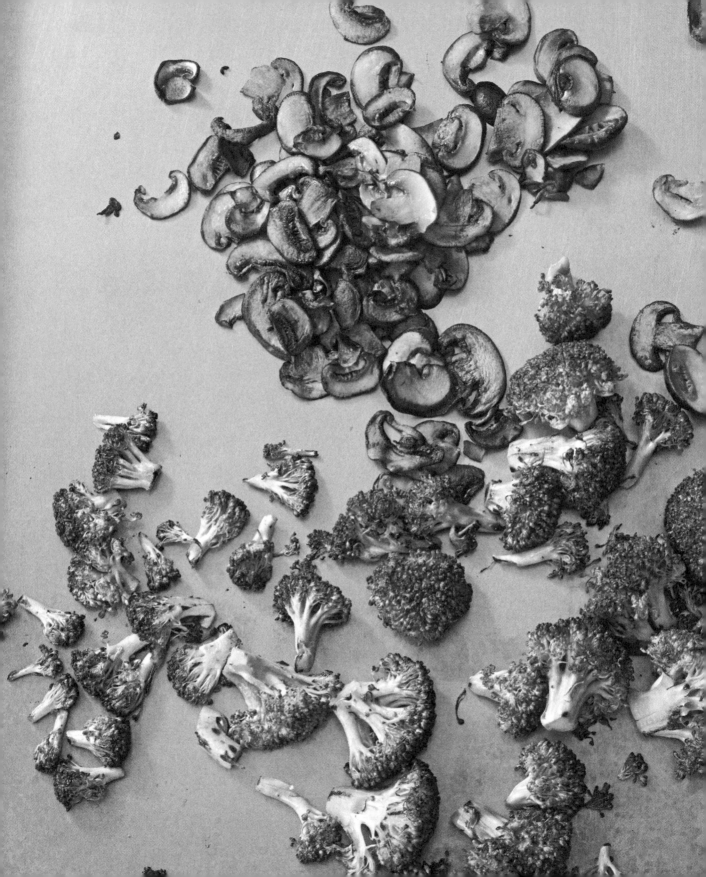

INDEX

Page numbers in *italics* refer to illustrations.

A

acacia fiber, 69

alcohol, 8, 35, 36, 259
    abstinence, 36

allergens, 31, 35

allergies, 18, 35, 36

Almond-Encrusted Flounder with Chopped Spinach and Clam Broth, 152–54, *153–55*

almond milk, 7, 82, 91
    homemade, 91

almonds, 6, 11–12
    Almond-Encrusted Flounder with Chopped Spinach and Clam Broth, 152–54, *153–55*
    Almond Vanilla Protein Smoothie, 90, *91*
    Apple, Cranberry, and Almond Bars, 200, *201*
    Apple and Cinnamon Breakfast "Risotto" with Oat Bran and Almonds, 100, *101*
    Cauliflower and Apples with Thai Almond Butter Sauce, 202, *203*
    Charred Thai-Style Broccoli Salad with Almonds and Lime, 120, *121*
    Chocolate and Almond Butter Truffles, 216, *217*
    Chocolate-Dipped Strawberries with Crushed Almonds, 218, *219*
    Cocoa-Dusted Almonds, 220, *221*
    Cucumber and Almond Rice Sushi, 198, *199*
    Eggplant and Almond Dip with Celery, 204, *205*
    Instant Almond Cake with Mixed Berries, 222, *223*
    Leafy Green Salad with Creamy Almond Dressing and Radishes, 148, *149*
    as negative calorie food, 11–12
    Red Ants on a Log, 208, *209*
    Roasted Cauliflower with Green Peppers, Almond Curry, and Lime, 180–81, *181*
    Shaved Brussels Sprouts with Warm Toasted Garlic, Almond, and Lemon Dressing, 138, *139*
    Strawberry and Spinach Salad with Almonds and Basil, 140, *141*

Almond Vanilla Protein Smoothie, 90, *91*

alpha-linolenic acid (ALA), 236

amino acids, 8, 16, 232

antibiotics, in food, 9, 21, 26, 27

Apple, Cranberry, and Almond Bars, 200, *201*

Apple and Cinnamon Breakfast "Risotto" with Oat Bran and Almonds, 100, *101*

Apple-Lime-Cilantro Protein Smoothie, 72, *73*

apples, 12
    Apple, Cranberry, and Almond Bars, 210, *211*
    Apple and Cinnamon Breakfast "Risotto" with Oat Bran and Almonds, 100, *101*
    Apple-Lime-Cilantro Protein Smoothie, 72, *73*
    Cauliflower and Apples with Thai Almond Butter Sauce, 202, *203*
    Crabmeat Salad with Apple, Celery, and Leafy Greens, 122, *123*
    Flank Steak Salad with Horseradish and Apple, 128, *129*
    Grate Salad Bowl with Chia Seed Dressing, 144, *145*
    Lemon-Ginger Smoothie, 80, *81*
    as negative calorie food, 12
    Peanutty Apple Slices, 206, *207*
    Rocco's Raw Applesauce, 212, *213*
    Spiced Apple Pie Smoothie, 92, *93*

Applesauce, Rocco's Raw, 212, *213*

arrowroot, 176

arthritis, 30

Asian Curry Mussel Soup, 136, *137*

Asian food, 248–49

avocado, 30, 259
    Avocado Toast with Spinach and Tomatoes, 110, *111*

B

bacteria, gut, 15

baharat, 172

Baked Chicken with Sweet-and-Sour Red Cabbage, 156, *157*

barbecue restaurants, 249

barley, 35

basil:
    Blueberry-Basil Smoothie, 94, *95*
    Breakfast Citrus Salad with Cucumbers and Basil, 104, *105*
    "Pappardelle" of Chicken with Winter Pesto, 177–78, *179*
    Spinach Pesto Pasta with Tomatoes, 191–92, *193–95*
    Strawberry and Spinach Salad with Almonds and Basil, 140, *141*

BCAAs, 232

beans and legumes, 54, 57, 258
  maintenance plan, 258
  in vegetarian diet, 232–34
  See also specific beans and legumes
beef, 4, 20, 26
  Beef-Stuffed Cabbage with Pepper and Tomato Goulash, 160–61, *161*
  Filet of Beef with Braised Kale and Black Olives, 167–68, *169*
  Flank Steak Salad with Horseradish and Apple, 128, *129*
  grass-fed, 20, 26
  hormones in, 21, 26, 27
  lean cuts, 20, 27
  Meatballs with Mushroom and Spinach Gravy, 174, *175*, 176
  organic, 20, 26, 27
  Sliced Pepper Steak with Swiss Chard and Mushrooms, 188, *189*, 190
  steakhouses, 254–55
  20-Day eating plan, 53, 57, 60
Beef-Stuffed Cabbage with Pepper and Tomato Goulash, 160–61, *161*
beets, 30
belly fat, 12, 20, 36, 263, 264
berries, 12–13
  Breakfast Bowl with Quinoa and Berries, 114, *115*
  Citrus-Berry Smash Smoothie, 96, *97*
  Citrus and Mixed Berry Bowl with Whipped Topping, 226, *227*
  Instant Almond Cake with Mixed Berries, 222, *223*
  as negative calorie food, 12–13
black pepper, 17, 172
beta-glucans, 18
blender, 61
blood clots, 263–64
blood pressure, 17, 263
  high, 17, 25, 30, 46, 243, 263
blood sugar, 5, 7, 13, 45, 233, 235
blueberries, 13
  Blueberry-Basil Smoothie, 94, *95*

Blueberry and Quinoa Porridge with Mint, 102, *103*
Breakfast Bowl with Quinoa and Berries, 114, *115*
Blueberry-Basil Smoothie, 94, *95*
Blueberry and Quinoa Porridge with Mint, 102, *103*
body mass index (BMI), 234–35
Bok Choy Stir-Fry, Shiitake and, 182, *183*
Bowl with Quinoa and Berries, Breakfast, 114, *115*
BPA, 27
brain, 7, 22, 35, 264
  fog, 35
  health, 264–65
bread, 4, 5, 7, 28
  Avocado Toast with Spinach and Tomatoes, 110, *111*
breakfast, 7, 50, 99–116, 237
  Apple and Cinnamon "Risotto" with Oat Bran and Almonds, 100, *101*
  Avocado Toast with Spinach and Tomatoes, 110, *111*
  Blueberry and Quinoa Porridge with Mint, 102, *103*
  Bowl with Quinoa and Berries, 114, *115*
  Citrus Salad with Cucumbers and Basil, 104, *105*
  Kale, Red Onion, and Tomato Frittata, 108, *109*
  maintenance, 259, 260
  Mexican Cauliflower Chili Scramble, 112–13, *113*
  Pizza with Mushrooms and Broccoli, 106–7, *107*
  restaurant, 247, 249–50
  Spinach and Mushroom Omelet, 116, *117*
  20-Day eating plan, 51–59, 61
  vegetarian, 237–39
broccoli, 7, 15, 30
  Breakfast Pizza with Mushrooms and Broccoli, 106–7, *107*
  Charred Thai-Style Broccoli Salad with Almonds and Lime, 120, *121*
  Grate Salad Bowl with Chia Seed Dressing, 144, *145*
  Green Goddess Smoothie, 74, *75*

Brussels sprouts, 15, 27, 30, 138
  Shaved Brussels Sprouts with Warm Toasted Garlic, Almond, and Lemon Dressing, 138, *139*

C

cabbage, 15, 30, 156
  Baked Chicken with Sweet-and-Sour Red Cabbage, 156, *157*
  Beef-Stuffed Cabbage with Pepper and Tomato Goulash, 160–61, *161*
  Grate Salad Bowl with Chia Seed Dressing, 144, *145*
  Shrimp and Cabbage Hot Pot with Chile Peppers, 184, *185*
caffeine, 36, 42
Cake with Mixed Berries, Instant Almond, 222, *223*
calcium, 23, 27
"Caldo Verde" with Chickpeas, Mixed Leafy Green Soup, 130, *131*
calories, 3–9, 257
  high vs. low quality, 3–7
cancer, 15, 30, 46, 138, 156
  lowering risk of, 263
canned foods, 40, 41
  20-Day eating plan, 54, 57, 60
Capers, Swiss Chard Turkey Salad with Golden Raisins and, 142, *143*
capsaicin, 18, 20
carbohydrates, 4, 5, 8, 45
  low-carb diet, 5
  processed, 6, 7, 8, 30, 33, 35
cardamom, 17
carnitine, 13, 14
cauliflower, 7, 15, 27, 30, 180
  Cauliflower and Apples with Thai Almond Butter Sauce, 202, *203*
  Grate Salad Bowl with Chia Seed Dressing, 144, *145*
  Grilled Shrimp with Marinated Cucumbers, Kale, and Cauliflower, 172, *173*
  Mexican Cauliflower Chili Scramble, 112–13, *113*
  Roasted Cauliflower with Green Peppers, Almond Curry, and Lime, 180–81, *181*

Cauliflower and Apples with Thai Almond Butter Sauce, 202, *203*
cayenne pepper, 17
celery, 13–14
	Crabmeat Salad with Apple, Celery, and Leafy Greens, 122, *123*
	Eggplant and Almond Dip with Celery, 204, *205*
	as negative calorie food, 13–14
	Red Ants on a Log, 208, *209*
celiac disease, 35
Celtic sea salt, 9, 178
cereals, 5, 7, 260
	20-Day eating plan, 53, 57
Charred Thai-Style Broccoli Salad with Almonds and Lime, 120, *121*
cheese, 54, 60, 237, 259
Chef Salad, Rocco's, 132, *133*
chemicals, 8, 15, 26–28, 29, 33
chia seeds, 235–36
	Grate Salad Bowl with Chia Seed Dressing, 144, *145*
chicken, 4, 8, 20–21, 26, 253
	Baked Chicken with Sweet-and-Sour Red Cabbage, 156, *157*
	Chicken with Mustard Greens, Quinoa, and Oranges, 162, *163*
	Chicken Soup with Escarole and Leeks, 124, *125*
	organic, 26, 27
	"Pappardelle" of Chicken with Winter Pesto, 177–78, *179*
	as protein source, 20–21
	20-Day eating plan, 53, 60
Chicken with Mustard Greens, Quinoa, and Oranges, 162, *163*
Chicken Soup with Escarole and Leeks, 124, *125*
chickpeas, 232
	Mixed Leafy Green Soup "Caldo Verde" with Chickpeas, 130, *131*
	in vegetarian diet, 232
childhood obesity, 242–43
chiles, 18
	Shrimp and Cabbage Hot Pot with Chile Peppers, 184, *185*
Chili Scramble, Mexican Cauliflower, 112–13, *113*

chocolate, 4, 259
	Chocolate and Almond Butter Truffles, 216, *217*
	Chocolate-Dipped Strawberries with Crushed Almonds, 218, *219*
	Cocoa-Dusted Almonds, 220, *221*
Chocolate and Almond Butter Truffles, 216, *217*
Chocolate-Dipped Strawberries with Crushed Almonds, 218, *219*
cholesterol, 12, 13, 16, 17, 18, 25, 77, 243, 263
Cilantro-Protein Smoothie, Apple-Lime, 72, *73*
cinnamon, 17
	Apple and Cinnamon Breakfast "Risotto" with Oat Bran and Almonds, 100, *101*
Citrus and Mixed Berry Bowl with Whipped Topping, 226, *227*
Citrus-Berry Smash Smoothie, 96, *97*
citrus fruits, 14–15
	Breakfast Citrus Salad with Cucumbers and Basil, 104, *105*
	Citrus-Berry Smash Smoothie, 96, *97*
	Citrus and Mixed Berry Bowl with Whipped Topping, 226, *227*
	as negative calorie food, 14–15
	Seared Tuna Tataki Salad with Citrus, Tofu, and Watercress, 134, *135*
	See also *specific fruits*
clams, 21
	Almond-Encrusted Flounder with Chopped Spinach and Clam Broth, 152–54, *153–55*
	as negative calorie food, 21
	as protein source, 21
Cocoa-Dusted Almonds, 220, *221*
cocoa powder, 9
coconut, 77
	milk, 27
	nectar, 9, 208
	Tropical Sunrise Smoothie, 76, *77*
coconut manna, 77

cod, 22
coffee, 36, 42
collard greens, 27
	Tropical Sunrise Smoothie, 76, *77*
condiments, 17, 51
	fat-burning, 17
	10-Day Negative Calorie Cleanse, 40, 42
	20-Day eating plan, 54, 58, 60
confidence, 46
configuration of eating, 62
conjugated linoleic acid (CLA), 20
corn, 30
crabmeat, 21, 122
	Crabmeat Salad with Apple, Celery, and Leafy Greens, 122, *123*
	as protein source, 21
Crabmeat Salad with Apple, Celery, and Leafy Greens, 122, *123*
cranberries:
	Apple, Cranberry, and Almond Bars, 210, *211*
	No-Sugar-Added Organic Cranberry Sauce, 200, *201*
	Red Ants on a Log, 208, *209*
cravings, handling, 42–43
Crepes Suzette with Oranges and Vanilla Cream, 224–25, *225*
cruciferous vegetables, 15, 30
Cucumber and Almond Rice Sushi, 198, *199*
cucumbers, 15–16
	Breakfast Citrus Salad with Cucumbers and Basil, 104, *105*
	Cucumber and Almond Rice Sushi, 198, *199*
	Cucumber-Strawberry Green Smoothie, 68, *69*
	Grilled Shrimp with Marinated Cucumbers, Kale, and Cauliflower, 172, *173*
	as negative calorie food, 15–16
	Shrimp and Cucumber Salad with Red Onion and Poblanos, 126, *127*
Cucumber-Strawberry Green Smoothie, 68, *69*
cumin, 17

Curry Mussel Soup, Asian, 136, *137*

D

dairy foods, 4, 237
    hormones in, 27
    sensitivity, 35
    20-Day eating plan, 54, 58, 60
delis, 250
dementia, 13, 15, 30
depression, 264–65
desserts, 214–27, 259
    Chocolate and Almond Butter
        Truffles, 216, *217*
    Chocolate-Dipped Strawberries
        with Crushed Almonds, 218,
        219
    Citrus and Mixed Berry Bowl with
        Whipped Topping, 226, *227*
    Cocoa-Dusted Almonds, 220,
        221
    Crepes Suzette with Oranges and
        Vanilla Cream, 224–25, *225*
    Instant Almond Cake with Mixed
        Berries, 222, *223*
detox, 6, 8, 33–43
    10-Day Negative Calorie Cleanse,
        8, 33–43
diabetes, 14, 16, 30, 36, 46, 243,
    264
dill, 78
"Dillicious" Green Smoothie, 78, *79*
DIM, 15
dinner, 50, 238
    maintenance, 259, 261
    restaurant, 247
    20-Day eating plan, 51–59, 61–62
    vegetarian, 237–39
    See also mains
dopamine, 22, 43, 265
drugs, 35

E

eating out. *See* restaurants
eczema, 30
eggplant, 18
    Asian Curry Mussel Soup, 136, *137*
    Eggplant and Almond Dip with
        Celery, 204, *205*
    Eggplant Roll-Ups, 164, *165*, 166

Flounder "a la Plancha" with
    Catalonian Eggplant Relish,
    170–71, *171*
Eggplant and Almond Dip with
    Celery, 204, *205*
Eggplant Roll-Ups, 164, *165*, 166
eggs, 21, 237, 260
    Kale, Red Onion, and Tomato
        Frittata, 108, *109*
    Mexican Cauliflower Chili
        Scramble, 112–13, *113*
    organic, 27
    as protein source, 21
    Spinach and Mushroom Omelet,
        116, *117*
    20-Day eating plan, 53, 57, 60
endocrine disruptors, 26–28
endorphins, 43
enzymes, 232
equipment, kitchen, 61
Escarole and Leeks, Chicken Soup
    with, 124, *125*
espresso, 36
estrogen, 15, 26, 27, 263
exercise, 6, 20, 33, 43, 262
    maintenance and, 262

F

family, 47, 241–45
    diet plan, 241–45
    meals, 244
    you're the only one on the diet,
        241–42
fast food, 28, 250
fat, 3–8, 12, 25, 30, 62, 237
    burn factor, 6–7
    low-fat diet, 5
fatigue, 34
fiber, 4, 7, 13, 14, 15, 16, 33, 34, 47,
    231
    acacia, 69
    insoluble, 15
    in vegetarian diets, 231–39
Filet of Beef with Braised Kale and
    Black Olives, 167–68, *169*
fisetin, 15
fish and shellfish, 4, 5, 8, 26, 122,
    253
    farm-raised, 26, 28
    as protein source, 21–23
    20-Day eating plan, 53, 57, 60

wild-caught, 26, 28, 31
    See also specific fish
Flank Steak Salad with Horseradish
    and Apple, 128, *129*
flounder, 21–22
Flounder "a la Plancha" with
    Catalonian Eggplant Relish,
    170–71, *171*
Flounder with Chopped Spinach
    and Clam Broth, Almond-
    Encrusted, 152–54, *153–55*
flour, white, 8, 30
Food and Drug Administration, 28
French food, 251
Frittata, Kale, Red Onion, and
    Tomato, 108, *109*
frozen foods, 40, 41
fruits, 4, 7, 9, 12, 13, 14–15, 25, 34,
    39, 45, 48, 237–39, 245, 260,
    264, 265
    citrus, 14–15
    local, 29
    organic, 26, 27–28, 30, 39
    10-Day Negative Calorie Cleanse,
        39, 41
    20-Day eating plan, 48, 50,
        52–53, 56, 59
    See also specific fruits
fullness factor, 7
fungicides, 26, 27–28

G

garlic, 17
    Shaved Brussels Sprouts with
        Warm Toasted Garlic, Almond,
        and Lemon Dressing, 138, *139*
ginger, 17, 31
    Lemon-Ginger Smoothie, 80, *81*
glutamate, 16, 18
gluten, 8, 28, 31, 35–36
    allergy, 35–36
GMO foods, 8, 25, 28–30, 36, 233
grains, 35–36
    maintenance plan, 258–59
    20-Day eating plan, 53, 57
    in vegetarian diets, 232–37
    See also specific grains
grapefruit, 14
    Breakfast Citrus Salad with
        Cucumbers and Basil, 104,
        105

Grate Salad Bowl with Chia Seed Dressing, 144, *145*
Greek food, 251
Green Goddess Smoothie, 74, 75
Greensicle Smoothie, Orange, 82, *83*
Green Smoothie, Cucumber-Strawberry, 68, *69*
Green Smoothie, "Dillicious," 78, *79*
green superfoods, 42
Grilled Shrimp with Marinated Cucumbers, Kale, and Cauliflower, 172, *173*

H
habaneros, 18
headaches, 35
healthier body, preparing for, 45–47
heart disease, 30, 46, 243, 264
heart health, 263–64
hemp, 27
    seeds, 232–33
herbs, 53, 57, 60
    10-Day Negative Calorie Cleanse, 40, 41
herring, 22
high-fructose corn syrup (HFCS), 27, 28, 30, 35
hormones, 13, 15, 16, 26, 263
    in food, 9, 15, 21, 26, 27
    obesogens, 26–28
    stress, 42
    thyroid, 21, 22, 26
horseradish, 17
    Flank Steak Salad with Horseradish and Apple, 128, *129*
hot peppers, 18–20
hummus, 232
hunger, 7, 20
    handling, 42–43
hydrogenated oils, 36
hypothyroidism, 21

I
immune system, 9, 263
Indian food, 252
indole-3-carbinol (I3C), 15

inflammation, 18, 30–31, 35, 36, 45, 263, 264
    avoiding, 30–31
    chronic, 30
Instant Almond Cake with Mixed Berries, 222, *223*
insulin, 16, 17, 36, 263
    resistance, 36, 236
iodine, 21, 23
iron, 20, 23
irritable bowel syndrome, 69
Italian food, 252, 254

J
jalapeños, 18
joint pain, 18, 46
juice cleanses, 33
junk food, 6, 8

K
kale, 16, 27, 30
    Cucumber-Strawberry Green Smoothie, 68, 69
    "Dillicious" Green Smoothie, 78, 79
    Filet of Beef with Braised Kale and Black Olives, 167–68, *169*
    Grilled Shrimp with Marinated Cucumbers, Kale, and Cauliflower, 172, *173*
    Kale, Red Onion, and Tomato Fritatta, 108, *109*
    Lemon-Ginger Smoothie, 80, *81*
Kale, Red Onion, and Tomato Fritatta, 108, *109*
kidney beans, 233
kidneys, 33
kitchen, setting up, 61

L
lactose, 31
    intolerance, 35
leafy greens, 16, 27
    Crabmeat Salad with Apple, Celery, and Leafy Greens, 122, *123*
    Leafy Green Salad with Creamy Almond Dressing and Radishes, 148, *149*

Mixed Leafy Green Soup "Caldo Verde" with Chickpeas, 130, *131*
    as negative calorie food, 16
    See also specific greens
Leafy Green Salad with Creamy Almond Dressing and Radishes, 146, *147*
Leafy Green Soup "Caldo Verde" with Chickpeas, Mixed, 130, *131*
leeks, 124
    Chicken Soup with Escarole and Leeks, 124, *125*
    Mushroom Bouillon with Leeks, Tofu, and Wasabi, 146, *147*
Lemon-Ginger Smoothie, 80, *81*
lemons, 14
    Lemon-Ginger Smoothie, 80, *81*
    Shaved Brussels Sprouts with Warm Toasted Garlic, Almond, and Lemon Dressing, 138, *139*
lentils, 233–34
leptin, 13, 20, 23, 26
limes, 14
    Apple-Lime-Cilantro Protein Smoothie, 72, *73*
    Charred Thai-Style Broccoli Salad with Almonds and Lime, 120, *121*
    Roasted Cauliflower with Green Peppers, Almond Curry, and Lime, 180–81, *181*
    Spinach, Pineapple, Lime, and Mint Smoothie, 70
    Tropical Sunrise Smoothie, 76, *77*
limonene, 14
liver, 6, 8 14, 33, 36
    detox, 6, 8
local foods, 29
lunch, 50, 238
    maintenance, 259, 260–61
    restaurant, 247
    20-Day eating plan, 51–59, 61
    vegetarian, 237–39

M
mackerel, 31
mains, 62, 150–95
    Almond-Encrusted Flounder with Chopped Spinach and Clam Broth, 152–54, *153–55*

mains (*cont.*)
  Baked Chicken with Sweet-and-
    Sour Red Cabbage, 156, *157*
  Beef-Stuffed Cabbage with
    Pepper and Tomato Goulash,
    160–61, *161*
  Chicken with Mustard Greens,
    Quinoa, and Oranges, 162, *163*
  Eggplant Roll-Ups, 164, *165*, 166
  Filet of Beef with Braised Kale
    and Black Olives, 167–68, *169*
  Flounder "A la Plancha" with
    Catalonian Eggplant Relish,
    170–71, *171*
  Grilled Shrimp with Marinated
    Cucumbers, Kale, and
    Cauliflower, 172, *173*
  Meatballs with Mushroom and
    Spinach Gravy, 174, *175*, 176
  "Pappardelle" of Chicken with
    Winter Pesto, 177–78, *179*
  Roasted Cauliflower with Green
    Peppers, Almond Curry, and
    Lime, 180–81, *181*
  Shiitake and Bok Choy Stir-Fry,
    182, *183*
  Shrimp and Cabbage Hot Pot
    with Chile Peppers, 184, *185*
  Shrimp with Mustard Greens,
    Mushrooms, and Miso, 186,
    187
  Sliced Pepper Steak with Swiss
    Chard and Mushrooms, 188,
    189, 190
  Spinach Pesto Pasta with
    Tomatoes, 191–92, *193–95*
  Vegetable Pot-au-Feu, 158–59,
    159
maintenance, weight, 257–65
  exercise, 262
  lifestyle, 263–65
  negative calorie cleanse, 261
  plan, 258–61
  sample meal configurations,
    259–61
meat, 4, 7, 8, 20–21, 50
  cutting back on, 237
  hormones in, 21, 26, 27
  organic, 20, 26, 27
  as protein source, 20–21, 23
  20-Day eating plan, 53, 57, 60
  See also specific meats

Meatballs with Mushroom and
    Spinach Gravy, 174, *175*, 176
memory loss, 13, 15, 30
menus, suggested, 51–59
  meatless, 238–39
metabolic syndrome, 14
metabolism, 4, 6, 7–8, 13, 21, 37
  fat burn factor, 6–7
  secrets revealed, 7–8
Mexican Cauliflower Chili Scramble,
    112–13, *113*
Mexican food, 254
Microplane, 61
milk, 27, 35, 54, 58, 60, 237
  almond, 27, 82, 83
  organic, 27
mint, 70
  Blueberry and Quinoa Porridge
    with Mint, 102, *103*
  Spinach, Pineapple, Lime, and
    Mint Smoothie, 70
miso, 134
  Shrimp with Mustard Greens,
    Mushrooms, and Miso, 186, *187*
Mixed Leafy Green Soup "Caldo
    Verde" with Chickpeas, 130, *131*
monk fruit extract, 9
mood improvement, 264–65
MSG, 27
muscle, 3, 6, 8, 262
Mushroom Bouillon with Leeks,
    Tofu, and Wasabi, 146, *147*
mushrooms, 16–18
  Breakfast Pizza with Mushrooms
    and Broccoli, 106–7, *107*
  Meatballs with Mushroom and
    Spinach Gravy, 174, *175*, 176
  Mushroom Bouillon with Leeks,
    Tofu, and Wasabi, 146, *147*
  as negative calorie food, 16–18
  Shiitake and Bok Choy Stir-Fry,
    182, *183*
  Shrimp with Mustard Greens,
    Mushrooms, and Miso, 186, *187*
  Sliced Pepper Steak with Swiss
    Chard and Mushrooms, 188,
    189, 190
  Spinach and Mushroom Omelet,
    116, *117*
mussels, 22
  Asian Curry Mussel Soup, 136, *137*
  as protein source, 22

mustard, 9, 17
mustard greens, 16, 162
  Chicken with Mustard Greens,
    Quinoa, and Oranges, 162, *163*
  Shrimp with Mustard Greens,
    Mushrooms, and Miso, 186, *187*

N

naringenin, 14
Negative Calorie Diet, 1–63
  eating plan essentials, 8–9
  eating real and losing weight,
    25–31
  family plan, 241–45
  good vs. bad calories, 3–7
  it's not about the calories, 3–9
  maintenance, 257–65
  metabolic secrets, 7–8
  protein, 20–23
  recipes, 65–225
  10-Day Negative Calorie Cleanse,
    8, 33–43
  10 negative calorie foods, 11–23
  20-Day All You Can Eat Plan, 8–9,
    45–62
  vegetarian, 231–39
Negative Calorie Lifestyle, 229–65
  family plan, 241–45
  maintenance, 257–65
  restaurants, 247–55
  vegetarian, 231–39
nervous system, 36
nightshades, 18–20
  allergy, 18
nonstick pans, 61
norepinephrine, 22
No-Sugar-Added Organic
    Cranberry Sauce, 200, *201*
nuts and seeds, 4, 6, 11–12, 30, 54,
    58, 60
  as protein source, 232–36
  See also specific nuts and seeds

O

oat Bran and Almonds, Apple
    Cinnamon Breakfast "Risotto"
    with, 100, *101*
obesity, 12, 257
  childhood, 242–43
obesogens, 26–28, 30

oils, 5
   olive, 5, 30
   20-Day eating plan, 54
olive oil, 5, 30
Olives, Filet of Beef with Braised
   Kale and Black, 167–68, *169*
omega-3 fatty acids, 21, 22, 23, 31,
   236, 264
Omelet, Spinach and Mushroom,
   116, *117*
onions:
   Kale, Red Onion, and Tomato
     Frittata, 108, *109*
   Shrimp and Cucumber Salad with
     Red Onion and Poblanos, 126,
     127
Orange Greensicle Smoothie, 82,
   83
oranges, 4, 14
   Breakfast Citrus Salad with
     Cucumbers and Basil, 104, *105*
   Chicken with Mustard Greens,
     Quinoa, and Oranges, 162, *163*
   Citrus-Berry Smash Smoothie,
     96, *97*
   Citrus and Mixed Berry Bowl with
     Whipped Topping, 226, *227*
   Crepes Suzette with Oranges
     and Vanilla Cream, 224–25,
     225
   Orange Greensicle Smoothie,
     82, *83*
   Sangrita Tomato, Orange, and
     Red Pepper Smoothie, 84, *85*
   Seared Tuna Tataki Salad with
     Citrus, Tofu, and Watercress,
     134, *135*
organic food, 9, 20, 21, 25–28, 30,
   39

P

papaya, 30
"Pappardelle" of Chicken with
   Winter Pesto, 177–78, *179*
pasta, 4, 5, 36, 252
Pasta with Tomatoes, Spinach
   Pesto, 191–92, *193–95*
Peanutty Apple Slices, 206, *207*
pea protein, 234
peas, 234
pectin, 12, 200, 201

peppers, 18–20
   Beef-Stuffed Cabbage with
     Pepper and Tomato Goulash,
     160–61, *161*
   Roasted Cauliflower with Green
     Peppers, Almond Curry, and
     Lime, 180–81, *181*
   Sangrita Tomato, Orange, and
     Red Pepper Smoothie, 84, *85*
   Shrimp and Cabbage Hot Pot
     with Chile Peppers, 184, *185*
   Pepper Steak with Swiss Chard and
     Mushrooms, Sliced, 188, *189*, 190
pesticides, 26, 27–30, 33, 39
phytochemicals, 31
Pineapple, Lime, and Mint
   Smoothie, Spinach, 70
pistachios, 234–35
pizza, 4
   Breakfast Pizza with Mushrooms
     and Broccoli, 106–7, *107*
Poblanos, Shrimp and Cucumber
   Salad with Red Onion and, 126,
   127
polyphenols, 12
popcorn, 5, 6
Porridge with Mint, Blueberry and
   Quinoa, 102, *103*
positive, focus on, 46–47
potato chips, 6
potatoes, 6, 258
Pot-au-Feu, Vegetable, 158–59, *159*
poultry. *See* chicken; turkey
processed foods, 6, 7, 8, 30, 33, 35
protein, 4, 5, 7–9, 20–23, 45, 47, 62
   Almond Vanilla Protein Smoothie,
     90, *91*
   Apple-Lime-Cilantro Protein
     Smoothie, 72, *73*
   organic, 26
   plant-based, 232–37
   10 best vegetarian, 232–37
   10-Day Negative Calorie Cleanse,
     40, 41
   10 favorite sources, 20–23
protein powder, 71

Q

quinoa, 233
   Blueberry and Quinoa Porridge
     with Mint, 102, *103*

   Breakfast Bowl with Quinoa and
     Berries, 114, *115*
   Chicken with Mustard Greens,
     Quinoa, and Oranges, 162, *163*
   in vegetarian diet, 235

R

radishes, Leafy Green Salad with
   Creamy Almond Dressing and,
   148, *149*
Raisins and Capers, Swiss Chard
   Turkey Salad with Golden, 142,
   143
raspberries, 13
   Breakfast Bowl with Quinoa and
     Berries, 114, *115*
Red Ants on a Log, 208, *209*
restaurants, 8, 50, 247–55
   American-style chain, 248
   Asian, 248–49
   barbecue, 249
   breakfast, 247, 249–50
   deli, 250
   fast food, 28, 250
   French, 251
   Greek, 251
   Indian, 252
   Italian, 252, 254
   Mexican, 254
   steakhouses, 254–55
   tips, 253
rice, 5
Roasted Cauliflower with Green
   Peppers, Almond Curry, and
   Lime, 180–81, *181*
Rocco's Chef Salad, 132, *133*
Rocco's Raw Applesauce, 212, *213*
rye, 35

S

salads, 4, 16, 34, 61, 118–49, 253,
   260
   Breakfast Citrus Salad with
     Cucumbers and Basil, 104, *105*
   Charred Thai-Style Broccoli Salad
     with Almonds and Lime, 120,
     121
   Crabmeat Salad with Apple,
     Celery, and Leafy Greens, 122,
     123

salads (*cont.*)
    Flank Steak Salad with
        Horseradish and Apple, 128,
        129
    Grate Salad Bowl with Chia Seed
        Dressing, 144, *145*
    Leafy Green Salad with Creamy
        Almond Dressing and Radishes,
        146, *147*
    Rocco's Chef Salad, 132, *133*
    Seared Tuna Tataki Salad with
        Citrus, Tofu, and Watercress,
        134, *135*
    Shaved Brussels Sprouts with
        Warm Toasted Garlic, Almond,
        and Lemon Dressing, 138,
        139
    Shrimp and Cucumber Salad with
        Red Onion and Poblanos, 126,
        127
    Strawberry and Spinach Salad
        with Almonds and Basil, 140,
        141
    Swiss Chard Turkey Salad with
        Golden Raisins and Capers,
        142, *143*
    10-Day Negative Calorie Cleanse,
        34, 37–39
salmon, 5, 22, 26, 31
    farmed vs. wild, 26
salt, 21, 23, 42
    sea, 9, 178
sandwiches, 260
Sangrita Tomato, Orange, and Red
    Pepper Smoothie, 84, *85*
satiety, 7, 13, 20
sauces, 54, 58
Seared Tuna Tataki Salad with
    Citrus, Tofu, and Watercress,
    134, *135*
sea salt, 9, 178
selenium, 23
serotonin, 23, 35, 43, 265
Shaved Brussels Sprouts with Warm
    Toasted Garlic, Almond, and
    Lemon Dressing, 138, *139*
Shiitake and Bok Choy Stir-Fry,
    182, *183*
shopping lists, 50, 51
    10-Day Negative Calorie Cleanse,
        39–42
    20-Day eating plan, 52–60

shrimp, 22–23, 26
    Grilled Shrimp with Marinated
        Cucumbers, Kale, and
        Cauliflower, 172, *173*
    as protein source, 22–23
    Shrimp and Cabbage Hot Pot
        with Chile Peppers, 184,
        185
    Shrimp and Cucumber Salad with
        Red Onion and Poblanos, 126,
        127
    Shrimp with Mustard Greens,
        Mushrooms, and Miso, 186,
        187
Shrimp and Cabbage Hot Pot with
    Chile Peppers, 184, *185*
Shrimp and Cucumber Salad with
    Red Onion and Poblanos, 126,
    127
Shrimp with Mustard Greens,
    Mushrooms, and Miso, 186,
    187
skin, 9, 33, 35
sleep, 43
Sliced Pepper Steak with Swiss
    Chard and Mushrooms, 188,
    189, 190
smoothies, 34, 50, 51, 61, 67–97,
    245, 260, 261, 262
    Almond Vanilla Protein, 90,
        91
    Apple-Lime-Cilantro Protein,
        72, *73*
    Blueberry-Basil, 94, *95*
    Citrus-Berry Smash, 96, *97*
    Cucumber-Strawberry Green,
        68, *69*
    "Dillicious" Green, 78, *79*
    Green Goddess, 74, *75*
    Lemon-Ginger, 80, *81*
    Orange Greensicle, 82, *83*
    Sangrita Tomato, Orange,
        and Red Pepper Smoothie,
        84, *85*
    Spiced Apple Pie, 92, *93*
    Spinach, Pineapple, Lime, and
        Mint, 70
    Strawberry Shortcake, 88, *89*
    10-Day Negative Calorie Cleanse,
        34, 37–39, 42
    Tropical Sunrise, 76, *77*
    Virgin Mary, 86, *87*

snacks, 6, 62, 196–213, 242
    Apple, Cranberry, and Almond
        Bars, 200, *201*
    Cauliflower and Apples with Thai
        Almond Butter Sauce, 202,
        203
    Cucumber and Almond Rice
        Sushi, 198, *199*
    Eggplant and Almond Dip with
        Celery, 204, *205*
    maintenance, 261
    No-Sugar-Added Organic
        Cranberry Sauce, 210, *211*
    on-the-go, 247, 253
    Peanutty Apple Slices, 206,
        207
    Red Ants on a Log, 208, *209*
    Rocco's Raw Applesauce, 212,
        213
    20-Day eating plan, 51–59, 62
    vegetarian, 238–39
soda, 28, 35
solanine, 18
soups, 34, 61, 118–49, 260
    Asian Curry Mussel Soup, 136,
        137
    Chicken Soup with Escarole and
        Leeks, 124, *125*
    Mixed Leafy Green Soup "Caldo
        Verde" with Chickpeas, 130,
        131
    Mushroom Bouillon with Leeks,
        Tofu, and Wasabi, 148, *149*
    10-Day Negative Calorie Cleanse,
        34, 37–39
soy, 27, 30, 236
    milk, 27
    protein, 236
Spiced Apple Pie Smoothie, 92, *93*
spices, 8, 16, 31, 51, 172
    fat-burning, 17
    10-Day Negative Calorie Cleanse,
        40, 42
    20-Day eating plan, 54, 57, 60
spinach, 16
    Almond-Encrusted Flounder with
        Chopped Spinach and Clam
        Broth, 152–54, *153–55*
    Avocado Toast with Spinach and
        Tomatoes, 110, *111*
    Meatballs with Mushroom and
        Spinach Gravy, 174, *175*, 176

Orange Greensicle Smoothie, 82, *83*
Spinach, Pineapple, Lime, and Mint Smoothie, 70
Spinach and Mushroom Omelet, 116, *117*
Spinach Pesto Pasta with Tomatoes, 191–92, *193–95*
Strawberry and Spinach Salad with Almonds and Basil, 140, *141*
Spinach and Mushroom Omelet, 116, *117*
Spinach Pesto Pasta with Tomatoes, 191–92, *193–95*
Spinach, Pineapple, Lime, and Mint Smoothie, 70
squash, 30, 258
starch, 7, 15, 232, 258
start date, for diet, 47
steakhouses, 254–55
Stir-Fry, Shiitake and Bok Choy, 182, *183*
strawberries, 13, 140
    Breakfast Bowl with Quinoa and Berries, 114, *115*
    Chocolate-Dipped Strawberries with Crushed Almonds, 218, *219*
    Cucumber-Strawberry Green Smoothie, 68, *69*
    Strawberry Shortcake Smoothie, 88, *89*
    Strawberry and Spinach Salad with Almonds and Basil, 140, *141*
Strawberry Shortcake Smoothie, 88, *89*
Strawberry and Spinach Salad with Almonds and Basil, 140, *141*
stress, 23, 30
    hormones, 42
    reduction, 30, 31
stroke, 46
sugar, 5, 7, 8, 15, 28, 30, 33, 35, 42
    addiction, 35
Sushi, Cucumber and Almond Rice, 198, *199*
sweeteners, 35, 40
    artificial, 40
    20-Day eating plan, 54, 57

Swiss chard, 16, 142
    Sliced Pepper Steak with Swiss Chard and Mushrooms, 188, *189*, 190
    Swiss Chard Turkey Salad with Golden Raisins and Capers, 142, *143*
Swiss Chard Turkey Salad with Golden Raisins and Capers, 142, *143*

T

tea, 28, 36
    green, 36, 42
    herbal, 36, 42
    maca, 36
10-Day Negative Calorie Cleanse, 8, 33–43, 261
    day-by-day meal plan, 38–39
    decontaminate your diet, 35–36
    follow the rules, 37
    handling hunger and cravings, 42–43
    kick out toxins, 34–35
    maintenance, 261
    preparation for, 37
    shopping list, 39–42
    smoothies, salads, and soups, 34–39
    with a friend, 243
10 negative calorie foods, 11–23
    almonds, 11–12
    apples, 12
    berries, 12–13
    celery, 13–14
    citrus fruits, 14–15
    cruciferous vegetables, 15
    cucumbers, 15–16
    green leafy vegetables, 16
    mushrooms, 16–18
    nightshades, 18–20
    protein, 20–23
Thai-Style Broccoli Salad with Almonds and Lime, Charred, 120, *121*
thermogenesis, 6–8, 13, 17, 18, 20
thylakoids, 16
thyroid, 21
    hormones, 21, 22, 26

tofu, 57, 60, 236
    "Dillicious" Green Smoothie, 78, *79*
    Mushroom Bouillon with Leeks, Tofu, and Wasabi, 146, *147*
    Seared Tuna Tataki Salad with Citrus, Tofu, and Watercress, 134, *135*
    in vegetarian diets, 236
tomatoes, 18, 25
    Avocado Toast with Spinach and Tomatoes, 110, *111*
    Beef-Stuffed Cabbage with Pepper and Tomato Goulash, 160–61, *161*
    Kale, Red Onion, and Tomato Frittata, 108, *109*
    Sangrita Tomato, Orange, and Red Pepper Smoothie, 84, *85*
    Spinach Pesto Pasta with Tomatoes, 191–92, *193–95*
    Virgin Mary Smoothie, 86, *87*
toxins, 6, 8, 30, 33
    kick out the, 34–35
trans fats, 36
triglycerides, 16, 28, 263
Tropical Sunrise Smoothie, 76, *77*
Truffles, Chocolate and Almond Butter, 216, *217*
tryptophan, 23, 265
tuna, 22, 23, 31
    as protein source, 23
    Seared Tuna Tataki Salad with Citrus, Tofu, and Watercress, 134, *135*
turkey, 23, 26
    as protein source, 23
    Swiss Chard Turkey Salad with Golden Raisins and Capers, 142, *143*
    20-Day eating plan, 57, 60
turmeric, 17, 31
turnip greens, 16
20-Day All You Can Eat Plan, 8–9, 45–62
    configuration of eating, 62
    essentials of, 47
    fruits and vegetables, 48, 50, 52–60
    how it works, 50–51
    making it your own, 60–62

20-Day All You Can Eat Plan (*cont.*)
    preparing for a healthier body,
      45–47
    shopping lists, 52–60
    start date, 47
    suggested menus, 51–59
tyrosine, 22

V

vanilla Cream, Crepes Suzette with
    Oranges and, 224–25, *225*
Vegetable Pot-au-Feu, 158–59, *159*
vegetables, 4, 7, 9, 13–20, 25, 27,
    34, 39, 45, 48, 50, 237–39,
    245, 258, 264, 265
    cruciferous, 15, 30
    GMO, 28–30
    leafy greens, 16, 27
    local, 29
    maintenance plan, 258
    nightshade, 18–20
    organic, 26–28, 30, 39
    starchy, 258
    10-Day Negative Calorie Cleanse,
      39–41

20-Day eating plan, 48, 50, 53,
    56–60
    See also specific vegetables
vegetarian diets, 27, 50, 231–39
    approach to, 236
    menu, 238–39
    personalized plan, 237
    planning meals, 237–38
    10 best proteins, 232–37
vinegar, 9, 54, 57
Virgin Mary Smoothie, 86, *87*
vitamins and minerals, 4, 23, 34,
    264
    B, 20, 21, 23, 265
    C, 14
    D, 16, 21
    in plant-based foods, 232–37

W

walnuts, 236–37
Wasabi, Mushroom Bouillon
    with Leeks, Tofu, and, 146, *147*
water, 7, 13, 28, 33, 35, 37, 42, 50,
    253, 261
    as negative calorie food, 13

Watercress, Seared Tuna Tataki
    Salad with Citrus, Tofu, and,
    134, *135*
weighing yourself, 37
weight loss, reasons for, 46
wheat, 35, 36
    crackers, 6
Whipped Topping, Citrus and
    Mixed Berry Bowl with, 226,
    227
white flour, 8, 30
whole foods,6, 7, 26–28, 30, 33,
    258

Y

yoga, 43
yogurt, 28, 54, 60
    Crabmeat Salad with Apple,
    Celery, and Leafy Greens, 122,
    123

Z

zinc, 20, 23
zucchini, 30

ABOUT THE AUTHOR

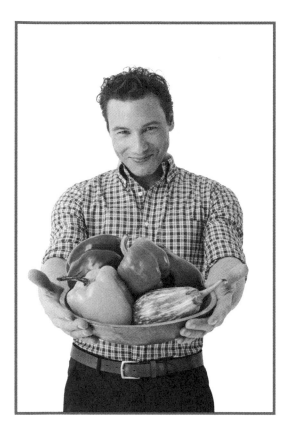

Rocco DiSpirito is a James Beard Award–winning celebrity chef and the author of eleven highly acclaimed books and three number one *New York Times* bestsellers, including *The Pound a Day Diet*. Rocco has starred on numerous television shows and is frequently featured as a food and weight-loss expert in print and online media. He is the founder of the Pound a Day Diet fresh-food delivery service and personally cooks for and coaches hundreds of clients to wellness as a passionate health advocate. He lives in New York City.

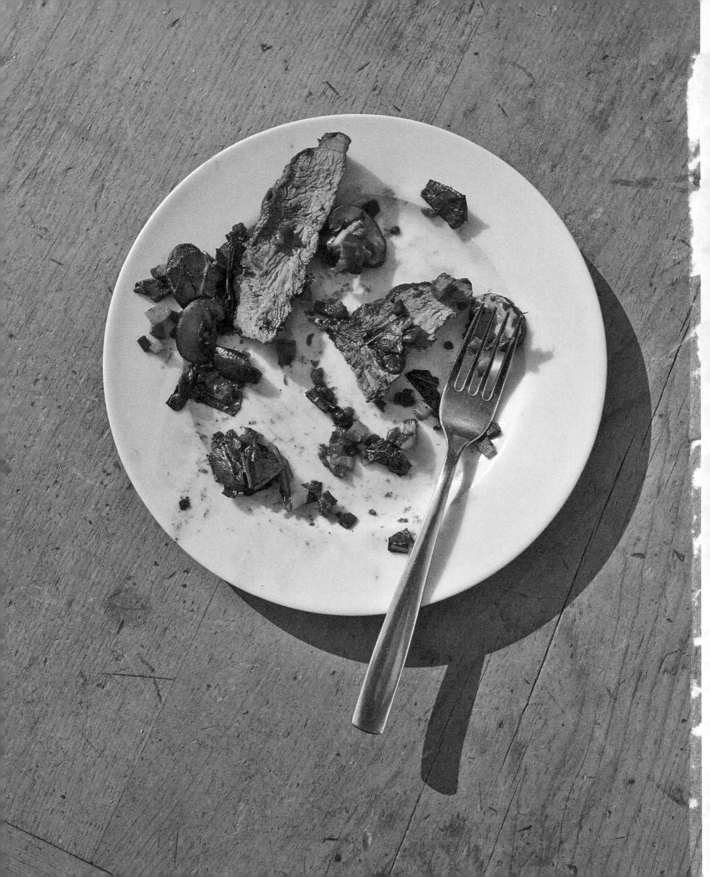